RURAL RESCUE AND EMERGENCY CARE

This textbook is intended solely as a guide to the appropriate procedures to be employed when rendering emergency care to or transporting the sick or injured. It is not intended as a statement of the standards of care required in any particular situation, since circumstances and patients' physical conditions can vary widely from one emergency to another. Nor is it intended that this textbook shall in any way advise emergency personnel concerning legal authority to perform the activities or procedures discussed. Such determinations should be made locally only with the aid of legal counsel.

The rescue series is written with the assumption that the reader has completed a basic EMT or first responder training course. The editors believe these levels represent the minimum level of medical training suitable for patient care in the rescue setting, but all rescue personnel are encouraged to attain the highest level of training available. Throughout this module, assessment and treatment skills are mentioned that require a higher level of training and licensure than are available to basic EMTs. In addition, there are wide variances throughout the United States in what rescue personnel are permitted by law to do. This textbook is intended for nationwide use, and we have sought to include various techniques that may be helpful in particular situations; it must fall to the instructor and the reader to determine what is acceptable within one's training and jurisdiction. Before using the advanced techniques presented in the textbook, the rescuer must review his or her scope of practice as well as the legal limits of his or her other training and authorization, so as not to exceed the limits of the law and to ensure the provision of the highest possible patient care.

THE RESCUE
AND EMERGENCY
CARE SERIES

RURAL RESCUE AND EMERGENCY CARE

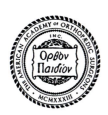

American Academy
of Orthopaedic Surgeons

Robert A. Worsing, Jr., MD
Chairman, Editorial Board

CREDITS

Executive Director: Thomas C. Nelson
Deputy Executive Director: Fred V. Featherstone, MD
Director, Division of Education: Mark W. Wieting
Director, Department of Publications: Marilyn L. Fox, PhD
Senior Editor: Lynne Roby Shindoll
Production Manager: Loraine Edwalds
Production Editor: Kathy M. Brouillette
Editorial Assistants: Susan Baim, Kathryn O'Brien

Book and cover design: Image House, Inc.
Consultants: Mary Ann Porucznik, Ann Kepler
Technical illustrations: Sheila Smith
Photography: Elizabeth Sawyer, Mark Hansen
Photo contributors: Rollin D. Schnieder, John Smith

American Academy of Orthopaedic Surgeons Board of Directors, 1992

Robert N. Hensinger, MD
Bernard A. Rineberg, MD
Bernard F. Morrey, MD
Robert E. Eilert, MD
Howard P. Hogshead, MD
Newton C. McCollough, III, MD
John B. McGinty, MD
Augusto Sarmiento, MD
James W. Strickland, MD

Edward V. Craig, MD
Joseph D. Zuckerman, MD
D. Eugene Thompson, MD
James G. Buchholz, MD
Gene E. Swanson, MD
Eugene R. Mindell, MD
Douglas W. Jackson, MD
Thomas C. Nelson, *ex officio*

First Edition

Copyright © 1993 by American Academy of Orthopaedic Surgeons

All rights reserved. No part of *Rural Rescue and Emergency Care* may be reproduced in any form or by any means, electronic or mechanical, including photocopying and recording, or by any information storage and retrieval system without prior permission, in writing, from the publisher. Address requests to American Academy of Orthopaedic Surgeons, 6300 N. River Rd., Rosemont, IL 60018.

ISBN 0-89203-075-5

Library of Congress Catalog Card Number 93-70198

Published and distributed by: American Academy of Orthopaedic Surgeons

10 9 8 7 6 5 4 3 2 1

This book is dedicated to all EMS personnel who follow the long tradition of farmers and ranchers helping their "neighbors," reaching out in times of need, danger, and distress.

ACKNOWLEDGMENTS

Editorial Board

Chairman

Robert A. Worsing, Jr., MD
Humana-Prime Health
Kansas City, Kansas

Principal Authors

Rollin D. Schnieder
Professor Emeritus
University of Nebraska-Lincoln
Lincoln, Nebraska

David L. Morgan, BS, EMT-A
Extension Safety Engineer
University of Nebraska-Lincoln
Lincoln, Nebraska

Contributing Authors

Emery W. Nelson
Professor Emeritus
University of Nebraska-Lincoln
Lincoln, Nebraska

Robert L. Zickler, MS, ED
Assistant Chief
Indianapolis Fire Department
Indianapolis, Indiana

FOREWORD

It is estimated that 27% of the population in the United States live in rural areas. Inherent in rural living is the difficult access to health and rescue services. Because of limited and inadequate transportation services, geographic isolation and distances from medical centers, emergency services in rural areas are generally more limited than in urban areas.

According to the National Safety Council, agriculture is second to mining in occupational death rates. In fact, in recent years, death rates in the agricultural industry increased while similar rates for other industries declined.

It has always been a tremendous challenge to manage a farm emergency. Living in a rural area and volunteering to serve on the local fire and ambulance service is gratifying, but it does not provide an opportunity to be fully prepared to deal with a farm accident. Generally speaking, every farm accident that we are called to will be a serious trauma call, as rescuers are generally called to a farm accident only after efforts to rescue a victim have failed. Suddenly, we find ourselves outside of that "normal world" we know. Only 10% of all "normal" ambulance calls are trauma calls and only 10% of those are serious.

The American Academy of Orthopaedic Surgeons is to be commended for the educational contribution made by their classic "Orange Book," *Emergency Care and Transportation of the Sick and Injured.* The training that has resulted from this textbook and others proved to make a positive difference in saving lives of patients by providing better patient care. Although most rescuers have received and seen the benefits of this training, those who respond to agricultural-rural emergencies quickly discover that they are not properly prepared to manage such emergencies. The tools and techniques used in extrication are not the same. There are unfamiliar hazards to overcome. It quickly becomes apparent that our good basic training prepares us for only about 90% of the emergencies that we are being called to and that we may need to prepare for the other 10% through separate efforts.

To continue the tradition and offer a part of the solution, the Academy embarked on a mission to develop various resources geared at expanding on those developed for basic courses. *Rural Rescue and Emergency Care* is one of those works designed for rescuers who will respond to agricultural-rural incidents.

Rural Rescue and Emergency Care is organized logically. It begins with the importance of preincident planning and rescuer preparation, and includes a section on the mechanics of farm accidents to help us understand the important differences between automobile extrication and extrication from under a tractor. Specific chapters related to the three major subheadings in agricultural-rural emergencies, i.e., emergencies involving farm machinery, farm structures, and agricultural chemicals, all give an overview of some of the hazards rescuers may be exposed to as well as some of the procedures for rescue and recovery.

No textbook can cover every aspect of every detail rescuers will need. That is why it is crucial to couple written information with a sound, proven training program. That is true with *Rural Rescue and Emergency Care*, when used as a resource for a sound training program in agricultural-rural rescue, such as the FARMEDIC Provider Course. With a textbook and training course in place, rescuers can begin to develop sound strategies to better manage agricultural-rural emergencies. With these strategies in place, we will then begin to see fewer deaths related to farm accidents and fewer injuries and deaths of rescuers at the scene of farm accidents, just the way we have seen fewer patient deaths and improved rescuer safety as a result of our prior training.

> Davis E. Hill
> Executive Director
> FARMEDIC National Training Center
> Alfred State College
> Alfred, New York

CONTRIBUTORS

Many thanks to the individuals at the FARMEDIC National Training Center at Alfred State College for their invaluable assistance both in reviewing the manuscript and volunteering their time to help us create many of the illustrations. Their attention to detail and commitment to excellence have contributed much to this text.

Davis E. Hill
Executive Director
FARMEDIC National Training
   Center

Richard A. Hoffman, Jr.
President
FARMEDIC Board of
   Directors

National FARMEDIC Faculty/Staff

David W. Ackroyd	Ted Fiorito, III	Douglas J. Nelson
John Bailey	Ted Halpin	David C. Oliver
Thomas Buckley	Ron Moore	Gerald R. Ray
Dennis G. Chapman	Larry Nagal	Anne Torrey
John A. Colegrove, Jr.		

TECHNICAL CONSULTATION

Brown Farm
Churchville Ambulance
Clifton Fire Department
Duane Johnson Farm
FARMEDIC National Training
   Center

Greenwood Fire and Rescue
Lamb Farm, Inc.
Mead Fire and Rescue
Noble Farm
S.C. Hansen, Inc.

REVIEWERS

Our thanks to the following individuals who, throughout the development of this project, either reviewed the entire manuscript or selected chapters of *Rural Rescue and Emergency Care*. Their comments and suggestions were extremely helpful to the editorial board.

Paul Anderson
Rural EMS Institute
Lincoln Medical Education
  Foundation
Lincoln, Nebraska

Captain Ben E. Blankenship
North Little Rock Fire
  Department
North Little Rock, Arkansas

David M. Habben
State EMS Training Coordinator
Boise, Idaho

Roger L. Hayes, NREMT-P
State EMS Training Coordinator
Webster City, Iowa

Davis E. Hill
Executive Director
FARMEDIC National Training
  Center
Alfred State College
Alfred, New York

George L. Lucas, MD
University of Kansas School of
  Medicine
Wichita/St. Francis Regional
  Medical Center
Wichita, Kansas

Jeffrey Mitchell, PhD
American Critical Incident Stress
  Foundation
Ellicott City, Maryland

Emery W. Nelson
Professor Emeritus
University of Nebraska-Lincoln
Lincoln, Nebraska

David C. Rector
Ottawa, Kansas

Joel Schroeder, Sr., FF/EMT-D
Belton, Missouri

Arden R. Shindoll, CPAg
Kirkwood Community College
Cedar Rapids, Iowa

Steven Stripe, MD, FAAFP
Humboldt, Nebraska

Ronald L. Williams, MD
University of Texas Health
  Science Center
San Antonio, Texas

Richard L. Withington, MD,
  FAAOS
Watertown, New York

Robert L. Zickler, MS, ED
Assistant Chief
Indianapolis Fire Department
Indianapolis, Indiana

CONTENTS

OVERVIEW 1

CHAPTER 1
Introduction   6

CHAPTER 2
Incident Command System   12

CHAPTER 3
Rescuer Preparation and Personal Safety   30

CHAPTER 4
The Mechanics of Extrication   46

CHAPTER 5
Extrication Tools   58

CHAPTER 6
Tractors   94

CHAPTER 7
Combines   120

CHAPTER 8
Agricultural Equipment   138

CHAPTER 9
Grain and Silage Storage Facility Rescues   176

CHAPTER 10
Animal Incidents   206

CHAPTER 11
Hazardous Materials   214

CHAPTER 12
Medical Care in the Rescue Setting   242

CHAPTER 13
Patient Assessment in Rescue Medical Care   252

CHAPTER 14
Common Medical Conditions and Injuries   260

CHAPTER 15
Patient Packaging and Litter Evacuation   302

CHAPTER 16
Vehicles and Transportation   316

CHAPTER 17
Crisis Intervention   326

APPENDIX
Selection, Storage, and Maintenance of Extrication Tools   338

GLOSSARY   353

INDEX   357

PREFACE

During the development of the third edition of *Emergency Care and Transportation of the Sick and Injured*, members of the agricultural community made their first request to the American Academy of Orthopaedic Surgeons for more agricultural-specific material. Though the number of individuals injured and killed in agricultural-rural settings was significant, EMT curriculum restraints prevented inclusion of agricultural-specific material in the third, fourth, and fifth editions.

When the rescue series was planned beyond the initial discussion stage, one of the important considerations was the inclusion of a module to address the issues confronting EMS and rescue personnel in rural and suburban agricultural settings. It has taken a lot of time and effort to pull all the ideas together and transform the information into a readable, understandable manuscript and illustrations. If the editors, contributors, reviewers, and others who participated in this project were successful, and if the information in this text saves even one or two of the 1,500 agricultural workers who sustain fatal injuries each year, all of the efforts of the project team will have been rewarded.

This text represents a small repayment from those of us who each day enjoy the bountiful fruits of the land to those who make American agriculture the envy of the world and to those dedicated individuals who help their neighbors.

The rescue series is written for those who have completed a basic EMT training course. The editors believe that this is the minimum level of medical training suitable for patient care in the rescue setting but encourage all rescuers to attain the highest level of training available. Throughout this text, assessment and management skills are mentioned that may require a higher level of training and licensure than are available to basic EMTs. This book is not designed to be a stand-alone training manual, but to serve as an integral component of a formal course of classroom and skills instruction in agricultural-rural rescue. Throughout the country, there are wide variances in what rescuers are licensed to do. So before learning and applying the advanced techniques occasionally presented in the text, you must review your personal scope of practice, the legal limits of what you are trained and authorized to do, and make sure that you do not exceed your scope of practice.

One topic not covered in this text is crime scene management. Though infrequent, agricultural-rural incidents may be attempts to cover up unlawful activity. Emergency medical and rescue personnel must be aware of this possibility so that suspicious incidents are immediately reported to law enforcement authorities. In questionable situations, rescuers must avoid actions and activities that might damage a crime scene or obscure possible evidence. Such activities must not deter you from providing necessary medical care to the patient nor should it delay transporting the patient to the hospital. Rescue personnel should confer periodically with local law enforcement officials so they may be aware of appropriate actions to take at a crime scene.

Rural Rescue and Emergency Care is a tribute to the perseverance, time, skills, and efforts of Rollin Schnieder and David Morgan. Without their technical expertise, this text would not exist. Their enthusiasm and expertise have been extremely important in the development of this text. I appreciate the wonderful education they have provided a "city boy" in the nuances of EMS and rescue operations in the agricultural-rural setting.

Without the support of the American Academy of Orthopaedic Surgeons' Board of Directors; Executive Director, Thomas C. Nelson; Deputy Executive Director, Fred V. Featherstone, MD; Division of Education Director, Mark W. Wieting; and the Academy's publications staff—particularly Marilyn L. Fox, PhD, director, and Keith Levine, marketing manager—this project might never have become reality. I appreciate their understanding and forbearance as we have navigated through this project.

Every author and editor needs a managing editor and I was extremely fortunate to work with Lynne Roby Shindoll, senior editor for the Academy's EMS publications. Also working hard to bring the manuscript and illustrations together into the finished product were Loraine Edwalds, production manager; Kathy Brouillette, production editor; and Susan Baim and Katy O'Brien, editorial assistants.

Especially appreciated are the three people who, once again, made my contribution to this project possible, my wife, Linda, and my children, Kalli and Ryan. They have had to endure years of "Daddy's got to work on 'the book' tonight." Their sacrifices represent the families of all of us who have heard the siren call of rescue and EMS. While we wear our rescue/EMS hats, we receive the vicarious thrills and "warm fuzzies" of saving lives and helping others. Meanwhile our families endure the cold, late dinners, phone calls in the wee hours of the morning, beepers disrupting important occasions, plans disrupted by extended operations, and the hassles of planning around call and duty schedules. With that in mind, the rescue series is dedicated to the families at home whose support, solace, and sacrifice enable our care in the field and allow lives to be saved and family and friends to be reunited.

Robert A. Worsing, Jr., MD
Kansas City, Kansas

Overview

Mental and/or physical isolation, entrapment, injury, illness, or other threats to the health and well-being of an individual can result in an *emergency* if the individual is unable to protect himself or herself. The goal of rescue is to *locate* and *access* the individual, *stabilize* the situation, and *transport* the person to safety, while caring for any injuries and avoiding additional risk or injury to the patient and rescuers.

RESCUE TERMS

This text uses certain standard rescue terms to avoid confusion. These terms and their definitions are listed below.

- *Victim*: An individual who needs to be rescued. Once a rescue operation begins, the victim is the *subject* of the operation, or a *patient* if he or she needs medical care.
- *Subject*: An individual who is being rescued. When the subject is ill or injured, he or she is called a *patient*.
- *Patient*: A subject with injuries or illnesses requiring medical intervention.
- *Operator*: An individual who is driving or operating a piece of farm equipment or machinery.
- *Extended Incident*: Any rescue operation lasting longer than 2 hours from the time of injury until the patient is delivered to definitive medical care. Many rescue operations in agricultural-rural settings are extended incidents because of the possibility of delayed notification, extended response or transport times, difficult access, or extrication problems that prolong the time at the scene. Extended incident is a broader, more generic term than "prolonged transport." It is also preferred to "delayed transport," which could imply that the rescue team is not working or cannot work in an efficient or timely fashion.

THE FOUR PHASES OF RESCUE

The four phases of rescue are commonly known as the **LAST** sequence: *locating* the victims at risk, *accessing* them to make an initial assessment of conditions and provide assistance, *stabilizing* them to prepare for transport, and finally, *transporting* them from the scene to safety or medical care.

In all of these phases, planning is critical in order to ensure that the quickest, easiest, and safest procedures are used during a rescue operation. Planning also involves developing and maintaining a written plan for response to and management of a rescue operation. The plan establishes who will be in charge and outlines the organization of the operation. In essence, planning defines procedures and makes decisions for conducting a rescue operation well before the incident occurs, when alternatives may be calmly discussed and logical decisions made.

Planning should also include provisions for critical incident stress debriefing (CISD). Many agricultural-rural rescue operations involve friends, neighbors, or relatives of rescuers. In addition, the relatively large number of agricultural-rural incidents that involve children and other young people increase the stress on the rescue team.

Locate Phase

The first step of a rescue operation is to locate the individual at risk. For most incidents in an agricultural-rural setting, the patient has been located before the initial call for assistance is made. The dispatcher requests the location of the incident, and the locate phase is restricted to finding the victim in a field, confined space, or farmstead.

A rescue response is activated on the **first notice**: a person is reported overdue; 911 is called about an abandoned vehicle, fire, or accident; distress signals are reported. Once the first notice is received, the name of the person reporting the emergency and a callback number must be obtained as part of the initial planning data.

Planning data are the pieces of information used to select the appropriate response for a rescue incident. Planning data include information requested at the time of first notice of the incident, such as the subject's physical and mental condition, location, type and brand of equipment, type of agricultural operation, nearby potential or actual hazards such as animals, electrical lines, agricultural chemicals, or confined spaces. Other data are the current and predicted weather, geographic information, structural diagrams or blueprints, available resources, and access routes. Knowing the current status of all factors is critical for rescuers to determine their response.

The person in charge then determines the **urgency** of the response to the situation by developing a priority system to rank such factors as age and condition of the subject, weather, and hazards. The urgency of the situation determines the speed, level, and nature of the response. Unfortunately, because of the size of the equipment involved, the potential for severe injury, and the time delay before rescuers are called, most agricultural-rural rescues require an urgent response.

As soon as possible, the person in charge initiates **scene confinement** to establish a safety zone to keep unauthorized persons out of the area.

Access Phase

During most agricultural-rural rescues, the rescue team will often be divided into two teams: the extrication team and the medical team. During the access phase, the primary responsibility of the medical team is to ensure that the patient sustains no additional injuries. The medical team may provide some assistance to the extrication team until patient assessment and management begins. After that point, the medical team should concentrate on patient management. Members of the extrication team may be asked to assist with patient management as necessary.

After locating the patient, the rescue team must *access* the individual to assess his or her condition and provide appropriate assistance. In an agricultural-rural setting, access methods may range from dismantling a PTO or removing the grain from a silo to entering an animal feedlot safely.

The **size-up** of the rescue scene requires gathering information on the subject, weather, resource capabilities, and limitations. A critical part of the size-up is an evaluation of the hazards facing the rescuers as well as those facing the subject.

Access techniques may change when patient and rescuer safety is threatened. If a location unexpectedly becomes hazardous, rescuers may have to alter medical protocols and remove the patient without stabilization. If the patient's medical condition is quickly deteriorating, accelerated rescue techniques may be necessary. Some examples of hazardous situations include the following:

- A surrounding atmosphere that is poisonous, flammable, explosive, or burning
- Unstable structures or ground
- Adverse weather conditions that threaten the safety of rescuers or subjects
- Leaking hydraulic fluid or battery electrolyte
- Agricultural chemicals

Patient care begins as soon as the rescue team arrives and makes the scene as safe as possible by eliminating as many environmental hazards as possible. This is an ongoing process, because environmental hazards may change. As part of their planning, many rescue units assign one member of the medical team responsibility for initiating patient assessment and providing initial emergency medical care. The other team members assist with patient management, packaging, and evacuation.

External influences may hinder all phases of the rescue effort, creating real hazards and obstacles during the access phase. Relatives, bystanders, and co-workers may interfere, particularly if they feel the rescue team is not doing enough (regardless of whether this is true or not). Anxious relatives and co-workers may feel compelled to contribute to the rescue effort, endangering themselves and other rescuers.

Curious neighbors or bystanders concerned about friends or looking for excitement may crowd the rescue scene; some people monitor rescue efforts on home scanners and may appear at the rescue scene.

An information officer who serves as a liaison to the family, media, or government officials may reduce problems caused by these external influences.

Stabilize Phase

Once rescue team members locate and access the subject, those assigned to the medical team begin primary assessment and patient management. In some cases, the primary assessment can begin as the extrication team begins accessing the patient. The primary assessment is an evaluation of ABCD (airway, breathing, circulation, disability). If necessary, basic life support—lifesaving procedures to deter failure of the respiratory or cardiovascular systems—is initiated. If the patient has possible spinal injuries, he or she must be carefully immobilized.

After the primary assessment is completed, and treatment of life-threatening conditions is initiated, the medical team can begin a secondary survey. This includes taking the patient's vital signs, determining the patient's level of consciousness, obtaining a brief medical history, and examining the patient for other injuries, wounds, or fractures. The patient is then stabilized and packaged for transport. The patient must be reassessed frequently during packaging and transport, so treatment plans can be adjusted depending on changes in the patient's condition.

Transport Phase

Transport is the fourth phase of rescue. It might be as simple as escorting a lost child to safety. Or it could be as complex as using an air medical helicopter to transport a patient while providing advanced life support during an agricultural-rural rescue.

Transportation involves several elements. **Packaging** is preparing the stabilized patient to be moved. It includes arranging the patient to allow necessary medical interventions, to provide as much patient comfort as possible, and to avoid additional injury by securing and protecting the patient during transport. Appropriate packaging of the patient depends on the injuries, the surrounding environment, the method (or type) of transport, and the time required for transport.

The choice of a specific transport method must be based on the patient's condition, the weather and terrain conditions, the types of transportation available, and human resources. The person in charge must always have an alternate method of transportation available in case the primary means of transportation cannot be used or becomes unavailable.

If continuing medical care is required, the transport phase of rescue should also be considered a continuation of the stabilize phase. Rescuers must continue to pay close attention to the patient's ABCDs and medical condition during transport, and must handle the patient carefully to avoid causing the patient additional injury.

During transport, rescuers must monitor the airway to ensure that it does not become blocked by the tongue, foreign objects, or vomitus. The patient must be packaged so that he or she may safely be turned to the side for airway management in the event of vomiting. If the patient is unconscious, an artificial airway should be used so the tongue does not block the natural airway.

The patient must maintain sufficient respiratory function for adequate oxygenation. If the patient cannot maintain adequate oxygenation independently, then rescuers must consider such alternatives as supplemental oxygen and ventilatory support.

Effective cardiac circulation must also be maintained. This may mean that rescuers use pressure dressings to control blood loss. If the patient's condition is more serious, it could mean providing circulatory support by using intravenous fluid therapy (IV) or pneumatic antishock garments (PASG). If circulation ceases, cardiopulmonary resuscitation (CPR) must be used.

Throughout the rescue operation, rescuers should work with plans that have been prepared in advance for each rescue phase. Using this process ensures that the rescue can be started, conducted, and completed in the most efficient, safe, and successful manner possible.

CHAPTER 1

Introduction

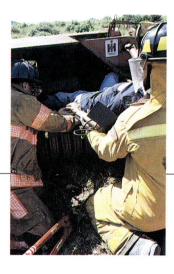

CHAPTER OUTLINE

Overview
Objectives
Agricultural-Rural Rescue
Safety Considerations at
  the Scene
Extrication Considerations

Equipment Construction
Scene Accessibility
Assistance Resources
Personal Safety
Preincident Planning
Summary

KEY TERMS

Agricultural-rural incident: incident involving farm equipment, animals, electricity, falls, fires, chemicals or pesticides, confined spaces, or natural events. These incidents may occur in isolated locations and may not be discovered for several hours.

Safety zone: area that encompasses at least 50' in all directions from the equipment in which rescuers extricate the patient and provide medical treatment. Bystanders are to be escorted out of the safety zone.

CHAPTER 1 Introduction

OVERVIEW

The purpose of this chapter is to outline the basic differences between agricultural-rural rescue situations and other rescue incidents. Rescuers working in an agricultural-rural setting may be called upon to respond to a variety of incidents. Rescue situations may involve large machinery, animals, confined spaces, toxic gases, or agricultural chemicals. Agricultural-rural incidents may be infrequent, but when they occur, they are likely to be extremely serious. Therefore, the importance of a carefully constructed preincident plan cannot be overemphasized. Rescuer safety is primary, because the patient's survival depends on a rescuer's ability to perform a swift and safe extrication, to administer proper medical treatment, and to provide transport to an appropriate medical facility. Agricultural-rural incidents are often not discovered for several hours, and frequently involve isolated locations. Reviewing and refining the preincident plan and frequent continuing education and training are important to enable rescuers to proceed swiftly and safely during rescue operations.

OBJECTIVES

After reading this chapter, the rescuer should be able to:
- identify the three basic differences between agricultural-rural rescues and other rescue situations.
- describe the major types of rescue situations in agricultural-rural settings.
- recognize the need for ongoing practice and training for agricultural-rural rescues.

AGRICULTURAL-RURAL RESCUE

Emergency personnel such as ambulance crews, rescue squads, and fire fighters who work in rural or exurban areas may be called upon to respond to a variety of agricultural-rural incidents. **Agricultural-rural incidents** may involve equipment, animals, electricity, falls, fires, vehicle overturns, chemicals or pesticides, confined spaces, or natural events. While "farming" sounds like a harmless occupation, the size and number of machines involved in agriculture today make it a dangerous occupation. There may be as many as 35 different machines or types of equipment on a farm, and each has the potential to cause a serious injury.

Historically, agriculture has been one of the most dangerous occupations in the United States. Ordinarily, 1,300 to 1,500 agricultural workers die annually in work-related accidents, twice as many as the next most dangerous occupation. In addition, approximately 170,000 people are injured in agricultural-rural incidents per year. The death rate among agricultural workers is approximately 45 to 54 per 100,000—five times the national average for all industries.

Most work-related accidents on farms usually involve some type of farm machinery. One reason for the danger in farming is the size of the equipment used; some of the largest tractors can weigh as much as 60,000 lb. If such a large vehicle overturns, the operator can sustain serious crushing injuries or death. Extricating an operator from such a large, heavy machine takes considerable care and practice.

Many farm machines are designed to cut, chop, pierce, compress, or otherwise process materials. These machines will treat people in the same way they treat ears of corn, heads of wheat, or bolls of cotton. The result is a serious injury.

SAFETY CONSIDERATIONS AT THE SCENE

The severity of injuries resulting from most agricultural-rural incidents requires that both rescue and emergency medical teams should respond to any incident. Oftentimes, rescue and emergency medical personnel are members of the same team, so notification of two separate teams is not necessary. In either case, rescuers should follow the same sequence of steps to ensure the safety of all individuals at the scene before beginning extrication or medical treatment. These steps are described below, and throughout the text as part of the extrication technique.

1. **Establish a safety zone.** The first step in any rescue operation is to establish a safety zone. As you approach the scene, look for potential hazards, such as downed power lines, fire, or a hazardous materials spill. Approach slowly from the front so you can size up the situation, and more importantly, so the patient can see you.

    The **safety zone** should encompass an area of at least 50' from the farm equipment in all directions (Figure 1.1). The safety zone should be expanded if there is spilled gasoline, agricultural chemicals, or if there is a possibility that large farm equipment may move unexpectedly. Do not permit any open flames, including smoking, around the scene. Plastic barrier tape and light stakes should be used to outline the safety zone.

2. **Escort bystanders out of the safety zone.** In many rescue operations, rescuers are called only after family and friends are unable to extricate the patient themselves. Escort neighbors, co-workers, family members, and other bystanders who are not participating in the

FIGURE 1.1

Inspect the area around the incident and then report any hazards to the incident commander. Mark the safety zone with barrier tape and stakes to limit unauthorized access by people not involved in the rescue operation.

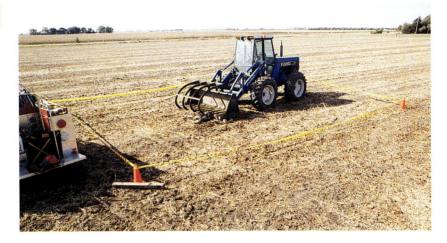

rescue effort out of the safety zone as soon as it is marked. Keep in mind that neighbors may be able to help with disassembly or explain how a particular machine works. It is particularly important for them to see the process completed and to feel like part of the process as the sense of community in rural areas is strong. One member of the rescue team should be assigned to communicate with the patient's family and friends throughout the rescue operation. Law enforcement personnel at the scene are often assigned this role. But regardless of who is assigned the role, remember that it is a crucial part of the operation.

3. **Turn off the engine and secure the machine.** Even if the engine does not appear to be running, make sure that the engine is shut off. Chock any wheels touching the ground. Use cribbing on the machine frame to prevent unwanted movement.

Specific directions appropriate for each situation are listed throughout the text, along with specific extrication and medical assessment instructions.

Regardless of how the team or teams are composed (a team may even include a neighbor or a farm equipment mechanic), a successful rescue operation relies on open communication, professional courtesy, and teamwork.

EXTRICATION CONSIDERATIONS

Extrication from farm equipment is similar to extrication from automobiles in many ways. There are, however, three major differences: equipment construction, scene accessibility, and assistance resources.

Equipment Construction

Rescuers must be familiar with the types of equipment found on farms and the safety rules for each type of equipment. A piece of farm equipment is both heavier and more sturdily constructed than an automobile. Standard rescue equipment used in automobile extrication, such as hydraulic rescue tools, may not work on farm equipment. Rescuers need to be especially careful about where and how they apply their tools. A machine may have to be disassembled to release a patient; therefore, the process will take much longer and be more involved than a similar operation for an automobile.

Scene Accessibility

Agricultural-rural incidents commonly occur in inconvenient locations such as in the middle of a muddy field or in a small equipment shed. If rescuers attempt to access the scene in a rescue vehicle, the vehicle may become stuck, or it may be in danger of overturning on the rough ground. There may also be limited space or dangerous atmospheric conditions, such as in a grain bin, manure pit, or animal confinement pen. These difficulties underscore the importance of preincident planning and of establishing one or even two alternative plans.

Assistance Resources

Finally, rescuers should not overlook two important sources of assistance: neighbors, who may be familiar with the way the equipment operates; and farm equipment mechanics, who will know how to disassemble the equipment quickly. These individuals may be able to make significant contributions to the rescue effort, if they are properly supervised by the rescue team, which gives primary consideration to the patient's safety and care.

PERSONAL SAFETY

In agricultural-rural incidents, as in other rescue situations, the safety of the rescue team is of primary importance. Rescue teams may be unfamiliar with the farm equipment involved, or may have little experience in agricultural-rural rescue. The size of the equipment, the speed at which it operates, and the severity of the patient's injuries require that rescuers take all possible precautions to ensure a safe, efficient rescue.

Personal safety begins with proper protective gear, along with training and practice. Because agricultural-rural incidents do not occur frequently, rescue teams must periodically review their preincident plans, including techniques for extrication and patient management.

Rescue teams must also familiarize themselves with the several different operating controls and procedures of the various types of farm equipment and with procedures for dealing with animals. Injuries sustained in agricultural-rural incidents are usually severe, so rescue teams must be ready to implement appropriate life support procedures. Rescuers must also be prepared to deal with their own emotions, especially if the injury is severe, or if a child is involved, or if the extrication is difficult and lengthy.

CHAPTER 1 Introduction

PREINCIDENT PLANNING

The importance of preincident planning for an agricultural-rural rescue operation cannot be overemphasized, but can be very difficult because these incidents occur so infrequently. Rescue and emergency medical teams should work together to develop a preincident plan and conduct joint practice drills in order to be prepared when an incident occurs. Of course it is impossible to plan exactly for every possible incident, but the preincident plan should adequately prepare a team to respond to any incident.

Because farmers often work alone, it may be several hours before they are missed or the incident discovered. There may be considerable distances involved from the rescue center to the incident site and from the incident site to the medical center. As a result, many agricultural-rural incidents do not result in an EMS response. It has been reported that over 70% of patients injured in agricultural-rural incidents transport themselves to a medical facility.

If extrication from farm equipment is necessary, the process may itself be lengthy. And while all this time is elapsing, the patient's condition may be deteriorating. Preincident planning can help the rescue operation proceed smoothly, efficiently, safely, and swiftly. Rescuers will have the proper equipment and a plan of action. Frequent practice sessions will enable the team to move quickly in an organized manner. They will also be prepared to implement alternate rescue plans if necessary, and to request additional medical or mechanical support.

Preincident planning should also include consideration of preserving potential evidence or other data in the event that the site is declared a crime scene. Agricultural-rural incidents offer certain unique opportunities to cover up criminal activity.

This text will help familiarize you with the types of farm equipment, with the types of injuries encountered, with basic extrication techniques, and with appropriate emergency medical care. Regular practice, review, and training will improve your skills.

SUMMARY

Agricultural-rural incidents, while not frequent, usually result in severe injuries. Extrication techniques may be similar to extrication from motor vehicles, but there are three basic differences: the size and construction of farm equipment, the location of the incident, and the potential resources for help. Preincident planning for an agricultural-rural rescue operation is important, as is frequent review and practice of rescue techniques, to ensure a safe rescue.

CHAPTER 2

Incident Command System

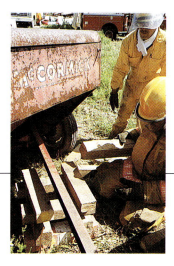

CHAPTER OUTLINE

Overview
Objectives
Managing Agricultural-Rural Incidents
 Preincident Planning
 Determining Urgency
 Notification
 A Resource Tracking System
The Incident Command System
 Mutual Aid in Agricultural-Rural Rescue
 Communications
Special Aspects of Agricultural-Rural Rescue
 Multi-Jurisdictional/Multi-Agency Incident Management
 Using Specialists Untrained in Rescue
 Air Medical Evacuation
 Extended Incidents
 Disasters and Mass Casualties
Obstacles to Overall Coordination and Leadership
 Loss of Communication
 Breakdown in Information Flow
 Disruption in Logistical Support
 Inadequate Leadership
 Loss of Span of Control
 Equipment Failure
 Change in the Nature of the Incident
 Personality Conflicts
Specific Problem Situations
 Problems With Initial Strategy and Tactics
 Injured or Deceased Rescuers
 Injury to Patient Caused by Rescuers
 When Rescuers Are Overwhelmed
Summary

CHAPTER 2 Incident Command System

KEY TERMS

Callout information sheet: document that provides the dispatcher with the information necessary to brief resources properly when they are requested to respond.

Disaster: any event that exceeds the capacity of local resources to respond effectively in an appropriate time frame.

Incident Command System (ICS): standardized emergency management system developed to organize and manage all functions required to handle an emergency situation.

Incident commander: the individual in charge of the rescue operation.

Mutual aid: system in which different agencies or organizations may be preassigned to various functional areas during a rescue operation.

Span of control: the optimum number of resources that can be effectively supervised by one person.

Step-up plan: plan that defines responsibilities for determining the need for and requesting additional resources.

OVERVIEW

The key to a successful rescue operation is a well-planned and carefully implemented incident management system. Rescue incidents require a flexible, adaptable management structure to prevent deterioration of the situation.

This chapter describes the Incident Command System (ICS) commonly used to organize and manage emergencies. Included are discussions of preincident planning, determining urgency, resource callout, and a resource tracking system. This chapter also outlines the organization of the ICS by functional areas with details of the incident command functions. It explains the incident action plan and discusses incident communications.

The ICS involves several functions, such as incident command, operations, planning, logistics, and finance. Incident command is responsible for the overall management of the rescue operation.

continued

The operations function carries out the actual rescue tactics. The planning function collects, evaluates, and distributes all incident information. The logistics function provides personnel, supplies, materials, and facilities to support the operation. And the finance function tracks all incident finances.

In addition to describing the optimal incident command system, this chapter presents instructions for handling exceptional situations, such as a multi-jurisdictional/multi-agency incident, an expanding rescue incident, special rescue situations, an extended incident, and disasters. Recommendations are also presented for coping with a response system that lacks coordination and leadership and other specific problems that may arise.

OBJECTIVES

After reading this chapter, the rescuer should be able to:

- define span of control.
- explain the need for a preincident plan.
- identify the principal components of a preincident plan for an agricultural-rural incident.
- describe how to use a callout sheet and a resource tracking system.
- list the requirements of an effective communications system.
- explain how to minimize potential conflicts in multi-jurisdictional/multi-agency responses.

MANAGING AGRICULTURAL-RURAL INCIDENTS

Agricultural-rural rescue and extrication can be the most difficult single-patient situation faced by emergency medical and rescue personnel. The isolated location, the difficulty of access and extrication, the rescuer's lack of familiarity with farm equipment, and the size of the equipment all contribute to the difficulty of agricultural-rural rescue. Of these, the most critical factor is time.

Farmers and ranchers often work alone in isolated locations, and several hours may pass before they are missed or the incident discovered. In rural areas, distances between the rescue center and the incident site, or between the incident site and a medical facility, may mean lengthy response and transport times. The size of the equipment, the rescuer's unfamiliarity with it, and the severity of the injuries may mean that extricating the patient could take hours.

In such situations, an effective Incident Command System is critical to success. The ICS can organize and manage the three basic components of a successful emergency operation: resources (personnel and equipment), communications (radio, telephone, person-to-person), and management (trained leadership) (Figure 2.1).

Frequently, the person in charge in an emergency attempts to supervise too many resources. The person in charge must maintain a manageable **span of control**, which is the optimum number of resources that can be effectively supervised by one person. The span of control for rescue operations is normally one person in charge for each three to seven subordinates or resources. The optimum ratio is one to five. Resources, safety factors, and the type, nature, and location of the incident determine the appropriate span of control for any incident.

Preincident Planning

Preincident planning is critical in order to ensure that the quickest, easiest, and safest processes are used in a rescue operation. Preincident planning also involves developing and maintaining a written plan for response to and management of a rescue. In most emergencies, supervisors try to make critical decisions based on limited information gathered very quickly at the time the incident is reported. The more information that can be gathered and analyzed *before* an incident, the quicker the rescue team can move from simply reacting to the incident to managing the incident.

Based on predictable problems or situations, incident commanders should have made as many decisions as possible before an incident occurs. In this way, they can later concentrate on the unique or unpredictable problems of the incident. Critical components of a preincident plan include incident command responsibilities, organization, management, and personnel requirements and qualifications.

First, the plan establishes who will be in charge and outlines the organization of the rescue operation. It should also include policies and procedures for responding to an incident, including an analysis of the kinds of incidents in the local area that may require rescue operations.

FIGURE 2.1

Resources, communications, and management are vital components of a successful rescue operation.

RESOURCES ——————— Personnel/Equipment
COMMUNICATIONS ——— Radios/Telephone/Person-to-person
MANAGEMENT ——————— Trained leadership

The responsibility for managing a rescue is often dictated by law or regulation. Sometimes, the responsibility for rescue is determined by the kind of incident. To avoid confusion or disagreement at the scene, the plan must specify who will be in charge of each type of rescue. Under the ICS, the individual in charge of the rescue operation is called the **incident commander.**

Areas under different ownership—private, municipal, county, state, or federal—may each have a different management philosophy. Preincident plans must contain options to resolve jurisdictional conflicts and accessibility problems. Alternate plans, often referred to in lay terms as "plans B and C," are important in the event that the initial plan becomes unworkable or dangerous to rescuers or the patient.

The preincident plan should also provide information about resources, including personnel, equipment, and a physical description of the area. It should list the personnel by name, type, capability, and location with telephone numbers, radio or pager numbers, or other methods for contacting them. This is especially important in agricultural-rural rescue operations, which frequently require specialized mechanical knowledge or extrication tools that are not part of the rescue team's standard equipment or expertise. Among these specialized resources are farm equipment dealers, farm equipment mechanics, heavy wrecker services, heavy machinery operators, and agricultural chemical dealers. Neighboring farmers, who are likely to be familiar with the way farm equipment operates, are often valuable resources. Some areas also have special silo rescue teams or hazardous materials response teams that can be called upon for backup. Because phone numbers, addresses, and personnel names change often, this listing should be contained in a separate resource locator file that can be easily updated without having to change the entire plan. Telephone numbers for evenings and weekends are critical. The resource list should be updated on a regular basis, at least four times a year.

The preincident plan must also include a **step-up plan** for expanding the rescue response if the size or complexity of the rescue operation increases. The step-up plan defines the responsibilities for determining the need for and requesting additional resources. The step-up plan should include previously negotiated mutual aid agreements.

The preincident plan should also include the following information:

- An evaluation of the rescuers' areas of responsibility, including access routes, terrain, hazards, potential base locations, staging areas, and helispots
- A farm layout map of the emergency response district
- A listing of resources needed to respond to a potential incident, including rescue and medical team personnel, farm equipment dealers, and a farm equipment mechanic. (If needed resources are not avail-

able to respond in time, additional personnel should be trained to meet the potential need.)

Information about the physical characteristics of the farms in a particular emergency response district is critical in ensuring quick response to the scene. Many farms have fields and woods that spread across a considerable area. A sketch of the farm with field numbers and road names is a logical first step in identifying the exact location of the incident. These maps should also identify barriers like water hazards, mud, and animal herds, which may complicate accessing the patient.

In addition, preincident planning should include information about the location of hazardous materials on a farm, possible hazardous materials spills, or other incidents that might require an evacuation. Most farms store pesticides and other hazardous materials, including explosives. The rescue team needs to know exactly where these materials are stored, what types of materials are stored, how much is stored, and in what season they are stored. Local chapters of community service agencies should be contacted to determine their capabilities and the conditions under which they will respond. These volunteer community agencies provide a wide range of services and can care for residents displaced from the affected area.

The preincident plan should be developed as a joint effort of all organizations that may be involved in a rescue operation. Representatives of each organization should participate in joint training exercises and periodic review and evaluation of the plan. Most farmers will cooperate with local emergency medical and rescue teams to use their farms for an interagency drill. The purpose of such a drill is to practice the preincident plan, evaluate the adequacy of the plan, and then make modifications as necessary.

Determining Urgency

Every incident requires some form of immediate response. The first hour is the most critical to the success of a rescue operation. A sound and tested preincident plan and early positive decisions often mean the difference between success or failure. It is most important that the right resources be called at the right time and given the right assignments.

The incident commander determines the urgency and type of response that will be needed when first notified of a potential incident. The incident commander gathers critical information on the location of the incident, the number of victims, their physical and mental conditions, potential hazards, scene accessibility, and current and predicted weather conditions.

In rural areas, family members, friends, or co-workers may attempt to rescue the subject before they call a rescue team. If the incident occurs in a field, a phone may be a considerable distance away. By the time the first notice is given, the condition of the subject is usually quite serious and requires an urgent response.

Notification

Notification is the process of contacting needed rescue resources and providing them with the information they need to get to the scene quickly, safely, and prepared for their assignments. While it is better to have too many resources than not enough, the incident commander should attempt to make the most efficient use of resources in performing the rescue. However, it is better to overreact to an incident than to underreact. In many cases, rescuers become overwhelmed because too few resources were called. It is always easier to cancel responding rescuers than to call them after the rescue operation gets into trouble.

Specialized resources for agricultural-rural rescues include farm machinery dealers, towing services, service managers at farm implement stores, experienced farm equipment mechanics, and county hazardous materials response teams. A mechanic, service manager, or neighbor who works with the same brand of machinery involved in the incident may be the best source of information on how to extricate the subject. Mechanics and service managers who repair competitive equipment are often familiar with other basic mechanical components and may be able to recommend a course of action.

When the required resources are identified, a **callout information sheet** is prepared. This sheet provides the dispatcher with the information necessary to brief resources properly when they are requested to respond. The callout information sheet should include the following:

- Type of incident
- Location of the incident
- Time of day
- Field conditions at the site (muddy, steep, etc.)
- Weather conditions
- Type of equipment involved in the incident
- Special access instructions
- Special equipment, clothing, protection required
- Estimated length of time rescuers will be involved in the operation

For extended en route travel times, rescuers should be assigned a specific radio frequency to monitor or be given specific times to check in by telephone with the dispatcher. The dispatcher can then provide updated information if the rescuers' services are no longer required. The demobilization planning should begin during the initial callout so that once the incident is concluded, units can be returned to their home base as quickly and economically as possible.

A Resource Tracking System

Once the resources are requested, the incident commander should maintain a method for resource tracking to monitor which resources are responding or assigned to specific tasks. A simple and inexpensive method is a T-card locator file, a plastic notebook with slots for the T-cards. With a T-card locator file, the incident commander can organize resources by function, assignment, capability, or location. Assignment changes can then be recorded by moving the T-card to the appropriate location in the file.

Using this resource locator system, each resource is assigned one of three current status conditions. *Assigned* means that a resource is actively performing a rescue-related task. *Available* means that a resource is ready to be assigned a task (for example, a resource in a staging area). *Out-of-service* means a resource is unavailable for assignment.

THE INCIDENT COMMAND SYSTEM

The **Incident Command System (ICS)** is a standardized emergency management system developed to organize and manage all the functions required to deal with an emergency situation. Using such a system will ensure that rescuers know what they must do, who is in charge, and where the resources are located. It is designed to allow the leader to *command the incident* and to prevent the incident from *commanding the leader*. The incident commander must be *proactive* to the incident, not *reactive* to it.

Mutual Aid in Agricultural-Rural Rescue

All rescue operations involve similar duties or tasks called functions. The ICS is organized into five functional areas, each with specifically defined responsibilities. The five major functional areas are listed below:

1. Incident command
2. Operations
3. Planning
4. Logistics
5. Finance

All of these functions, along with several subordinate functions, are performed on almost every rescue operation, though they may not be performed as separate entities. Whether one person or several people carry out specific responsibilities, this structure provides the flexibility to respond to the demands of the incident and grows when the size or complexity of the incident increases. In agricultural-rural areas, the incident command system may incorporate a system of **mutual aid,** which means that different agencies or organizations may be preassigned to various functional areas.

Incident command provides overall management of the incident, and includes the incident commander, the information officer, the liaison officer, and the safety officer. In a small incident, all of these roles may be performed by a single person, the incident commander. In a large operation, however, the roles of safety officer, liaison officer, and information officer are delegated to other qualified staff members so that a proper span of control (three to seven persons) is maintained.

The incident commander initially establishes incident objectives, goals that must be achieved to successfully complete the rescue operation. Based on these objectives, the incident commander develops tactics, the specific actions the rescuers will use to complete the rescue operation.

Communications

Because there are so many different kinds of communication codes, all rescue communication should be in plain English. No ten codes or other codes should be used, except to report fatalities if communication channels are not secure. Radio networks are rarely needed for agricultural-rural rescue operations. Communication problems are generally the result of "holes" that make it difficult to contact dispatch or medical control. Alternate communications plans for such situations should be incorporated in rescue planning, such as cellular phones or satellite communications.

In a rescue operation where several agencies work together, all personnel must communicate using commonly understood terms. The ICS uses standard terms to ensure that everyone involved completely understands all communications (Table 2.1).

SPECIAL ASPECTS OF AGRICULTURAL-RURAL RESCUE

Agricultural-rural rescue situations present specific problems in organizing and managing a rescue operation.

Multi-Jurisdictional/ Multi-Agency Incident Management

One of the most common problems in emergency response occurs when more than one jurisdiction or agency is involved in an incident. In many rural areas, mutual aid agreements defining roles and responsibilities minimize the potential for disagreements and problems and speed the operational response to an incident. Interagency training that tests and refines the preincident plan will likely result in a coordinated rescue effort when an incident actually occurs.

Using Specialists Untrained in Rescue

Agricultural-rural rescue operations often require specialists such as farm equipment mechanics, physicians, paramedics, or engineers. These resources may not be trained to handle the particular rescue environment. Nevertheless, rescue leaders can still safely and effectively use them.

In some cases, these specialists may be used as advisers. Neighbors, farm equipment mechanics, and service managers may be more familiar with the equipment than the rescue team, and may be the best sources of information on how to extricate the victim. Even though these individuals may not have specific rescue training, they can contribute to the operation, yet remain a safe distance away from the incident. If their as-

TABLE 2.1 List of ICS Terms

Branch	The organizational level having functional/geographic responsibility for major segments of incident operations. The Branch level is organizationally between section and division/group.
Clear text	The use of plain English in radio communication transmissions. No ten codes or agency specific code are used when using clear text.
Command	The act of directing, ordering, and/or controlling resources by virtue of explicit legal, agency, or delegated authority.
Command staff	The command staff consists of all personnel within the command function who report directly to the incident commander, such as the safety officer, the liaison officer, and the information officer.
Committed resource	A resource checked-in and assigned work tasks on an incident.
Coordination	The process of systematically analyzing a situation, developing relevant information, and informing appropriate command authority (for its decision) of viable alternatives for selection of the most effective combination of available resources to meet specific objectives. The coordination process (which can be either intraagency or interagency) does not in and of itself involve command dispatch actions. However, personnel responsible for coordination may perform command or dispatch functions within limits as established by specific agency delegations, procedures, legal authority, and so forth.
Dispatch	The implementation of a command decision to move a resource or resources from one place to another.
Division	That organizational level having responsibility for total operations within a defined geographic area.
Element	Any identified part of the incident command system organization structure.
Group	A division with functional responsibilities only for certain field operations such as air support, rescue, law enforcement, and so forth. Often not constrained by geographic areas on an incident (see also division).
Incident	Any situation man-made or natural, regardless of size or complexity, that requires action to protect life and property.
Incident action plan	The action plan, which is initially prepared at the first planning meeting, contains general objectives reflecting overall incident strategy, and specific rescue, fire suppression, or law enforcement actions for the next operational period. When complete, the incident action plan will have a number of attachments.

continued

TABLE 2.1 List of ICS Terms, *continued*

Incident commander	The individual responsible for the management of all IC activities at a specific incident.
Incident command post	The location from which the command functions are executed, usually co-located with the incident base.
Jurisdictional	The agency having jurisdiction and agency responsibility for a specific geographic area.
Operational period	The period of time scheduled for execution of a given set of actions as specified in the incident action plan.
Out of service	Resources assigned to an incident, but unable to respond for mechanical, rest, personnel, or other reasons.
Personnel pool	Unassigned personnel who may have reported to the incident without an assignment. They do not belong to a company, a strike team, or a task force.
Planning meeting	A meeting, held periodically during an incident, to select specific strategies and tactics for incident control operations and for service and support planning.
Rescue	Systematic removal of person(s) from a hazardous situation.
Resources	All personnel and major items or equipment available, or potentially available, for assignment to incident tasks and on which status is kept.
Section	The organizational level having responsibility for an entire incident specialty function, such as operation, planning, logistics, and finance.
Staging area	A location near an incident where available incident resources are grouped together waiting for specific assignments.
Strike team	Specified combinations of resources consisting of like units with a leader, personnel, and a common communications.
Task force	A group of unlike resources with a leader, personnel, and common communications assembled for a specific mission.
Technical specialist	Personnel with special skills who are activated only when needed. Technical specialists may be needed in the areas of fire behavior, water resources, environmental concern, resource use, or training.
Unit	The organizational element having functional responsibility for a specific incident or activity with the larger functions of planning, logistics, or finance.

sistance in extricating the patient is required at the site itself, they may assist in disassembling the machinery, but only under the guidance of the rescue team to help protect the patient, specialist, and rescue team. Part of the preincident plan should include contacting farm equipment dealers and mechanics for support during an incident.

If specialists are needed at the site to help with the extrication, they should be escorted to the scene by a trained rescuer. The rescuer must closely supervise and assist the specialists to handle the rescue environment safely by properly equipping and instructing them about potential hazards at the scene. However, this method removes trained rescuers from activities directly involved in rescuing the patient. The advantages and disadvantages of both methods must be carefully weighed before a decision is made on how untrained specialists can best be used.

Air Medical Evacuation

The severity of injuries encountered in agricultural-rural incidents and the time and distances involved in transport to a medical facility may mean that the rescue team will use an air medical helicopter. (See chapter 16 for a complete discussion.) Stabilization and evacuation of the patient should be established as part of the preincident plan. The plan should also include notifying medical and rescue resources and receiving hospitals, and preparing for all possible medical contingencies for the patient and rescuers. Alternate transportation plans should be included in every preincident plan in the event that weather, mechanical problems, or other missions make the aircraft unavailable.

The types of helicopters used for air medical operations vary, but the dangers are the same. Rescuers must stay a safe distance from the helicopter whenever it is on the ground and the rotors are spinning. In addition, rescuers should never approach the helicopter from the rear. If it is necessary to move from one side to the other, rescuers should walk around the front of the aircraft.

When approaching the helicopter, rescuers should walk in a crouched position until they are at the helicopter door. Secure all loose clothing, hats, equipment, and long hair before approaching the aircraft. If the helicopter must land on a grade, rescuers must approach the helicopter from the downhill side only. Do not move a patient to the helicopter until the crew signals they are ready to receive the patient. When accompanying a flight, rescuers must follow the directions of the flight crew exactly.

Extended Incidents

Most rescues are completed within a few hours or, at most, within a day. However, a small percentage of incidents last more than a day. Most commonly, these will be hazardous materials incidents or natural disasters requiring evacuation and scene containment. These extended efforts challenge rescuers' abilities to organize and manage the incident.

The incident commander must ensure that there is advance planning for replacements of exhausted personnel and for logistical support such as food, water, shelter, sanitary facilities, transportation, and special equipment. The extended incident may require a larger and more experienced management team than would be needed for a smaller or shorter duration incident. In the initial stages of an incident, the incident commander must anticipate and plan for the additional requirements of an incident that is expected to last more than 8 to 12 hours.

Disasters and Mass Casualties

A **disaster** is any event that exceeds the capacity of local resources to respond effectively in an appropriate time frame. An incident need not involve widespread destruction or hundreds of casualties to be a disaster. A chemical release is an example of a human-caused disaster, while a flood is an example of a natural disaster. Each disaster may cause different specific problems, but the overall effect on rescuers is the same. Personnel and equipment resources are inadequate, transportation systems are congested, medical facilities are overwhelmed, and communication systems are overloaded or damaged.

One common problem during disasters is the uneven distribution of patients to medical facilities. Hospitals close to the incident receive the majority of patients, including the "walking wounded" and become overloaded. Before a rescue team begins to transport multiple casualties, the disaster medical coordinator or the receiving hospitals must be consulted. One primary goal is to avoid transferring the disaster from the incident site to the medical facility.

OBSTACLES TO OVERALL COORDINATION AND LEADERSHIP

Areas of emergency response that continue to cause problems in organizing and managing on-scene activities include the following:

- Lack of a preincident plan
- Lack of well-defined authority
- Lack of adequate communications (especially among different agencies)
- Lack of a staging area to assemble and control the flow of equipment and personnel
- Inappropriate use of specialized resources
- Inability to identify and track responders at the scene
- Failure of responders to complete their assigned tasks

For an effective rescue operation, the incident commander must establish an on-scene organization to provide coordination and leadership and to manage these problems. The incident commander should address each of the following elements on every incident:

- Someone must be in charge of the overall scene and of each task.
- Responders must be able to identify leaders easily.
- An incident command post must be established in a safe, accessible, and visible location, if the size of the response warrants.
- A staging area must be established in an accessible and controlled location that does not impede incident traffic flow.
- Functions must be delegated to maintain a manageable span of control.
- Functions should be preassigned whenever possible to help coordinate the operation.
- Organizational staffing must be stepped up early to stay ahead of incident requirements.
- Responders must know what they are expected to do and where and to whom they report.
- Decisions must be made carefully, based upon the best information currently available, and then reevaluated as more information becomes known or as the situation changes.
- The incident action plan must be updated and revised as necessary.

Critical decisions must not be delayed in the hope that more information will make the decision easier or that the problem will solve itself. To delay a decision is to decide to continue the status quo. Most preincident plans are not perfect, but they are a map showing where to start.

Decisive leadership, a well-organized response, and proper delegation of responsibility all improve the incident commander's ability to manage effectively. When problems arise, the incident commander must not lose sight of the incident objectives. He or she must deal only with the problems that directly affect the overall success of the incident, and not get bogged down in unimportant details that can be delegated to others. Problems should be solved and actions taken at the lowest appropriate organizational level. If a unit or team leader can solve the problem, the incident commander should delegate it to that person.

The incident commander must evaluate problems when they occur and determine the best response based on the specific situation. Planning for commonly encountered problems and possible solutions eases the stress on the incident command staff.

Loss of Communication

Modern emergency response has a critical dependence on electronic communications. When these communications are lost, the rescue effort may be crippled, so planning should identify backup communication methods. In rural areas, radio communication is often limited by "blind spots" caused by the terrain. In these situations, radio relays can be established on high points of land to communicate messages between the incident and the communication center. In a disaster, telephone lines may be downed or overloaded. Even some base station radios will be lost because they are linked to transmitter towers by land lines.

Provisions for replacing these communications must be made in the emergency plan. Cellular phones with satellite linkage are possible substitutes for loss of land lines.

Breakdown in Information Flow

The breakdown of the information flow in a rescue organization will hinder the operation and endanger both patients and rescuers. The critical areas where information flow may break down occur in both large and small operations:

- Failure to report changes in the situation from field teams to incident command
- Inaccurate reporting of conditions from field teams to incident command
- Failure to report changing objectives or tactics from incident command to field teams
- Untimely and inaccurate recording of events
- Lack of communication between sections of the rescue organization
- Interference in the chain of communication such as radio personnel who fail to pass along portions of messages or who add their own interpretation to messages
- Inaccurate briefing of significant events by shift personnel to their replacements

Communications between incident command and the field teams can be improved by briefing upon assignment, debriefing when the assignment is completed, requiring regular check-in reports from the field teams, and if appropriate, conducting operational period briefings. The incident commander must insist that all rescuers know and adhere to reporting requirements and procedures.

Disruption in Logistical Support

If critical resources are not available when needed, even the most well-organized rescue operation will quickly deteriorate. When there is a disruption in logistical support, the incident commander must quickly identify the source of the problem. Adequate lead time is important for good logistical support of any rescue operation and must be stressed to the staff. The major reason for disruption in logistical support in agricultural-rural rescue operations is that resources are not currently available or cannot be acquired. If the problem is a lack of available resources, the incident commander must develop and carry out an alternate plan that does not require those resources. If the logistics staff is not performing satisfactorily, the incident commander should add trained staff or replace ineffective personnel.

Inadequate Leadership

If leadership deteriorates during an incident, the responsible individual must be replaced or assigned an assistant capable of providing the necessary leadership. A rescuer working for an individual with inadequate leadership skills should tactfully provide assistance, or, if the lack of leadership interferes with group performance, inform a higher supervisor.

The preincident plan must specify leadership needs for the organization and determine how appropriate leadership will be provided. Rescuers should have or obtain training and experience to assume command and provide effective leadership.

Loss of Span of Control

For rescue operations, the acceptable span of control is one supervisor for every three to seven subordinates or resources. The optimum span of control is one supervisor for every five subordinates. When the number of subordinates exceeds a supervisor's ability to manage the assigned task, the supervisor should appoint subordinate supervisors and delegate them the necessary authority to accomplish the task.

Equipment Failure

Equipment failure can be minimized by instituting the following precautions:

- Using the right tool for the right purpose
- Maintaining and properly caring for equipment
- Promptly repairing equipment and returning it to service
- Discarding damaged or irreparable equipment

Rescue teams should always have backup equipment available to replace broken equipment. Additionally, rescuers should be able to improvise equipment with available materials. For example, some teams use pneumatic tools connected to SCBA bottles to assist in rapid dismantling of heavy farm equipment. The logistics section must ensure that adequate supplies are always available, that they are in good working order, and that backups, especially for specialized equipment, are available.

Change in the Nature of the Incident

At times, the initial plan may fail because the nature or scope of the incident changes dramatically. For example, the weather may change and endanger both the patient and rescuers. In such a situation, one or two alternate plans should be in place, or even in progress, to fit the new developments. The incident commander is responsible for informing the rescue team of any changes in the plan. Developing alternate plans not only allows for quick, efficient changes to be made, it also helps to relieve the frustration that often occurs if the initial plan fails.

Personality Conflicts

Personality conflicts commonly occur in stressful situations and often keep rescuers from performing at their highest potential. Personality conflicts must be handled early. If two individuals cannot work out their problems, the supervisor must quickly mediate. If mediation is unsuccessful, the individuals should be separated or removed from the scene.

SPECIFIC PROBLEM SITUATIONS

Problems With Initial Strategy and Tactics

An incident commander must be able to recognize *when* the chosen strategy and tactics are not working and be willing to change them. The incident commander must continually reevaluate the progress of the rescue operation in terms of successfully meeting the incident objectives, and should always have alternate plans for completing the operation. The incident action plan can then be adjusted or modified to meet changing needs. Alternate plans should be in place as part of the original preincident plan for two important reasons: first, if the initial plan fails, well-planned alternates are already in place; second, with alternates in place, rescuers will not be forced to scramble under stress to devise an alternate plan.

Injured or Deceased Rescuers

The safety of the rescuers is a higher priority than the safety of the patient. An injured rescuer cannot assist in the rescue, and the injury adds another incident that diverts resources from the original objective. Safety must always be a primary concern of the incident commander.

If a rescuer is injured or killed during a rescue effort, the incident commander must review the incident objectives, reevaluate priorities and tactics, and develop alternate plans to meet the changing needs. The incident commander must first ensure that no other rescuers will be injured. While the injured rescuer is treated, the cause of the injury must be identified and specific steps taken to eliminate the unsafe situation. If the rescuer is killed, the scene must be protected. An investigation will be necessary to determine the cause of injury or death. Whenever there is injury or death to a rescuer, trained individuals should monitor the stress levels of the other rescuers and their ability to function. A critical incident stress debriefing (CISD) session may need to be held at the scene. Whatever the circumstances, the stress levels of the rescue team must be taken into account when making assignments.

Injury to Patient Caused by Rescuers

Additional injury to the patient caused by the rescuers is managed in the same way as a situation in which there is an injured rescuer. The rescuers must first take action to prevent another occurrence and then treat the patient for the injury. An investigator should be assigned to determine the cause of the accident, document the accident scene, the actions of the rescuers, and the equipment in use, and then obtain statements from the rescuers and the patient.

When Rescuers Are Overwhelmed

When rescuers reach the scene and face the reality of performing emergency medical care and rescue, they may be overwhelmed by the size or complexity of the tasks to be performed. After evaluating the overall situation, the incident commander must establish objectives and priorities for resolving the incident. If additional rescuers or specialized resources are required to manage the incident, they should be ordered immediately. Initial on-scene rescuers should be assigned the highest priority tasks, such as scene safety, scene control, triage, and priority care of the patients. The incident commander should initiate plans to expand management organization to accommodate the resources required to accomplish the rescue. Rescuers who arrive on-scene later must be assigned, tracked, and supervised to effectively perform their assignments.

SUMMARY

A well-organized preincident management plan is essential to carry out a successful rescue operation. The Incident Command System (ICS) is such a plan.

The first step in establishing an ICS is developing a preincident plan, which enables rescue managers to make as many decisions as possible before the actual rescue operation. This plan should be a joint effort, in both planning and practicing, of all the organizations that may be involved in a rescue operation.

The ICS uses an incident action plan, a general strategy on how to conduct the rescue. Incident objectives are developed and tactics selected to achieve the objectives.

During a rescue operation, communications are extremely important and are managed by a communications plan. If several agencies are working together, all personnel must communicate using commonly understood terms.

The ICS minimizes jurisdictional conflicts by using the unified command concept. Each agency having jurisdiction identifies a representative to meet with other representatives and prepare a joint operational plan. Planning the management of these situations is vital to avoid conflicts and problems.

To prevent loss of control when an incident expands, the incident commander must maintain the span of control by providing a controlled step-up of the organization, adding modules to the command structure to keep the core intact whatever the size of the incident.

An extended incident presents special considerations. There must be advance planning to ensure logistical support and to replace exhausted rescuers.

As a rescue operation gets underway, the incident commander must be certain that there is an on-scene organization to provide coordination and leadership to prevent or manage any problems. A well-organized response, strong leadership, and proper delegation of authority also help the incident commander manage effectively when things go wrong.

CHAPTER 3

Rescuer Preparation and Personal Safety

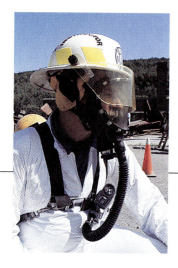

CHAPTER OUTLINE

Overview
Objectives
Physical Threats
   Types of Threats
Exposure to Blood-Borne
   Pathogens
   Universal Precautions
Protective Clothing
   Types of Clothing
   Minimum Clothing
      Requirements

Headgear
Protection From Dust and
   Contaminants
Footwear
Hand Protection
Skin Protection
Gear
   Lighting
   Litters
Summary

KEY TERMS

Outer layer: a shell of windproof, waterproof material that resists wind and precipitation.

Thermal layer: a second layer of clothing worn on the outside of the transport layer to provide insulation.

Transport layer: a thin layer of clothing worn next to the skin that wicks moisture away from the skin to keep the wearer dry and warm.

CHAPTER 3 Rescuer Preparation and Personal Safety

Turnout gear: protective clothing garments designed for use in structural fire-fighting environments.

Universal precautions: protective measures that emphasize infection control and urge caution when dealing with equipment subject to breakage or accidental puncture of the skin.

OVERVIEW

Protecting rescuers is one of the primary goals of a successful rescue operation. Injuries or other hazards in emergency operations can jeopardize the successful outcome of a rescue operation. Therefore, the primary responsibility of the rescue team is to avoid injuring themselves or other rescuers while protecting the patient from injury or additional injury. Avoiding potential threats and selecting appropriate protective clothing and gear is vital to the successful outcome of a rescue operation. This chapter describes different types of clothing and other personal gear that protects rescuers from environmental elements.

Rescuers must be prepared for a rescue operation at all times. Part of this preparation is a plan or checklist for all the protective clothing and gear that might be needed at the scene. Because even experienced rescuers sometimes forget pieces of equipment or appropriate protective clothing during the rush of callout, a checklist of all the necessary gear should be reviewed when the team is called out.

OBJECTIVES

After reading this chapter, the rescuer should be able to:

- describe universal precautions and protection from blood-borne pathogens.
- describe ways to become prepared physically for rescue operations.
- choose appropriate protective clothing and gear for rescue operations.

PHYSICAL THREATS

The primary responsibility of all members of the rescue team is to avoid injuring themselves or other rescuers and to protect the patient from additional injury. Injury, illness, stress, and the other hazards common in rescue situations reduce the effectiveness and efficiency of rescuers in caring for the patient. These problems may also jeopardize the rescue operation or result in injury or loss of life of the patient and/or other rescuers.

The best way to reduce these risks during a rescue operation is by preparing physically and mentally and by avoiding physical threats. Knowledge and awareness of potential hazards are the tools rescuers use to reduce the threats inherent in rescue activities.

Types of Threats

Rescuers are exposed to different situations and environments that may pose a physical threat to their survival. The most common physical threats are described below.

Atmosphere One of the greatest physical threats to rescuers is the contamination of the atmosphere. This is particularly a problem when rescuers must work in confined spaces and when they are exposed to the different gases and chemicals common in agricultural-rural settings.

Temperature Another physical threat is extreme temperature. The human body functions efficiently within a narrow temperature range. Therefore, when rescuers must work outside of buildings or vehicles, they must depend on appropriate clothing for protection from extreme heat (sun and exertion) and extreme cold (cold, wind, and precipitation).

Hydration Adequate fluid intake or hydration is important for proper functioning of the human body. Because the body is composed mostly of water, maintaining a high level of fluid in the body is essential for efficiency and survival.

In many environments, dehydration is a common problem for both rescuers and patients. When people leave their usual environment, they often fail to maintain an adequate fluid intake. Remember that dehydration is not unique to hot, dry environments. It is also a problem in cold environments, since drinking cold liquids is not appealing. Fluids are lost more rapidly with greater altitude and decreased humidity in the air.

The simplest way to replenish fluids is by drinking. Any nonalcoholic, noncaffeinated fluid is suitable. Water is most often available and is absorbed faster by the body than any other fluid. Fluids with high levels of sugar and carbohydrate should be avoided as they can actually slow the absorption rate and cause stomach discomfort and vomiting.

One convenient indicator of hydration is urination. Infrequent urination or urine that has a deep yellow color is an indication of dehydration. Drink enough fluid to keep your urine appearing either clear or light yellow.

Nutrition The human body must also have adequate nutrition to function efficiently. Food is the fuel on which the body runs. The physical exertion and physical stress of rescue require a high energy output. Therefore, rescuers must have a ready supply of energy, otherwise they may become weak, uncoordinated, irritable, or even more susceptible to environmental conditions such as hypothermia. Without an adequate fuel supply, rescuer performance will be impaired, which during a rescue operation could endanger the rescuer or the patient. Therefore, it is recommended that rescuers carry an individual supply of high-energy food to help maintain energy levels.

Overeating may also reduce physical and mental performance. After a large meal, the blood required by the body to digest food is not available for other body activities. Eating several small meals throughout the day is usually more effective than eating a few large meals for keeping the body's energy resources at constant high levels.

Exercise Every rescuer should participate in a regular program of exercise. Physical conditioning enables the body to use body fuel more efficiently to produce energy and to delay exhaustion. A well-conditioned rescuer is better prepared to cope with the physical demands and mental stress encountered during a rescue operation.

EXPOSURE TO BLOOD-BORNE PATHOGENS

In many situations, rescuers will be exposed to blood and other bodily fluids. As a result, there is significant potential for exposure to blood-borne pathogens. Rescuers must be aware of current requirements for minimizing exposure and practice universal precautions, based on the assumption that all patients are potential carriers of blood-borne pathogens.

Universal Precautions

Federal regulations require all healthcare workers, including rescue/EMS personnel, to assume that all patients in all settings are potentially infected with HIV (AIDS), HBV (hepatitis B virus), or other blood-borne agents. These regulations mandate the use of barriers and other protective equipment to prevent parenteral, mucous membrane, and skin exposure to the blood and certain body fluids of all patients.

The Centers for Disease Control (CDC) **universal precautions** also emphasize infection control measures and urge caution when dealing with equipment subject to breakage or accidental puncture of the skin of a healthcare worker.

The primary assumption underlying the CDC's universal precaution recommendations is that protective barriers can be expected to reduce the healthcare worker's risk of exposure to blood, body fluids containing blood, and other body fluids. The CDC notes that the type of barrier chosen depends on the clinical situation. In general, the selection of the type of protective barrier, protective equipment, or work practice should include consideration of (1) the probability of exposure to blood and body fluids, (2) the type of body fluid contacted, and (3) the amount of blood or body fluid likely to be encountered.

Because it is often not possible to know when a patient may be infected with HIV or other blood-borne agents, adoption of universal precautions represents one effective way to reduce the risk of transmission of HIV and other blood-borne agents in the healthcare setting. Thus, rescue and EMS personnel, regardless of HIV caseload, should always use universal precautions.

The CDC recommendations, amended in 1987, 1988, 1989, and in 1991, specifically provide the following:

1. All health care workers should routinely use appropriate barrier precautions to prevent skin and mucous membrane exposure when contact with blood or other body fluids of any patient is anticipated. Gloves should be worn for touching blood and body fluids, mucous membranes, or nonintact skin of all patients, for handling items or surfaces soiled with blood or body fluids, and for performing venipuncture and other vascular access procedures. Gloves should be changed after contact with each patient. Masks and protective eye wear or face shields should be worn during procedures that are likely to generate droplets of blood or other body fluids to prevent exposure of mucous membranes of the mouth, nose, and eyes. Gowns or aprons should be worn during procedures that are likely to generate splashes of blood or other body fluids.
2. Hands and other skin surfaces should be washed immediately and thoroughly if contaminated with blood and other body fluids. Hands should be washed immediately after gloves are removed.
3. All health care workers should take precautions to prevent injuries caused by needles, scalpels, and other sharp instruments or devices during procedures; while handling sharp instruments; during disposal of used needles, and whenever manipulating needles by hand, such as when removing them from disposable syringes, purposely bending or breaking them, or not recapping them. After they are used, disposable syringes and needles, scalpel blades, and other sharp items should be placed in puncture-resistant containers for disposal; the puncture-resistant container should be located as close as

CHAPTER 3 Rescuer Preparation and Personal Safety

practical to the use area. Large-bore reusable needles should be placed in a puncture-resistant container for transport to the reprocessing area.

4. Although saliva has not been implicated in HIV transmission, to minimize the need for emergency mouth-to-mouth resuscitation, mouthpieces, resuscitation bags, or other ventilation devices should be available for use if the need for resuscitation is predictable.

The CDC guidelines have been adopted by the Occupational Safety and Health Administration (OSHA) and the National Fire Protection Association (NFPA). Rescuers should routinely review current recommendations and regulations in this area.

PROTECTIVE CLOTHING

Regardless of the environment, the first line of self-protection is clothing and gear appropriate to both the task and the environment. It is important that rescuers become familiar with available clothing and gear and understand the specific functions of each type. This knowledge will enable rescuers to select the proper clothing and gear for each rescue situation and adapt or change them as the situation and environment change.

Protective equipment is only safe when it is in good condition. Rescuers are responsible for determining the safety of their equipment before using it for a rescue operation. If the condition of protective equipment is not known, it should be considered unsafe and should not be used until it is inspected.

Types of Clothing

A layered system of clothing provides the greatest flexibility in protection from the cold or heat. Opening layers of clothing or adding or removing layers can help control body temperature. A cold weather system of layered clothing consists of at least three layers (Figure 3.1). A thin, inner layer next to the skin, sometimes called the **transport layer**, wicks moisture away from the skin to keep the wearer dry and warm. Underwear made from polypropylene or polyester works well for the transport layer except where flame is a possibility. Next comes a **thermal layer** of bulkier material that acts as insulation. Wool is traditionally used as the thermal layer, but it is being replaced by other materials such as polyester pile. The **outer layer** is a shell of windproof, waterproof material to resist chilling winds and precipitation. The two outer layers should have front zippers to aid in venting body heat to prevent overheating. Some designs also have pit zips, which are zippers in the garment's armpits, to dissipate additional heat.

FIGURE 3.1

An inner transport layer, a thermal layer, and a protective outer layer of clothing provide adequate protection from the weather.

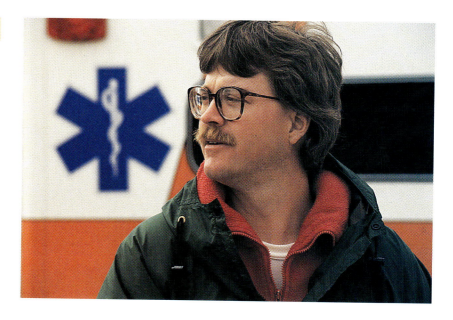

Clothing Construction The type of material used is very important in determining how well the clothing protects the wearer from the weather. Because it wicks moisture and heat away from the body, cotton is a good material for warm environments. However, cotton should be avoided when chilling from wetness is a possibility because when it becomes saturated, cotton wicks heat away from the body instead of insulating it. Cotton also tends to absorb moisture thoroughly. For example, if a rescuer wears cotton jeans and walks through wet grass, the cotton will wick the moisture from the cuffs up to the upper legs and chill the rescuer.

Down-filled clothing can be very warm as long as the down retains its loft, which acts as insulation. But if down gets wet, it loses its loft and its ability to retain warmth.

An outer layer of plastic-coated nylon provides waterproof protection, but it may also prevent the venting of body heat and perspiration. Newer permeable materials allow perspiration and some heat to escape while retaining their water resistance. Avoid flammable or meltable synthetic materials where there is a possibility of fire.

Minimum Clothing Requirements

For each rescue environment, there is a minimum level of protective clothing that is required. Fire-fighting equipment is generally not appropriate for a rescue operation in a confined space. Likewise, requirements for a silo rescue in Texas in August differ from those used for rescue from a manure pond in Minnesota in January.

A suggested minimum protective clothing level for rescuers would include a long-sleeved shirt and pants or jumpsuit, steel-toed, steel-shanked work boots, helmet with face shield, leather gloves with dis-

FIGURE 3.2

a. Minimum protective clothing includes coveralls, a helmet with a face shield, goggles, gloves, and steel-toed boots.

b. Full turnout gear protects the rescuer from heat of fire, reduces trauma from impact or cuts, and keeps water away from the body.

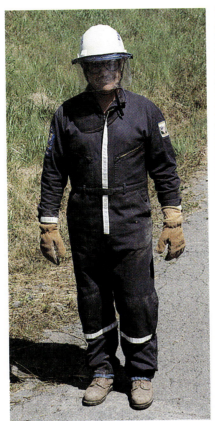
a.

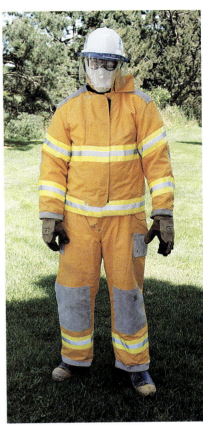
b.

posable latex or vinyl inner liners, and goggles (Figure 3.2a). Standard eyeglasses do not constitute adequate eye protection from flying particulates nor do they meet the OSHA requirements for blood-borne pathogens. To this basic minimum, additional equipment may be added for specialized rescue operations. The minimum protective clothing level applies not only to the rescue team, but should also be required of emergency medical personnel who are inside the safety zone.

Fire Fighting Turnout or bunker gear is a fire service term for protective clothing garments designed for use in structural fire-fighting environments (Figure 3.2b). Turnout gear provides head to toe protection and uses different layers of fabric/material to provide protection from the heat of fire, to reduce trauma from impact or cuts, and to keep water away from the body. As with most protective clothing, turnout gear adds weight and reduces range of motion to some degree.

The exterior fabrics used provide increased protection from cuts and abrasions and act as a barrier to high external temperatures. In cold weather, an insulated thermal inner layer of material that helps retain body heat is recommended.

High-angle/Confined Space Clothing worn for high-angle/confined space rescue in an agricultural-rural setting must be appropriate for the activity and the environment. Usually, loose-fitting clothing is recommended to permit the fullest range of movement. Part of the rescue team will be working outside the structure, so clothing must provide protection against possible chill and wetness caused by the weather. Additional clothing and protective equipment may be needed in specialized situations.

Electrical Hazards Most electrocutions and electrical injuries in an agricultural-rural setting are due to direct contact or proximity arcing from overhead power lines. If such a hazard is present, the local power company should be contacted immediately to turn power off and provide scene assistance. Do not approach the scene until the power has been disconnected, and the power company has confirmed that no auxiliary power sources have kicked in and re-energized the line.

If electrical hazards are a possibility, all rescuers should wear helmets with chin straps and face shields. The shell of the helmet should be constructed of a certified electrical nonconductor. The chin strap should not stretch and should be securely fastened so that the helmet will stay in place under the worst of conditions. The face shield must be lockable to protect the face and eyes from flying sparks.

A bunker jacket offers minimal protection from electrical hazards, but may provide protection from heat, fire, possible flashovers, and flying sparks. The opening of the bunker jacket must be properly secured with the front opening fastened and the collar up and closed in front to protect the neck and upper chest. Ordinary fire-fighting gloves and boots do not provide adequate protection against electrocution; rescuers should wear rubber-soled footwear and nonconductive gloves.

Cold Water A full-body encapsulated flotation suit may be used for emergency entry into water during a rescue operation. It can be put on over street clothes and covers the body from the top of the head down to and including the feet. Although not totally waterproof, the suit provides excellent flotation and thermal protection. When this suit is used in rescue work, it must have a harness built in or added to provide for easy attachment of safety lines.

Headgear

Helmets All rescuers should wear helmets, especially when working in a fall zone. The helmet should offer both top and side impact protection and have a secure chin strap and face shield. Objects frequently fall in a series; therefore, a helmet with an inadequate chin strap is likely to be knocked off after the first impact, leaving the rescuer without protection from the following objects.

Most construction-type helmets are not adequate for use in a rescue environment. Modern fire helmets offer impact protection but those with a projecting rear brim may encumber a rescuer. Helmets certified by the Union of International Alpine Associations (UIAA) offer the kind of protection required for high-angle work.

Patients in fall zones must also wear helmets unless they have injuries that require the use of other shielding. Patients may also need additional shielding. Items used for shields include back boards and inverted litters. Plastic litter shields are also available to protect the upper torso of the patient.

In cold weather, a major portion of body heat is lost without adequate protection for the head. Insulating hats are made from a variety of materials from wool to synthetics. For very cold weather, wear a hat that can be pulled down over the face and base of the skull to reduce heat loss.

Eye Protection Rescuers must protect their eyes and their patients' eyes against injury from foreign objects and the environment (e.g., plants, insects, pesticides). Whenever tools are being used during extrication, face shields and goggles must be worn. Prescription eyeglasses or sunglasses alone do not provide sufficient eye protection. **Rescuers must also wear eye protection when there is a possibility of exposure to blood or other body fluids.**

Exposure to sunlight at high altitudes for long periods of time may cause serious eye damage. Sunlight reflects on snow and can result in snow blindness, a temporary but painful condition. Wear glasses or goggles that fully protect the eyes against exposure to ultraviolet rays when working at high altitudes and in snow or white sand.

Clear vision is imperative, regardless of temperature extremes and physical demands, and vision restrictions should be minimized. Goggles must be adaptable to the weather and the physical demands of the rescue operation. However, goggles that perform well for one rescuer may be useless for another. At the very least, a rescuer's goggles should fit over prescription eyeglasses and should perform well at various light intensities.

Ear Protection Farm and rescue equipment can be quite loud, so ear protection should be used to reduce the noise level as much as possible until the equipment can be turned off. Soft foam industrial-type earplugs usually provide adequate protection. High winds can also be extremely uncomfortable to the ears and hearing of patients and rescuers. This discomfort may directly affect safety and morale. Again, earplugs may provide suitable protection.

Protection From Dust and Contaminants

Rescuers must protect their eyes, ears, and respiratory tract from contamination by dirt, dust, and wind. Therefore, eye protection, earplugs, and some type of simple respiratory protection must be kept in the rescuer's gear bag and in the patient packaging system at all times.

Footwear

Footwear should protect the rescuer's feet from injury, cover and protect the ankles, keep stones and other material out, be water resistant, fit well, and be supple so they are comfortable for walking. Footwear must also protect the feet from the cold.

While leather is one of the best choices for footwear, footwear made at least partially of synthetic materials such as Gore-Tex is increasingly being used.

Socks warm and protect the feet from blows to the boots. In cold environments, wearing two pairs of socks is generally preferable to wearing one pair of thick socks. A thin inner sock next to the foot helps to wick perspiration away to the thicker outer sock.

Protective footwear for structural fire fighting is designed for this special environment. Fire-fighting boots have varying levels of foot support and protection. Many rescuers now use short (ankle to lower calf area) fire-fighting boots in combination with other protective turnout gear. This reduces the size and weight of the boot worn yet still provides adequate protection.

Boots should have the maximum amount of puncture resistance, toe protection, and foot support that is available from the manufacturer. It may be difficult to obtain a good fit on fire-fighting boots, so shoe inserts or sock layering may be needed for a comfortable fit. The loose fit of some fire-fighting boots may hinder rescuers working in mud or other materials that tend to pull the boot off of the foot. The top (throat) of the fire-fighting boot must be "sealed off" (i.e., covered by pant legs or tight against the thigh) to keep rain, snow, glass, or other materials from entering the boot.

Fire-fighting boots often develop leaks from chemical or mechanical damage sustained during fire suppression activities. Therefore, these boots must be checked frequently for deterioration of the exterior boot skin (checkering, cracking, peeling, or flaking). Any opening in the exterior barrier must be sealed according to the manufacturer's recommendations. These boots may not be the best choice for all environments and rescue situations. In all rescues involving machinery extrication, rescuers must wear steel-toed work boots with a steel shank and nonslip soles. It is important to remember that ordinary fire-fighting boots will not provide adequate protection from electrical hazards.

Hand Protection

All rescuers need protection for their hands and wrists. Latex gloves must be worn at all times when there is a potential for exposure to blood or other body fluids. In many agricultural-rural rescue situations, latex gloves will be worn as liners under leather gloves. Leather gloves provide mechanical protection from metal and glass; special chemical-resistant gloves are needed when working around agricultural chemicals. Select gloves that provide maximum protection for the specific rescue operation.

Structural fire fighting requires good hand and wrist protection. The gloves designed for structural fire fighting minimize the effects of heat, cold, and cuts on the hands and wrists, but reduce manual dexterity. In rescue situations, gloves must provide the dexterity necessary to operate rescue tools, provide medical care, and perform other assigned duties. Additionally, ordinary fire-fighting gloves do not provide adequate protection from electrical hazards.

During any incident in which rescuers may be exposed to blood or other body fluids, rubber gloves must be worn to avoid direct skin-to-fluid contact.

Skin Protection

Sunburn is a threat, not simply an annoyance, in any outdoor environment because it is considered at least a first-degree thermal burn. Long-term, excessive exposure to the sun can result in premature aging of the skin and skin cancers. Severe sunburn can be debilitating to rescuers.

In areas that are very reflective, such as sand, water, and snow, the risk of sunburn is increased. The reflected sunlight may burn areas of the body that are normally not exposed, such as under the chin, inside the ears and nose, and around the eyes. At higher altitudes, the solar radiation is much stronger than at sea level; therefore, rescuers must be particularly careful about sunburn on the lips and nose.

When working outdoors, at high altitudes, or on a reflective surface, rescuers must protect their skin by applying a sun block with an appropriate rating. Wear sun block even on a cloudy day because it is the ultraviolet rays that cause sunburn. In addition to a sun block, protective hats are also helpful.

Sun is not the only threat to the skin when working outdoors. Insects and agricultural chemicals may also irritate the skin; therefore, rescuers should ensure their skin is protected with long sleeves, long pants, and/or insect repellant, when necessary.

GEAR

Rescuers are responsible for maintaining the safety of their personal gear and equipment. In an agricultural-rural rescue operation, the team will most likely know ahead of time the type of machinery involved and will be able to estimate the type and quantity of equipment necessary for the rescue. However, if the equipment taken to the scene proves to be inadequate, rescuers should call for additional help or equipment. A complete discussion of tools is provided in chapter 5.

Any single agricultural-rural incident may involve several hazards. In a machinery accident, there may be danger from fire, hydraulic fluid spills, chemical or pesticide spills, or overhead power lines. A confined space rescue from a silo may involve exposure to dust, spore molds, or other allergens or to toxic gases. Rescuers must have adequate personal safety gear for all of these situations.

Lighting

Agricultural-rural accidents often occur in the middle of fields where there is no electricity. Therefore, rescuers must provide their own light source for travel and for attending a patient during a rescue operation at night.

Flashlights may be reliable sources of light, but they are also limiting because they are hand held. Therefore, a headlamp that either clips to a helmet or attaches to a headband is recommended. Always carry spare batteries and light bulbs for each light source. In the total darkness of a confined space such as a closed silo, headlamps are an absolute necessity. Although it is not always practical, alternate sources of lighting should be available. Weather conditions can greatly reduce the effective operating life of some battery operated illuminating devices.

Litters

In many rescue situations, rescuers must transport patients in litters. Litters used for extended transports, such as from the middle of a field, or from the bottom of a ravine, must protect the patient from environmental hazards, immobilize the patient, and be easily used in a variety of rescue situations and vehicles.

Stokes Litter The Stokes litter is one of the most commonly used litters for patient transport. These litters are manufactured in a variety of materials and are constructed in many different ways.

Older models use a woven wire basket in which the frame and carrying rails are constructed of metal tubing (Figure 3.3). If this type of litter is subjected to high forces, such as those that occur in hauling, lowering, or attaching rescuers, the frame and rails should be constructed of steel. This type of litter is also very uncomfortable for the patient unless the wire basket is padded. The unpadded woven wire has sharp ends that snag clothing, damage equipment such as air splints and pneumatic antishock garments (PASG), and may pierce the skin of the patient or rescuers. If the litter has a leg divider, the patient's groin must be protected with padding.

A particular disadvantage to using the woven wire litter is that the bottom of the basket is open, exposing the patient to cold and wetness, as well as to injury from stones or tree branches. If a wire basket litter is used, then the patient must be protected from environmental hazards, such as weather and terrain. If exposure to wetness is a possibility, pro-

FIGURE 3.3

The woven wire basket is an older model of the Stokes litter. Place a pad in this type of litter for patient comfort and protection.

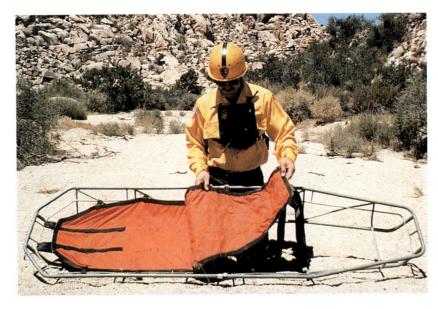

FIGURE 3.4

A body-shaped spine board may be used for full body immobilization in litters that have leg dividers.

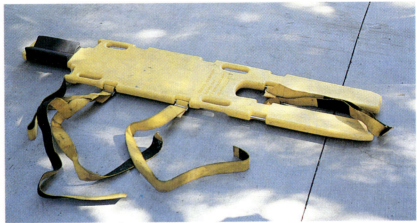

tect both the top and the bottom of the patient by lining the bottom with a tough waterproof material and placing padding on top.

If chilling is a possibility, the patient should be placed between blankets or in a sleeping bag that is accessible from all sides. After the patient is in the litter, an additional waterproof layer should be placed on top and tucked in so that no water will run down onto the patient.

Since a full spine board will not fit most woven wire litters, a conforming short board device may be needed for cervical and spinal immobilization. A body-shaped spine board (Figure 3.4) may also be used in litters with leg dividers. In some difficult rescue situations, such as confined space, vehicle extrication, high angle, or high altitude, it may be initially easier to immobilize the patient with a conforming short

FIGURE 3.5

Newer models of the plastic Stokes litter will accommodate a full back board. They slide across snow and rocks easily. However, they should not be used for air medical transports because of aerodynamic instability.

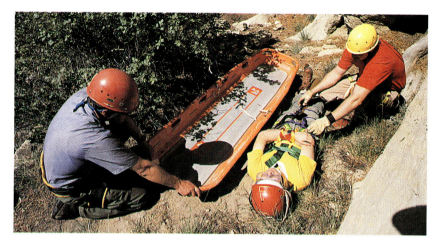

FIGURE 3.6

The semirigid conforming litter is constructed of flexible plastic that envelopes and protects the patient's body.

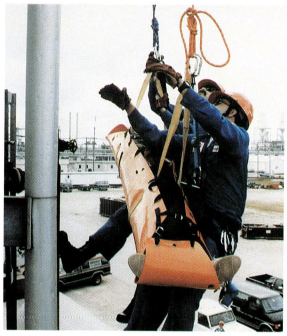

spine board device. However, full body immobilization should be initiated as soon as possible with a long spine board.

The plastic-type Stokes litter is a more recent design in which the main body is made of a single piece of plastic riveted to a large diameter aluminum carrying rail. Current models do not have a leg divider so they can accommodate a full back board (Figure 3.5). Because sunlight damages plastics, these litters should not be exposed to prolonged sunlight or stored on top of vehicles exposed to the sun.

Both metal and plastic Stokes litters are available in two-piece versions that may be separated for easier carrying.

If a patient must be transported by helicopter, rescuers should discuss with the pilot the type of litter that is acceptable for use in fixed-line fly-away operations (i.e., short distance transports in which the litter is slung under the aircraft). Certain types of litters, such as solid plastic Stokes litters, have aerodynamic characteristics that make them unacceptable for such operations because of the high risk of patient injury or death.

Semirigid Litters These litters have been designed for rescue operations in confined spaces, but they have also been adapted to other difficult rescue environments. One of the oldest designs is the Neill-Robertson litter, which has a narrow, rigid central spine board running from head to feet. Fabric sheets containing wooden laths are attached to the board and can be wrapped around the patient and secured with buckles. A more recent version, the modified Neill-Robertson litter, provides greater protection because it uses stainless steel runners lengthwise under the central spine board and has an attached helmet.

A recent development is the semirigid conforming litter, constructed of a large piece of flexible plastic that envelopes and protects most of the patient's body (Figure 3.6). This litter also has attachment points, carrying handles, and lifting straps. Because it does not add bulk, the semirigid conforming litter works well in confined spaces.

SUMMARY

All members of the rescue team must be equipped with the proper protective clothing and gear for each rescue operation. Protective clothing, including headgear and footwear, must shield the body and help control body temperature.

Outdoors, sunburn is a threat. Rescuers should carry and apply a sun block with an appropriate rating. Eyes and ears require protection from both the environment and from foreign objects. In addition, eyes, ears, and the respiratory tract must be protected from dust, dirt, and wind.

Rescue gear must meet professional standards and must be kept in safe and top-performing shape.

CHAPTER 4

The Mechanics of Extrication

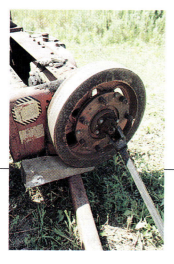

CHAPTER OUTLINE

Overview
Objectives
Simple Machines
  Lever
  Inclined Plane
Laws of Motion
  First Law of Motion
  Second Law of Motion
  Third Law of Motion

Law of Gravity
Friction
Stability
  Mechanics of Vehicle Stabilization
  Mechanics of Vehicle Lifting
  Elasticity of Solids
Summary

KEY TERMS

Center of gravity: the point in any body at which all of the body's weight is said to be concentrated.

Equilibrium: when objects are balanced or at rest.

Friction: the force resisting the relative motion between two surfaces.

Inclined plane: simple machine consisting of a ramp, wooden wedge, or screw thread.

Inertia: a body at rest remains at rest until acted upon by a force.

Joule (J): unit of measure of work.

CHAPTER 4 The Mechanics of Extrication

Lever: simple machine consisting of a rigid bar that rotates about an axis.

Machine: device that converts energy into work by transferring energy to a body or an object.

Mechanical advantage (MA): the ratio of effort applied to move a given load.

Moment of force (torque): special type of work when a force rotates around a pivot point or fulcrum.

Momentum: a body in motion remains in motion until it is acted upon by an outside force.

Power: the rate at which work is done.

Pulley: specialized wheel that uses the mechanical advantage of the lever.

Stress: distorting forces within a body, such as compression, tension, and shear.

Universal gravitation: another term for the law of gravity.

Work: the application of a force over a distance.

OVERVIEW

Before a rescuer is called to an incident involving a rear overturn, entanglement in a PTO, or entrapment in the snapping rolls of a combine, it is important for the rescuer to understand basic mechanics of extrication. The purpose of this chapter is to introduce basic terms and concepts of mechanics and how they relate to extrication. This chapter will also define and explain how simple machines work, how to estimate the stability of upset or overturned equipment, and how mechanics affects lifting vehicles and equipment.

OBJECTIVES

After reading this chapter, the rescuer should be able to:
- define basic terms used in mechanics of extrication.
- describe how a simple machine works.
- identify two simple machines.

continued

- describe the three laws of motion.
- explain the two components of stability.
- explain the process of "TOS"ing a vehicle.
- describe the mechanics involved in lifting a vehicle.

SIMPLE MACHINES

A **machine** is a device that converts energy into work by transferring energy to a body or an object. **Work** is defined as the application of a force over a distance and is measured in **joules**. **Power** is defined as the rate at which work is done. For example, the horsepower rating of a machine is the amount of work the machine can do in a specific unit of time. A knowledge of simple machines and their use helps rescuers select and use all extrication tools more effectively. Inappropriate or ineffective use of extrication tools is often a result of a lack of understanding of the simple concepts of the lever, inclined plane, gravity, friction, and stability.

All machines are really based upon the two simplest machines: the lever and the inclined plane.

Lever

A **lever** is a rigid bar that rotates about a point or axis called the fulcrum. The basic principle of the lever is that *the longer the arm of the lever to which the effort is applied, the less effort needed for a given amount of work*. **Mechanical advantage (MA)** is the ratio of effort applied to a given load. It is the ratio of the load divided by the effort:

$$MA = L/E$$

The application of levers appears in everyday life. Levers help carry out many basic tasks. A pry bar is an example of a lever, as is a wheelbarrow.

Pulleys are used to change the direction of a force or increase the mechanical advantage. A fixed pulley is anchored to a point and allows the rope/chain/cable attached to a load to change the direction of the force. There is no mechanical advantage to a fixed pulley. The effort required to move the load with a fixed pulley is the same as the resistance force or weight that is being moved (actually a little more effort because of the friction of the pulley).

A pulley that is rigged to move with the load offers mechanical advantage. Though the total work required to move the load remains the same, less effort is applied over a greater distance. The reduced effort is stated as the mechanical advantage. The mechanical advantage equals the number of lines attached to the movable pulley (Figure 4.1).

CHAPTER 4   The Mechanics of Extrication

FIGURE 4.1

Three feet of line must be pulled to move the load one foot.

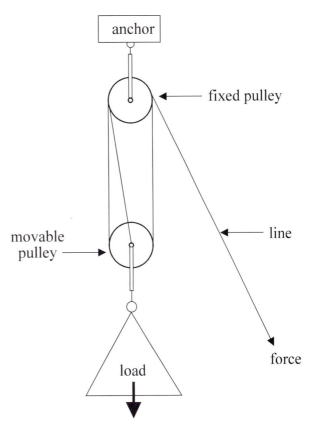

Inclined Plane

The second type of simple machine is the **inclined plane**, which is often seen in the form of a ramp, wooden wedge, or a screw thread (Figure 4.2). A screw thread is a continuous incline wrapped around a cylinder. For example, an automobile winding around a mountain road travels a greater distance than an automobile that travels straight up the side of the mountain. However, the automobile may not be able to travel straight up the side of the mountain because of the force of gravity acting upon it. The road wrapped around the mountain allows the energy of the car to be used more effectively.

FIGURE 4.2

If the weight of each vehicle is the same, less force is required to pull the vehicle up ramp A, but the vehicle must be pulled further along the ramp to reach the same height as on ramp B.

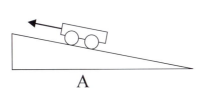
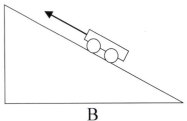

LAWS OF MOTION

Sir Isaac Newton was an early physicist who described three basic laws of motion—inertia, momentum, and reaction.

First Law of Motion

A body at rest remains at rest until acted upon by a force. This is known as **inertia**. An example of inertia is a golf ball resting on a tee. The ball rests on the tee until it is hit with the club.

Second Law of Motion

A body in motion remains in motion (traveling in a straight line) until it is acted upon by an outside force. This is known as **momentum**. For example, if a golf ball is hit, there are two forces that act upon it—gravity and wind resistance. When the ball is hit "with" the wind, it will travel farther; when the ball is hit "against" the wind, it will not travel as far.

Third Law of Motion

For every action there is an equal, but opposite reaction. An example is seen in a rowboat. The oar applies a backward force on the water, moving the boat forward.

LAW OF GRAVITY

Another physical law important to the rescuer is the law of gravity, also sometimes called **universal gravitation**. The law of gravity says that every particle attracts every other particle with a force proportional to their mass and inversely proportional to the square of the distance between them. There are no exceptions to the law of gravity.

The laws of physics apply in every rescue situation. Lifting, moving, and stabilizing objects (vehicles) require that the rescuer *understand and account for the effects of inertia, momentum, reaction, and gravity.*

FRICTION

Another important element to consider during extrication is friction. **Friction** is the force resisting the relative motion between two surfaces. Frictional force is generated by contact between two surfaces. The direction of the force is parallel to the two surfaces.

Three basic concepts about friction are important to remember when working at an incident. First, the smoother the two contact surfaces, the less friction there will be. A metal surface, such as that of a tractor, will generate less friction against another metal surface than against a concrete surface. Second, liquids generally reduce the friction between surfaces. Thus, when a combine has come to rest on its side on a wet, grassy slope, there is less friction between the combine and the ground.

Third, there is usually less friction if materials with rounded surfaces can break the contact between the vehicle and the ground because the

CHAPTER 4 The Mechanics of Extrication

rounded surfaces act as "little wheels." This changes sliding friction, such as between two surfaces, to rolling friction.

Friction may be the outside force acting on an object that is helping to maintain equilibrium. It is possible to change the amount of friction holding a vehicle in place, allowing the force of gravity to exceed the force of friction. This is particularly true when the vehicle is found on a slope or incline. Therefore, when estimating and preparing to stabilize a tractor or any other object on a slope, the rescue team must consider the resistance to rolling offered by the surface as well as the gravitational pull on the tractor.

STABILITY

One important concept of extrication is stability. Stability has two components: center of gravity (CG) and base of support. All objects have a center of gravity. The **center of gravity** is the point in any body at which all of the body's weight is said to be concentrated. In other words, the point in a body where all the gravitational forces are equal. Rescuers must be able to estimate the location of the center of gravity of an overturned tractor, or a combine resting on its side. They must also think of the perpendicular line from the center of gravity to the ground, and the perpendicular line from the center of gravity to any point of force application as lever arms. The longer the lever arms, the greater the potential for instability.

The other component of stability is the base of support of the object. Several components contribute to determining the base of support. First is the footprint of the vehicle. The footprint is similar to a dot-to-dot drawing in that it is an imaginary figure drawn by straight lines connecting the points of ground contact. For an upright pickup truck, the footprint is a rectangle through the four tires (Figure 4.3). For a row crop tractor, it would be a triangle. For an overturned combine, it would be an irregular shape defined by each point of ground contact. The second component of base of support is the surface on which the object is resting: flat or inclined, the composition of the surface, and the condition of the surface.

FIGURE 4.3

"Footprint" of a pickup truck. The dotted lines indicate the footprint area.

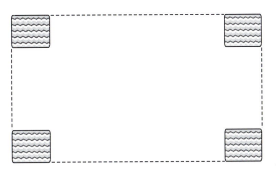

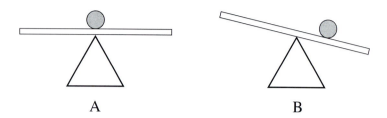

FIGURE 4.4

a. The ball and plank are in equilibrium.
b. Very little force is needed to move the ball to an unstable position.

When objects are balanced or at rest, they are said to be stable or in **equilibrium**. Equilibrium can be a fragile state. Depending on the circumstances, a minimal outside force can quickly move an object from equilibrium to instability. For example, a pickup truck is found resting on its side on a level field. The center of gravity is well above the surface, and the base of support is narrow compared to the truck's height. The distance from the center of gravity of the truck to the highest point on the truck is a lever arm. Remember that the longer the lever, the less the effort is needed to move an object (Figure 4.4).

Mechanics of Vehicle Stabilization

Triangle of Stability (TOS) It is an essential skill for all rescuers to be able to use the principles of mechanics to systematically assess stability, particularly during the initial survey of the scene. One way to assess stability is to imagine two triangles–one over the end, and one over the side of each vehicle, implement, or object involved in the incident. This is known as "TOS"ing a vehicle. Based on the information derived from "TOS"ing a vehicle, the rescue team can develop a plan to safely stabilize the vehicle, implement, or object, and then proceed with extrication. (Note: Though this discussion focuses on vehicular stability, the concepts apply to any implement or object.)

There are four components to the triangle of stability—three sides and a central area. The bottom is the base of support; the right side is the estimated weight of the vehicle or load; the central area is the estimated center of gravity; and the left side is the moment of force (Figure 4.5). The triangle of stability may be determined by following the four steps listed below:

1. The base of the triangle of stability—estimating the base of support includes an assessment of both the position and type (tires or metal surface) of vehicle contact with the ground. This step includes the following:
   a. Determining the orientation or footprint of the vehicle: on its side, top, or tires
   b. Assessing the type of ground surface: grass, mud, pavement, dry, wet
   c. Estimating the vehicle's weight relative to the vehicle suspension system (suspension systems allow the vehicle to rock and a shifting of the vehicle may put it into a state of potential instability)

FIGURE 4.5

A tractor on its wheels is stable because of its broad base of support.

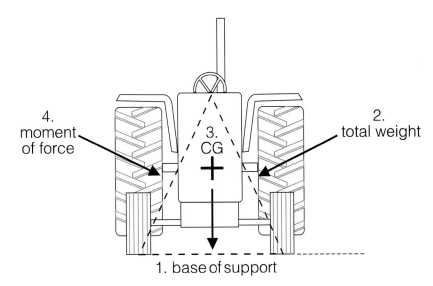

d. Determining the angle of the grade or slope on which the vehicle is resting
2. The right side of the triangle of stability—estimating the total weight of the vehicle or load. This step includes the following:
   a. Memorizing general weight classifications for farm equipment and implements
   b. Asking the operator, if conscious and knowledgeable
3. The central area of the triangle of stability—estimating the center of gravity requires knowledge of the vehicle weight, the load, and the location of the load. This step includes the following:
   a. Considering both the side and the end of the vehicle when estimating the location of the center of gravity
   b. Dropping an imaginary vertical line from the estimated center of gravity to the ground (CG line) (In theory, the entire vehicle can be balanced upon the single point of contact where the CG line meets the ground.)
   c. Extending the CG line upward through the uppermost portion of the vehicle (The point on this vertical line that intersects with the highest point on the vehicle is the apex of the triangle of stability (Figure 4.6). The CG line is not fixed within the triangle. The base and the two legs of the triangle will change position and size with each incident. They may also change during an incident as different forces are applied during the extrication process. "TOS"ing is ongoing during the rescue operation.)
4. The left side of the triangle of stability—estimating the moment of force. A **moment of force** (distance times weight) is created when the center of gravity moves around a fulcrum. Rescuers must estimate the distance from the center of gravity to the base of support. The greater the distance, the greater the moment of force. A narrow

FIGURE 4.6

The highest point on the tractor is the apex of the triangle of stability.

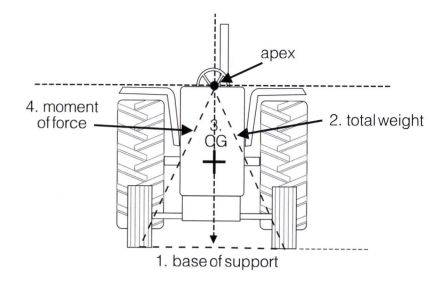

FIGURE 4.7

A tractor on its side has a much smaller base of support, a higher apex, and is less stable.

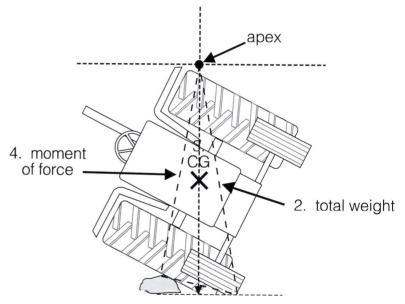

base of support such as that found on a tractor on its side can rapidly become a fulcrum or pivot point for the vehicle. This step includes the following:

a. Considering that the higher the center of gravity, the wider the base of support needs to be to maintain equilibrium
b. Considering that a vehicle with a relatively high estimated center of gravity and a narrow base of support (e.g., a pickup truck on its side) to be in a state of relative instability

This means the moment of force of the vehicle's own weight or a small external force (rescuer pushing on the vehicle to test its stability) may cause the vehicle to roll over or move to another position of equilibrium (Figure 4.7).

Estimating External Forces Wind is an external force that can affect the stability of a vehicle. The wind can be generated by weather conditions or by moving vehicles and aircraft (helicopter landing at the scene). A vehicle with a relatively high estimated center of gravity and a narrow base of support can easily move out of its current position by wind currents. This is particularly true of vehicles that have large exposed surfaces for the wind to act upon. Similar consideration must be given to vehicles at rest in flowing water.

A second external force rescuers must consider is the possibility of shifting loads. This might be seen in a leaking overturned grain trailer, or a truckload of cattle scrambling to get out of the only open escape route.

Developing an Action Plan Once the TOS has been estimated, an action plan for vehicle stabilization should be initiated:

1. Vehicle attachments should be stabilized above the estimated position of the center of gravity. The vehicle and vehicle load are better controlled when chains or cable are attached or positioned above the vehicle's estimated center of gravity.
2. Widen and extend the vehicle's base of support in the presence of the following conditions:
    a. The distance from the base of support to the estimated center of gravity is greater than the width of the base of support.
    b. The vehicle is showing any signs of rocking or swaying, or other potential instability.
    c. There is any possibility that the center of gravity may change or shift position. Examples of this include cattle suddenly changing positions in an overturned semitrailer tractor or wind currents pushing against the top of an unstable grain trailer.
    d. There is a need to keep the CG line well within the base of support if the vehicle must be lifted or moved as part of the extrication process.
3. Chock the tires/wheels of all upright vehicles to prevent rolling or sliding. Also chock any wheels in contact with the ground in an overturn incident.

For an object on an incline, the effects of gravity change the percentage of the vehicle weight that must be restrained by the rescuers during the stabilization process (Table 4.1).

For example, a 5,000-lb tractor on a 15 degree slope must be restrained by a chain rated for at least 1,250 lb. For the same tractor on a 45 degree slope, the chain must be rated at 5,000 lb.

TABLE 4.1 Estimated Vehicle Resistance on a Grade or Slope

Degree of Grade/Slope	Percent of Vehicle Weight to Be Considered
45°	100%
35°	60%
25°	40%
15°	25%

Mechanics of Vehicle Lifting

Consider the following example: an air bag is inflated, and the vehicle rotates as the wheels lift off the ground. The rotation is caused by the outside force of the air bag acting on the vehicle. This means that the rescuer did not properly estimate the location of the center of gravity. The center of gravity in this example has become the fulcrum (pivot point), the air bag the effort, and the vehicle the lever. The solution is to move the air bag (effort) closer to the CG line (fulcrum). The closer the air bag is placed to the CG line the less chance the vehicle will rotate because of the shorter lever arm.

To review these concepts, consider another example. Imagine the steps required for lifting a long, empty grain trailer lying on its side:

1. Estimate the center of gravity, the fulcrum, and the lifting (effort) point.
2. Consider the trailer as a lever, the same as a wheelbarrow. The load (center of gravity) is in the middle, the fulcrum is one end, and the effort (air bag) is the other end.
3. Remember that as the trailer begins to rotate onto the fulcrum (downside tires), the trailer (as with the wheelbarrow) is free to move. Friction against the ground may prevent the trailer from slipping sideways, and the friction of the brakes (if they are working) or chocks may prevent the trailer from rolling forward or backward.
4. Consider the trailer to be in equilibrium when the center of gravity of the trailer lines up over the fulcrum or pivot point, and the balance point has been reached (Figure 4.8). Once in this critical area, the trailer can be made unstable by a small amount of outside force (wind or the hand of a rescuer).

When the center of gravity gets past the fulcrum, the trailer will tip until it reaches a new equilibrium, with the center of gravity within the base of support.

Elasticity of Solids

All bodies have some degree of elasticity. If the force on the body is great, the body will exceed its elastic limit. This means that the body

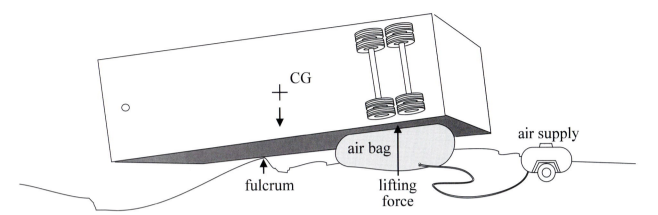

FIGURE 4.8

The trailer is stable in this position but would become unstable if raised too high.

will no longer return to its original shape when the outside distorting force is removed. Once the outside forces exceed the overall strength of the body, the body will break. These distorting forces are called **stress**. The stress within the body can be of three types: compression (pressure slightly higher than normal); tension (a stretching force); and shear (cutting through).

Vehicles that collide distort when the elasticity of the vehicle has been exceeded. But remember that many vehicle parts retain their elasticity and may be held in a distorted configuration because of continued outside forces acting upon them. Therefore, rescuers must remember that cutting, pushing, pulling, lifting, and disassembly during extrication may release this stored elastic energy with devastating results. The patient and the rescue team must be protected with barrier protection, such as wooden back boards and heavy blankets, to guard against such injuries. Vehicle parts that are moved during extrication must be held in place by the extrication tool causing the movement, or be blocked and cribbed with other objects, such as wood, to prevent the recoil of the vehicle parts.

SUMMARY

Understanding the basics of mechanics is essential before attempting to extricate a patient trapped in or under a vehicle. With large farm equipment, such as tractors and combines, quick, efficient extrication is necessary due to the severity of patient injuries.

Rescuers should have working knowledge in the use of simple machines, such as levers and inclined planes, in order to understand how extrication tools work. Also important when extricating a patient trapped under a tractor or any large, unstable vehicle is the ability to estimate the vehicle's stability. This includes identifying the vehicle's center of gravity and then assessing the triangle of stability before applying any extrication tools or attempting to lift the vehicle.

CHAPTER 5

Extrication Tools

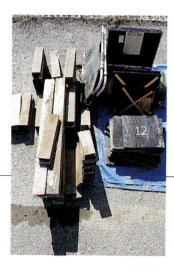

CHAPTER OUTLINE

Overview
Objectives
Basic Rigging
   Pulleys
   Slings
   Loading Effects
Manual Effort Tools
   Cutting Tools
   Spreading Tools
   Pulling Tools
   Disassembly Tools
Ropes and Related Equipment
   Types of Rope
   Rope-Related Equipment
Chains and Hooks
   Chains
   Hooks

Pneumatic Tools
   Pneumatic Tool Systems
   Pneumatic Chisels
   Pneumatic Impact Wrenches
   Pneumatic Cutting Tools
Air Bags
   High-Pressure Air Bags
   Low-Pressure Air Bags
Hydraulic Systems and Tools
   Hydraulic Cylinders
   Hydraulic Valves
   Hydraulic Fluids
   Hydraulic Hoses and Couplings
   Operating Hydraulic Tools
Summary

KEY TERMS

Block and tackle rigging: a configuration of rope and pulleys used to gain mechanical advantage for lifting, pulling, or moving a load.

CHAPTER 5   Extrication Tools

Come-along: commonly used manual effort pulling tool consisting of rope, hooks, blocks, and pulleys.

Dogs: two catch levers on the come-along.

Hydraulic power: type of energy transmission that uses a closed fluid system to transform energy to work.

Kernmantle: rope design consisting of a tightly woven outer sheath that helps protect the inner core that supports most of the load.

Lifting force: the amount of air pressure in the bag multiplied by the number of square inches of bag surface contact area.

Purchase point: point at which rescuers can apply a tool or insert air bags.

Shock load: a load resulting from a rapid change of movement of a static load.

Sling: a length of synthetic rope, wire rope, chain, or webbing that attaches to a load or anchor for the purpose of stabilizing, lifting, pulling, or moving objects.

Strike zone: an area of potential injury from a moving tool or object.

OVERVIEW

Rescuers must have a basic understanding of the mechanics of extrication in order to stabilize vehicles and other equipment, such as tractors and combines. Coupled with this knowledge should be familiarity with various types of extrication tools. These tools aid in the extrication process by cutting, lifting, spreading, disassembling, pushing, pulling, and stabilizing heavy farm equipment. This chapter describes basic tools rescuers are likely to use in agricultural-rural rescue. Also discussed are the principles of rigging, along with various types of manual tools, and pneumatic and hydraulic tool systems. Ropes, slings, blocks, chains, and pulleys are also discussed. High-pressure and low-pressure air bag systems are described as well. A rescue tools inventory checklist is presented at the end of the chapter.

> ## OBJECTIVES
>
> After reading this chapter, the rescuer should be able to:
>
> - identify the components of a basic rigging system.
> - describe the loading effects of angles on pulleys and slings.
> - identify situations in which basic manual effort tools should be used.
> - describe how to rig a wire rope come-along.
> - compare and contrast the properties of rescue rope, wire rope, and utility rope.
> - explain the principles by which pneumatic tools operate.
> - list the basic components of a pneumatic tool system.
> - compare and contrast the capabilities of high-pressure and low-pressure air bag systems.
> - explain the principles by which hydraulic tools operate.
> - list the basic components of a hydraulic tool system.
> - describe the functions of hydraulic fluid.
> - discuss safety considerations for each of the tool systems described in the chapter.

BASIC RIGGING

Rigging for use during agricultural-rural incidents includes the following equipment: synthetic rope, wire rope, chains, and pulleys (blocks) to lift, stabilize, move, or pull loads, vehicles, or attached equipment.

Pulleys

A pulley is a wheel that turns on an axle. A fixed pulley (one that does not move) acts like a lever with equal arms on either side of the center pin (axle). The force applied on one side of the pulley by pulling on the rope is equal to the load (resistance force) on the other side of the pulley. This means that there is no mechanical advantage. The movement of the rope through a fixed pulley changes the direction of the force, but does not provide a mechanical advantage.

A movable pulley (one that moves with the load) has two ropes supporting the load. The load is distributed to both ropes, creating a theoretical mechanical advantage of two. **Block and tackle rigging** is the configuration of rope and pulleys used to gain mechanical advantage for lifting, pulling, or moving a load. Blocks have two or more wheels (sheaves) fitted in a frame with a hook or shackle attached to the frame. The mechanical advantage of a block is equal to the number of rope returns through the block.

Slings

A **sling** is a length of synthetic rope, wire rope, chain, or webbing that attaches to a load or anchor to stabilize, lift, pull, or move objects. There are endless loop slings and straight slings. Slings generally have hooks, shackles, or eyes for termination points so that connections can easily be made to the load or anchor. Both endless loop and straight slings can be rigged in a variety of hitch configurations, including the following: the single vertical (or horizontal) hitch; the single and double basket hitches; the single and double choker hitches; and the double-, triple-, and four-legged bridle hitches.

The single vertical/horizontal hitch supports a load with a single line (leg) of rope, chain, or webbing, which means that the full load is carried by one straight piece of rope, chain, or webbing. This sling configuration should not be used if the load is hard to balance, the estimated center of gravity is difficult to determine, or the load is loose or extends well past the point of attachment, such as a tractor on its side.

The single basket hitch supports a load by attaching one end of the sling to a hook, wrapping the sling around the load, and then returning the other end to attach to the same hook. But like the single vertical/horizontal hitch, the single basket hitch has problems keeping the load balanced. The double basket hitch uses two single slings wrapped in the same manner at separate locations on the load, which makes it more stable than the single basket hitch. The double basket hitch allows the rescuer to place the center attachment hook over the estimated center of gravity, and then wrap the two slings to either side of the estimated center of gravity. This keeps the load more stable and balanced.

The basket hitch can be modified with a double wrap to help secure loose loads. The double-wrap basket hitch makes contact all the way around the load surface. This hitch configuration is good for cylindrical loads such as culvert pipes.

The single choker hitch attaches one end of the sling to a hook, wraps the sling around the load, and secures it back onto itself. As with other single-legged hitches, the rescuer must monitor the stability and balance of the load. The double choker hitch has two single slings spread apart around the load, instead of the one sling of the single choker hitch. The choker hitch does not make full contact with the load surface as does the double-wrap basket hitch. As with the basket hitch, the choker hitch can be double wrapped to help control and hold the load. The double choker hitch, with its two points of wrap around the load, provides better lifting, pulling, stabilizing, and moving than the single choker hitch.

The bridle hitch is made using two, three, or four single slings secured to a single point that is usually in line between the center of gravity and the anchor/lifting point. The bridle hitch can provide very stable lifting, stabilizing, moving, and pulling because the load is distributed onto multiple slings. Attention must be paid to the length of each sling so that the load is distributed evenly onto each leg of the sling.

Loading Effects

Rescuers must be concerned with the angle created by the incoming and outgoing lines of a fixed pulley, because a fixed pulley changes the direction of the synthetic/wire rope. The downward load placed on the fixed pulley and the anchor/pulley changes as the angle changes. Remember that the greater the angle, the less the downward load on the anchor/pulley. For example, a load of 1,000 lb with an angle of 120° between the incoming and outgoing lines places a load of 1,000 lb on the anchor/pulley. At an angle of 90°, this same load places 1,410 lb of load on the anchor/pulley. A similar effect occurs in rigging a sling with two or more legs. Try to keep the legs of the sling perpendicular to the load surface. The smaller the angle between the legs of the sling, the smaller the load distributed to each leg. As a general rule, make sure that the angle is 45° or less. Each leg of a two-legged bridle hitch, holding a 1,000-lb load, would carry about 700 lb at 45°.

MANUAL EFFORT TOOLS

Manual effort tools are used to cut, pull, lift, spread, and disassemble heavy equipment. Many manual effort tools increase available effort because they have extended handles or assemblies that provide leverage.

Cutting Tools

Manual cutting tools include bolt cutters, wire cutters, tin snips, hacksaws, hook bill knives, webbing cutters, axes, panel cutters, and chisels (Figure 5.1).

The hook bill (or linoleum) knife can be used to cut thin wire, thin metal, seat belts, seat cushions, and even the adhesive around fixed windows.

Webbing cutters can also cut seat belts. However, rescuers should not always cut the seat belt immediately, because the seat belt is a restraint device and may be helping to immobilize the patient or an injured body part. It may be necessary to package the patient before cutting and removing the seat belt.

Spreading Tools

Manual spreading tools include such flat-bladed tools as axes, pry axes, and pry bars. The pry bar is an effective tool to develop leverage when needed (Figure 5.2). The flat-bladed pry bar, for example, is a practical tool for gaining access in the door latch area for placement of hydraulic spreading tools. This is called gaining a **purchase point**. Force the flat blade into an open space and then move the bar up and down parallel to the side of the vehicle. This motion creates an opening large enough for

FIGURE 5.1

Manual cutting tools are used to cut, pull, lift, spread, and disassemble heavy equipment.

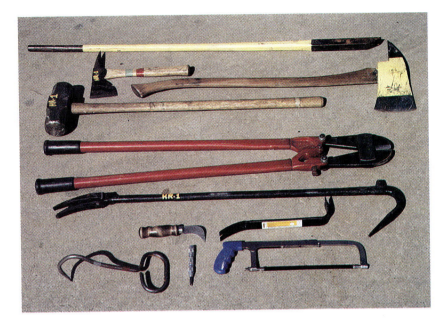

FIGURE 5.2

A pry bar and crowbar can be used to create a larger opening for the insertion of other types of spreading tools.

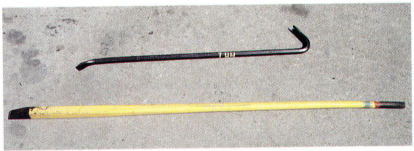

other types of spreading tools to be inserted for more extensive application of force.

Pulling Tools

The most commonly used manual effort pulling tool in extrication is the hand winch or **come-along** (Figure 5.3). The come-along for farm equipment extrication should include at least 20' of wire rope with matched capacity hooks, blocks, and pulleys. The minimum capacity for a farm equipment extrication come-along should be 2,000 lb in a straight, single-part line pull configuration. The handle of the come-along should be designed to bend before the wire rope breaks. This will warn the rescuer and offer a margin of protection before the wire rope breaks.

A come-along is used in a straight, single-part line pull configuration to allow the maximum reach of the available cable. However, a single-part line pull does not provide mechanical advantage. A two-part line pull using a rig with a pulley moving toward the come-along does pro-

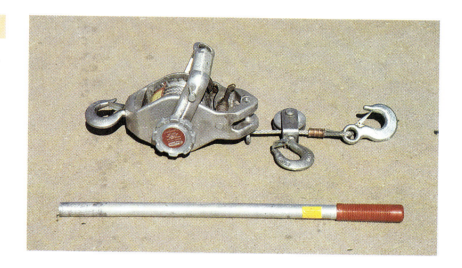

FIGURE 5.3

The wire rope come-along is the most commonly used manual effort pulling tool in farm equipment extrication.

vide mechanical advantage. A come-along rigged with a single-part line pull and a fixed pulley provides only a change of direction or redirection of the pull.

A chain-type come-along is not as popular as a wire rope come-along, because the chain type is usually heavier and is designed primarily to be rigged for straight pulls. In addition, the chain-type come-along does not work as well as the wire rope come-along when the chain is pulled over cribbing or other obstacles.

Using the Wire Rope Come-Along Rigging chains (webbing or wire rope slings) should be equipped with hooks (either slip or grab hooks) or rings (weldless rings are called master links) to quickly shorten the chain, if necessary. The rigging chains should be rated at double the strength of the come-along. Having at least two different lengths of chain (6' and 12') allows faster rigging for pulling heavy farm equipment.

Use wood cribbing any place the cable, rigging chains, or come-along touches the equipment. This reduces the extent of structural collapse to parts of the equipment, which could decrease the effectiveness of the pull.

The come-along should be placed on the tractor, combine, or other equipment so that rescuers can use their leg muscles to push up on the handle. If the come-along is placed too far from the edge of the equipment, rescuers are forced to use the weaker muscles of the arms and the lower back. However, if the come-along is placed too close to equipment components, the range of movement of the handle can be decreased. This makes it difficult to release the bottom catch lever of the come-along when taking the tension off the machine.

The come-along has two catch levers called **dogs**. The bottom dog is the catch lever that fits into the sprocket of the cable drum to prevent the cable drum from reversing more than one notch at a time and releasing cable tension. The top dog is the catch lever that moves with the handle of the come-along. It also fits into the sprocket of the cable drum. The top dog transfers the effort of the handle to the cable drum to tighten the cable. The top dog pushes the bottom dog away from the sprocket during the tension-release cycle to release tension on the cable. The release cycle requires greater forward movement of the handle than does the tension cycle. Therefore, it is important to ensure that there is enough space between the body of the vehicle/implement or other obstructions and the come-along to allow full forward motion of the handle during the release cycle. If an equipment component is to be displaced, ensure that the come-along has enough space to move freely without obstruction.

Apply or release tension (load or unload) on the wire rope of the come-along with smooth motions of the legs. Lift the handle up and forward. Rapid, jerking movements tend to shock load the dogs, the hooks, the handle, the sprocket assembly, and the rescuer's back and legs. A **shock load** is a load that results from a rapid change of movement of a static load.

Watch the cable as it moves through the pulley wheel. It is common for the angle of the pull to move the wire rope off the pulley wheel. The cable then falls between the pulley wheel and the side wall of the pulley block. If the wire rope becomes caught between the side wall and the wheel, it binds, disabling the pulley and possibly damaging the cable.

When the extrication is completed, the come-along wire rope should be respooled onto the drum under slight tension, so that it is tight and compact on the drum. If the wire rope is respooled unevenly, it can pinch and damage itself. That is, the rope can grab a loose piece or loop as it is being respooled, which places excessive pressure on that small area of the rope.

Disassembly Tools

Disassembling parts of a tractor, combine, or other farm equipment components with manual effort tools is often overlooked by rescuers in favor of using power hydraulic tools. Disassembly tools include wrenches, socket sets and appropriate accessories, hay hooks, sledge hammers, and punches. The deformity of the equipment and the location of the patient may not always allow for effective use of larger power hydraulic equipment. Removing a few bolts or other fasteners that hold parts of a tractor or other equipment together may be all that is needed to quickly extricate the patient.

ROPES AND RELATED EQUIPMENT

Types of Rope

Rescue Rope Rescue rope should be of a static design, meaning it has little stretch. This lack of stretch gives rescuers better control of the rope. Static rope is constructed with a tightly woven outer sheath that helps protect an inner core that supports most of the load on the rope. This kind of construction is known as **kernmantle** or **kermantle**.

Rescue rope is most commonly used in diameters of 7/16" (11.1 mm) or 1/2" (12.5 mm). Larger ropes will not fit most rescue hardware, are difficult to handle, and are heavier to carry long distances. The specific rope diameter should be determined on the basis of local rescue needs while maintaining an acceptable safety factor. Table 5.1 lists characteristics of several types of rescue ropes.

Rope and other equipment used in rescue operations must have an adequate safety factor for the rescue work anticipated. The safety factor is the ratio of the highest likely load that might occur during a rescue to the strength of the equipment. A safety factor of 10:1, for example, means that if the highest expected load on a rope is 1,000 lb, the rope should have a strength of 10,000 lb. In agricultural-rural settings, a minimum safety factor of 15:1 should be used. Table 5.2 lists safe working capacities for several types of ropes.

Rescue rope can be purchased in almost any length desired. In agricultural-rural rescue situations, ropes of 100', 150', or 300' are usually

TABLE 5.1 Characteristics of Rescue Ropes

	POLY-P	POLY-E	NYLON	DACRON Polyester
Moisture regain	0%	0%	to 9%	Less than 1%
5/8" diameter strength	6,200 lb	5,600 lb	10,400 lb	10,000 lb
Elongation break in rope	24%	22%	35%	20%
Change of strength	No change	No change	Less than 10%	No change
Floatability	Yes	Yes	No	No
Resistance to rot, mildew, and attack by marine organisms	100% resistant	100% resistant	100% resistant	100% resistant
Resistance to surface abrasion	Good	Good	Very good	Excellent
Acids	Excellent	Excellent	Fair	Very good–Excellent
Alkalis	Good	Good	Excellent	Very good
Solvents	Good	Good	Excellent	

Reprinted with permission from the second edition of the IFSTA *Essentials of Fire Fighting*, copyrighted by the Board of Regents Oklahoma State University.

TABLE 5.2 Safe Working Capacities For Ropes

Diameter	Nylon (new)	Nylon (used)[1]	Dacron (new)	Dacron (used)[1]	Polypropylene (new)	Polypropylene (used)[1]	Braided Nylon Cover Nylon Core (new)	Braided Nylon Cover Nylon Core (used)[1]
3/8"	363	181	492	246	408	204	840	420
1/2"	726	363	803	401	731	365	1,500	750
5/8"	1,122	561	1,100	550	1,122	561	2,400	1,200
3/4"	1,485	742	1,496	748	1,644	822	3,400	1,700
7/8"	2,145	1,072	1,980	990	1,921	960	4,740	2,370
1"	2,640	1,320	2,695	1,347	2,856	1,428	5,700	2,850
1 1/4"	3,960	1,980	3,795	1,897	3,859	1,929	8,800	4,400
1 1/2"	5,610	2,805	5,610	2,805	5,525	2,762	13,000	6,500
1 3/4"	8,250	4,125	6,710	3,355	7,684	3,842	19,200	9,600
2"	9,845	4,927	(11%)[2]	(5.6%)[2]	9,197	4,598	21,000	10,500
	(11%)[2]	(5.6%)[2]			(17%)[2]	(8.5%)[2]	(20%)[2]	(10%)[2]

[1] Persons using synthetic rope should consult the manufacturer for their interpretation of "used" rope.
[2] Based on manufacturer's recommendations for new rope.

Reprinted with permission from the second edition of the IFSTA *Essentials of Fire Fighting*, copyrighted by the Board of Regents Oklahoma State University.

used. These lengths provide enough flexibility for the different heights encountered on farms and ranches, such as ditches, silos, and other tall or below-ground structures. At least one rope should be twice the longest length that may be needed for access into the largest structure in the area.

As with all safety equipment, rescue rope must be inspected thoroughly and carefully after each use, with a *sight* and *feel* inspection. The rope should be visually inspected and then run through bare hands. Look and feel for the following characteristics:

- Lumps, depressions, and changes in circumference that may indicate damage to the rope core
- Broken sheath bundles, exposed rope core, or sheath bundles in which over 50% of the bundle is broken
- Discolorations that indicate damage from acids and other substances
- Glossy marks indicating heat damage

If any of these conditions are found, the rope should be removed from rescue service, or the bad section cut out, leaving two shorter sections of good rope. Rescue ropes are life safety equipment and must be treated as such. Protect them from damaging activities and substances.

FIGURE 5.4

Edge rollers help protect rope from abrasion against a rough surface.

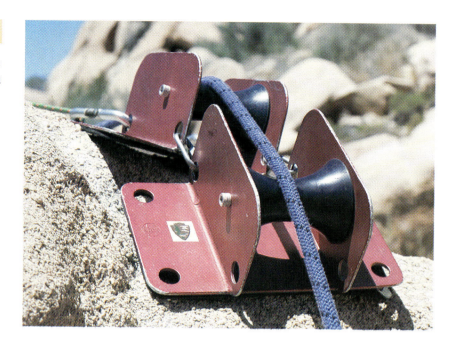

Abrasion, which occurs when a rope is run over a rough surface, commonly causes rope damage. Putting a weight on the rope, or loading it, also increases abrasion. Rope pads or edge rollers will help protect a rope from abrasion (Figure 5.4). Ground-in grit and dirt can damage load-bearing fibers, so avoid walking on or driving over rescue lines. Be careful that two ropes do not run over each other, as when a lowering or hauling rope runs over an anchor rope. This can cause heat fusion and result in a cut rope.

Protect ropes in use and in storage from acids and other damaging substances. Acids in storage batteries are obvious, but wet concrete may also contain damaging acids. Soot and bleaches can also damage ropes.

Wire Rope The type of extrication dictates whether wire rope, sometimes called wire cable or cable, can or should be used. The strength, size, length, grade, construction, and type of wire rope used will depend upon the application and the environmental conditions. Rescuers should consider the following criteria before using a wire rope.

1. The ultimate load strength should provide a safety factor of 5:1. A safety factor of 10:1 is preferred in incidents in which human life is dependent on the rope.
2. It should resist corrosion.
3. It should withstand repeated bending without failure from fatigue.
4. It should keep its shape, and resist crushing or distortion.
5. It should have reasonable resistance against abrasion.
6. It should be able to tolerate rotational stress.

CHAPTER 5 Extrication Tools

Wire rope design incorporates six basic elements: the number and pattern of wires in each strand; the type of lay or twist in the wire; the grade of wire; the type of wire; the core; and the required performance standards. The performance standards are the requirements established by the end user, based on how the rope is to be used and the working environment. (The Appendix provides more detailed information.)

Utility Rope Utility rope is any rope used to secure equipment, tow vehicles, or lift equipment. Utility rope should never be used for life support or rescue activities. Rescue rope should be used only for life support activities, not towing vehicles or lifting heavy equipment. Rescue rope may be downgraded to utility rope, but then should never be used again for rescue work.

In agricultural-rural rescue operations, both utility and rescue ropes may be required, but these ropes must not be confused. Rescue ropes should be a different color than utility ropes, be tagged for life support only, and be stored separately from utility ropes.

Store ropes in loose coils inside hanging bags or in a protected place (Figure 5.5). Do not store ropes in areas where they might be exposed to sunlight or in overheated rooms. Allow ropes to dry completely before storing them to avoid mildew.

FIGURE 5.5

Store ropes separately in bags to avoid entanglement and to facilitate quick retrieval.

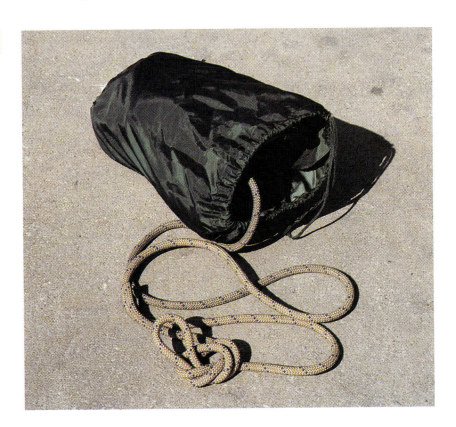

Rope-Related Equipment

Webbing Webbing is a woven fabric used instead of rope in certain situations. It is flat, is more comfortable against the body than rope, and is used for rescue harnesses or for securing patients in litters. Webbing comes in two basic designs: flat, as found in seat belts; and tubular, a woven tube of material that is more supple and comfortable than flat webbing (Figure 5.6). Webbing used for rescue operations is usually 1" wide.

Harnesses Harnesses must be worn by the patient and all rescuers in a high-angle rescue operation. The harness must be tied to either a main line or a safety line. Although chest and seat harnesses are available, a full body harness should be used in agricultural-rural rescue operations. They provide the security needed when working in any confined space.

Carabiners Carabiners are metal snap links that connect the individual elements of a high-angle rescue. They may be used to connect a harness to a rope, or to attach a rope to an anchor system. The basic parts of a carabiner are the *spine*, the *gate*, the *hinge*, and the *latch*. The spine is the C-shaped main body that supports most of the load. So that the carabiner can be attached, the gate swings open on the hinge. A spring in the end of the gate at the hinge keeps the gate closed. At the opposite end, the latch helps keep the gate closed when the carabiner is loaded (Figure 5.7).

Locking carabiners are a more secure design. They have a sleeve that rotates up a threaded area on the gate to secure it closed. For most rescue situations, the added security of locking carabiners is preferred.

FIGURE 5.6

Tubular webbing is commonly used to secure a patient in a litter.

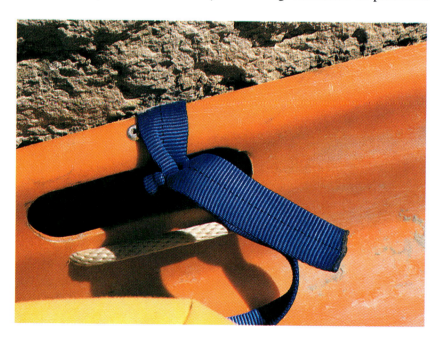

FIGURE 5.7

Carabiners are metal snap links used in a high-angle extrication to connect a harness to a rope or attach a rope to an anchor system.

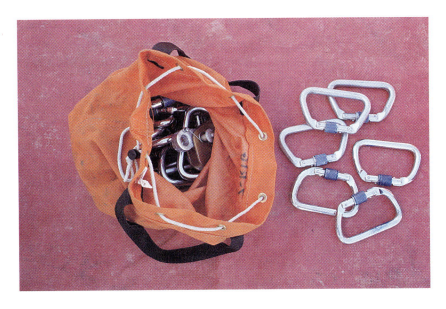

However, locking carabiners may accidentally become unlocked if the locking sleeve rolls open as it rubs against a building face, or is jarred by vibrations. Locking carabiners must be frequently checked to ensure the gates are locked.

Carabiners are made from either steel or aluminum alloys. Steel carabiners generally have higher tensile strength, but some aluminum carabiners have an adequate safety factor for rescue operations. However, the locking mechanism on steel carabiners will usually outlast the mechanism on aluminum carabiners, and steel locking carabiners usually withstand heavy shock loading better than aluminum carabiners. The sudden shock loading of a fallen climber, while frequent in recreational climbing, rarely occurs in rescue situations. When severe shock loading does occur in rescue situations, all involved rope and equipment should be retired from service. With the significant weight difference between steel and aluminum carabiners, rescuers who carry equipment for long distances may prefer aluminum carabiners.

CHAINS AND HOOKS

Chains

Chains are multi-purpose tools in extrication: they withstand rough handling, do not knot easily, are easy to store, grip loads well, and can take a reverse bend without damage. Chains also resist abrasion, corrosion, and sharp bends better than wire rope.

However, chains do not tolerate shock loads as well as wire rope. The failure of a chain can be sudden and dramatic. A chain may give warnings of potential failure by stretching under severe loads, or by elongating and narrowing the links to the point that the links bind. But be advised that chains can fail without warning should a weld be defective or other damage (a welder's torch weakening the chain) be present that decreases the strength of the chain.

The National Association of Chain Manufacturers (NACM) has agreed upon a grading system for welded chain that makes it easier to evaluate and select chain. The grading system uses grades 30, 40, 70, and 80. Only 80 grade chain should be used for rescue operations.

Hooks

There are a number of hooks available for use with chains, including the grab hook, the slip/sling hook, the sorting hook, and the plate hook. Other accessories used with chains include oval and round master links, shackles, coupling links, and swivel connectors. Grab hooks, slip/sling hooks, and master links are most likely to be used when rigging chains for extrication operations.

Grab hooks and slip/sling hooks are manufactured with two types of ends: the clevis-type end and the eye-type end. The clevis-type end has a pin that slips through the chain and the top of the hook to make the attachment to the chain. The eye-type end is attached to the chain by a welded link. Each type of end has the same strength rating, when properly installed and matched to the chain.

The grab hook is designed to hook onto a matched chain between the links. It is normally attached to the master link, connected to the end(s) of the chain, or joined to another grab hook with a short piece of chain. Two grab hooks can be used to connect two separate pieces of chain. The grab hook is commonly used to hook back into the chain between the links after wrapping an object, to connect separate pieces of chain, and to permit the rescuer to shorten the chain by hooking back to the grab hook.

The slip/sling hook is designed with a wider throat, which is the space between the tip and the back of the hook, than the grab hook. This allows items such as webbing, chain, master links, or shackles to be placed into the hook. Safety catches must be installed on all slip/sling hooks to ensure that the items placed on the hook do not slip out when there is no weight holding them in place. The grab hook does not need a safety catch.

PNEUMATIC TOOLS

The pneumatic tools normally used for heavy equipment extrication are the percussive-type tools, such as the rivet hammer, and the rotary-type tools, such as the pneumatic impact wrench and the die cut-off saw.

The basic principles of percussive pneumatic tools are based upon the velocity and mass of the piston and the number of blows struck per second.

Another principle of pneumatic tools is the transfer of potential energy to rotary mechanical energy. This principle is seen at work in the pneumatic motor. All pneumatic motors operate as a result of the difference of pressure across a driving member. This pressure difference transmits energy by the development of torque or rotation.

Pneumatic Tool Systems

Pneumatic hand tools perform a wide range of tasks in extrication. The tools are lightweight and highly maneuverable. Parts and support are readily available because of their wide use in industry. The disadvantages include the noise and vibration often associated with their operation and the need for a pressurized air supply. There are five basic components of a pneumatic tool system: a pressurized air source; an air pressure regulator; air hoses with matched fittings/couplings; the pneumatic tool; and various supporting components and tool attachments.

Pressurized air sources for pneumatic tools include apparatus air brake systems (air taken from one of the brake system storage tanks), air cascade systems (multiple tanks of compressed air), self-contained breathing apparatus (SCBA) tanks, self-contained underwater breathing apparatus (SCUBA) tanks, and fixed or portable compressors pumping into storage tanks. Vehicle-based air supplies, cascade systems, or air compressors provide larger volumes of air for extended use but do limit where tools can be used. Portable air bottles and tanks allow for easy transport to remote locations, but these sources have a limited capacity.

Use of a pressurized air supply requires the ability to monitor and regulate the air pressure. There are two types of regulators used for extrication: the adjustable diaphragm-type and the adjustable piston-type. Both types allow the rescuer to monitor incoming and outgoing air pressures and adjust the outgoing pressure. The piston-type regulator is generally more durable than the diaphragm-type regulator. Some models have the capacity for incoming pressures in excess of 5,000 psi and outgoing pressures in excess of 300 psi.

The air hose and the couplings must be matched to the fittings on the regulator and on the pneumatic tool. The pressure rating for the hose and fittings must exceed the working pressure of the tools to be used. The inside diameter of the air hose, the working pressure, and the cubic feet per minute (cfm) of the air all affect the ability of the hose to deliver the needed pressure for effective air tool operation. A 25' section of 1/4" inside-diameter air hose with 90 psi flowing at about 6 cfm will have a pressure drop of 29 psi at the tool. A 25' section of 5/16" inside-diameter air hose will only lose about 10 psi. Small inside-diameter air hose lines often allow the tool to run away from its air supply. This means, for example, that the cutting effectiveness of an air hammer is reduced, and air is wasted during ineffective cutting time. Using short bursts of air will help alleviate this problem, particularly with pneumatic chisel operations. Ensure that the type of coupling, the operating

Pneumatic Chisels

pressure of the tool, and the flow requirements are stated when consulting with a supplier about purchase of an air hose.

Of the several pneumatic tools used in agricultural-rural extrication, the one most commonly used is the pneumatic (or air) chisel (Figure 5.8). It "cuts" through plastic, sheet metal, and other materials. The principal parts of the air chisel are as follows: the user control valve (trigger) set into the pistol grip tool body; the barrel or cylinder; the piston that slides back and forth in the barrel; directional valves that move air alternately from the back to the front of the piston and out the exhaust ports; and the chisel retainer.

Chisel retainer styles include the wire beehive, a threaded quarter turn, the chisel shank/threaded collar, and a quick-release (rotating and nonrotating chisel types) retainer. The wire beehive retainer is the least expensive, but is also the least acceptable for heavy equipment extrication. The wire beehive allows for quick interchange of chisel bits, but does not provide good control and retention of the chisel during critical operations. The threaded quarter turn retainer is permanently attached to the barrel of the air hammer. It uses the pressure of ball bearings to hold the chisel bit in place. The chisel shank/threaded collar requires that each chisel bit have its own retaining collar. With this system, the rescuer must actually change both the chisel and the retainer when changing chisel bits. The quick-release (pull back to release) retainer can be designed to allow for rotation of the attached chisel or for the chisel to remain in a fixed position once inserted. Many rescuers prefer the ability to rotate the air hammer around the chisel to provide better hand and body positioning. Rotating and nonrotating chisel retainers are a user preference for extrication because they do not affect the performance of the tool.

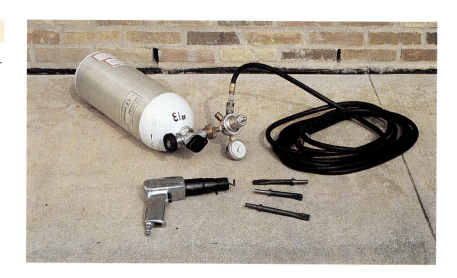

FIGURE 5.8

The principal parts of a pneumatic chisel are the control valve, the barrel, the piston, retainer directional valves, and the chisel retainer.

Not all pneumatic chisels function well for agricultural-rural extrication. Therefore, rescuers should field-test a pneumatic chisel on various types of farm equipment, including sheet metal and pillars, before making a final selection.

Chisel Tips Although there are many chisel shapes and lengths from which to choose, three primary styles are used for extrication: the flat chisel, the sheet metal chisel, and the cold chisel. The flat chisel (sometimes called a spot weld splitter) has a curved, half-moon tip and ranges in length from 6" to 18". The flat chisel is used to cut pillars, door pins, and other multiple-layered sheet metal components or plastic.

The cold chisel also ranges in lengths up to 18" long and has a stocky, blunted tip that is normally not much wider than the shank. This chisel is used to cut off bolts and rivets and to cut through heavier materials than the flat chisel can handle.

The sheet metal or panel cutter chisel is designed to stay on the surface of the metal and to make long continuous cuts. The single panel cutter has a flat surface extending from a rounded chisel shank. The flat surface helps to keep the chisel from digging into the sheet metal and binding up the cutting operation. Extending down from the flat surface is the bottom of the "T" or the cutting tooth. The bottom of the "T" does the actual cutting of the sheet metal.

A second style of sheet metal chisel is the double panel cutter, which does not have the wide flat surface of the single panel chisel. This chisel actually has two cutting edges. Some chisel manufacturers add a bull point at the end of the double panel cutter to allow the user to make a quick puncture of the sheet metal for faster cutting starts. The trade-off with the double panel cutter chisel is that it is easier to push the chisel through the sheet metal and bury or hang up the tool, thus slowing the cutting operation.

Chisel bits with shorter shafts are stronger but lack the reach that may be required for some operations. Rescue units should have more than one length and width of the flat chisel bits. Chisel selection should be based on the grade of metal used in the bit. Higher performance and durability are found in the heat-treated, tooled steel chisel bits.

Pneumatic Impact Wrenches

Although the pneumatic wrench is not currently widely used in agricultural-rural extrication, it does allow rapid disassembly of some equipment. The nature of rescue work requires that case-hardened steel sockets (both metric and standard) and heavy-duty impact wrenches be selected from the types available for commercial applications, not from those designed for light duty or home use. Manufacturers normally indicate the intended application in the sales literature. Be sure to purchase heavy duty or commercial equipment.

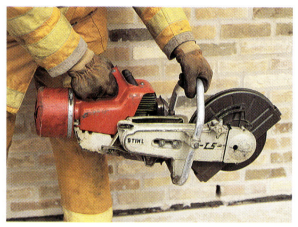 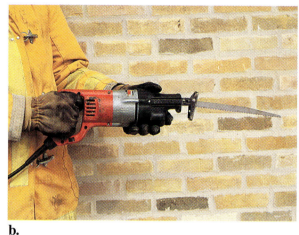

FIGURE 5.9 High-speed circular saws (**a**) and pneumatic reciprocating hacksaws (**b**) are used to cut such materials as light metal, sheet metal, plastic, and fiberglass.

Pneumatic Cutting Tools

Two other pneumatic tools, the high-speed circular cut-off saw and the pneumatic reciprocating hacksaw (Figure 5.9), while not used extensively in agricultural-rural extrication, are excellent tools for cutting light metal, plastic, lexan, fiberglass, and sheet metal. The high-speed circular cut-off saw is available with a gear drive or air vane drive. The gear drive does not bind up as fast as the air vane type and will handle heavier material. However, the air vane type is often the tool of choice when working right next to the patient's body. It is often better in tight, confined spaces to have a tool that may stop or bind up rather than continue to cut regardless of the material encountered. This tool is particularly useful when dealing with plastic and fiberglass on the interior of passenger vehicles and semitrailer tractors.

As with the other pneumatic tools, check the manufacturer's specifications for the air consumption (cfm), size of the air inlet port, the minimum recommended air hose, and the rpm. There are a number of different types of blades available for cutting different types of materials. Fiberglass, plastic, and metal are the three most common materials that the rescue team will need to cut with the high-speed circular saw.

The reciprocating hacksaw is another valuable tool for confined space rescue operations. The small, hand-held reciprocating hacksaw can be used in tight quarters with little potential to harm the patient.

AIR BAGS

Inflatable air lifting bags were introduced in the United States rescue market in the early 1970s. The bags are categorized two ways. The first

CHAPTER 5 Extrication Tools

way is to use the inflated appearance. In this category, the air cushion appears like a cylinder with the sides clearly visible when inflated. The second category is known as an air bag. The air bag looks like a pillow when inflated, but there are no visible vertical sides on an inflated air bag. This section will focus on this second category.

Air bags are classified in three ways, based on their air pressure classification: high pressure, medium pressure, and low pressure. Table 5.3 illustrates the basic features of each type of air bag.

The basic components of all three systems include the following: a pressurized air supply similar to those for pneumatic tools, plus manual air pumps, and high-volume, low-pressure air pumps; air hose lines with matched fittings/couplings; an air pressure regulator to reduce high-pressure air sources to a more functional working pressure; pressure relief valve(s); and air control valve(s) to control flow to and from the air bags.

All three systems work on the same basic principles. The air pressure in the bag is multiplied by the number of square inches of bag surface contact area. The air pressure times the bag surface area results in **lifting force** available for rescue work. Most air bags are marked and rated by tons of force (psi × bag surface area) ÷ 2,000 = tons of force.

High-Pressure Air Bags

High-pressure air bags (80 to 120 psi) are made with butyl or nitrile rubber or neoprene. A hot vulcanization or heat/mold process is used to produce a multi-layered material, reinforced with strands of steel wire or kevlar, to form the top and bottom of the air bag. This reinforcement is added to the top and bottom, but not the sides of the air bag. The outside layer of rubber or neoprene usually has a textured surface to reduce slippage and to help place the bag for maximum lift. The working temperature range for most high-pressure air bags is from below zero to 150°F. An additional reinforcement and a receptacle for the air inlet/discharge fitting is placed at one of the corners of the air bag to maximize strength.

The high-pressure air bag is about 1" thick with a square or rectangular shape (Figure 5.10). The larger the surface area of the air bag, the greater the lifting capacity. The lifting capacity and the working pres-

TABLE 5.3 Types of Air Bags

Type	Maximum Lifting Force	Air Pressure	Maximum Lifting Height
High	75 tons	80 to 120 psi	Low
Medium	17 tons	14 to 16 psi	High
Low	10 to 12 tons	7 to 8 psi	Low

FIGURE 5.10

A high-pressure air bag system can lift between 2,000 and 150,000 lb.

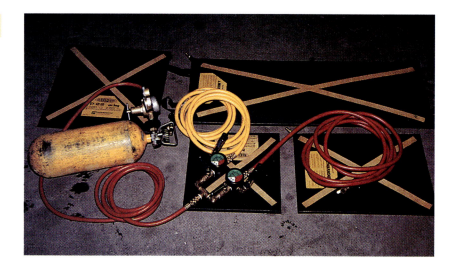

sure of the air bag should appear on the air bag label. Most manufacturers use a 4:1 safety margin for high-pressure air bag systems. This means that the bursting pressure is designed to be four times greater than the working pressure. Check the manufacturer's specifications for the working capacity, the safety margin, and proof testing (quality control test that helps the manufacturer detect defects) before selecting a high-pressure air bag system.

Advantages of a high-pressure air bag system include the following:

1. The bags are strong and durable, not easily damaged in normal extrication work.
2. The purchase point required for air bag placement is small, often less than 1".
3. The bags use a low volume of air to provide lift. For example, a bag containing 2.5 cubic feet of air can lift 10 tons.
4. A variety of air sources can be used, including SCBA or SCUBA tanks, truck air brake systems, compressed air cascade systems, manual pumps, or air compressors.
5. The bags inflate quickly. For example, a 10-ton air bag can be inflated in 3.8 seconds.
6. Two air bags can be stacked for greater lifting height.
7. The bags work well in rubble and on soft or uneven ground.
8. The lifting capacity of the bag and the point at which maximum lift has been obtained can be monitored by a pressure gauge.
9. The bags provide a quiet, highly controlled form of energy that works well with other extrication tools to improve speed in the extrication process.

Disadvantages of high-pressure air bag systems include the following:

1. Maximum lifting height is less than that of medium- or low-pressure air bags.
2. The bags are not repairable in the field.
3. The high working pressures can crush objects or surfaces rather than lift. For example, high-pressure air bags on unbraced sheet metal will often collapse or push through the sheet metal rather than lift or spread.

Stacking High-Pressure Air Bags An advantage to using high-pressure air bags is the ability to stack two bags for greater lifting height. The lifting capacity of two bags stacked and inflated is the maximum capacity of the smallest bag. For example, inflating a 10-ton capacity air bag placed on top of a partially inflated 20-ton capacity air bag provides a maximum lifting capacity of 10 tons, not 20 or 30 tons. The lifting capacity of two air bags placed side by side and lifted together is the combined capacity of the two bags. When used side by side, two 20-ton capacity air bags can theoretically lift 40 tons.

When using two bags, ensure that the smallest bag has the capacity to lift the entire load. When using high-pressure air bags of dissimilar size, *always place the larger air bag on the bottom and keep the air pressure in the larger bag lower than that in the smaller bag, so that the smaller bag is cradled by the larger bag and cannot slip free* (Figure 5.11). It is important to maintain as much surface contact as possible between the bags, as well as between the load and surface of the top bag. Inflating both bags to the maximum pressure reduces the air bag surface contact areas, resulting in less lifting capacity and greater insta-

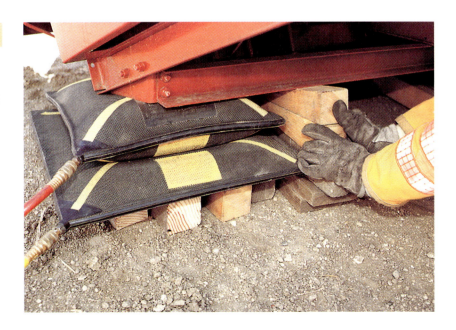

FIGURE 5.11

Stack high-pressure air bags so that the smaller bag is on top, cradled by the larger bag on bottom.

bility between the (rounded) air bags. To lower the load safely, reverse the lifting sequence.

Stability Considerations There are a number of stability considerations to keep in mind when using high-pressure air bag systems. Always estimate the location of the center of gravity of the load to determine the best placement of the air bag(s). The location and needs of the patient may dictate placement of the air bags. Improved stability can be obtained by using two or more air bags placed on either side of the estimated center of gravity or by placing a single air bag at a right angle to the estimated center of gravity.

A solid base of support is needed under the air bag(s) to achieve maximum lifting capacity and optimum safety. Wood cribbing is an effective base for high-pressure air bags. Wood cribbing should be set up to provide a near solid surface of wood in contact with the air bag. The base of support for the air bag must be equal to or greater than the surface of the air bag. A base of support area that is smaller than the surface of the air bag reduces the lifting capacity of the air bag and provides an unstable surface. Extra cribbing may need to be added to make sure that the gaps between the wood are as narrow as possible.

Remember that the lifting capacity of high-pressure air bags varies depending on the surface contact of the load. High-pressure air bags may only have 20% load contact at 90% inflation. This means that there is considerably less lifting capacity for the rescue operation when maximum inflation is used. This same principle holds true for loads with a potential surface area that is smaller than the air bag. The amount of contact surface area between the air bag and the load affects the lifting capacity of the air bag.

Safety Considerations A strike zone of at least 25' in line with the air bag should be included when establishing the safety zone for the incident. A **strike zone** is an area of potential injury from a moving tool or object. Air bags can lose contact with the ground or the load and pop out from under the load. Pay particular attention when the air bag is on wet grass, uneven ground, loose gravel, soybeans, ice, or oil, and with smooth or rounded load surfaces.

Only one person should give commands for the lifting operation. This person must be in sight of the air bags and should receive information continuously from both the rescuer operating the air bag controls and the safety officer monitoring the overall rescue operation, including load stability. A shifting load can kick the lifting air bags out with great force.

Barrier protection (mud flaps or a commercial air bag protector) should always be placed over air bags whenever they are not in full sight, or whenever there is a risk of puncture from antennas, glass, sharp metal edges, or hot surfaces. As a rule, try to keep exposure of air bags to temperatures under 150°F. Temperatures below zero can also have an adverse effect on air bag safety. In addition, air bags should not be used if there is potential or actual exposure to chemicals that may damage the air bag material. Check the manufacturer's specifications for a listing of adverse chemicals.

Make sure that there is a pressure relief valve for each air bag in use in the rescue operation. Pressure relief valves reduce the possibility of air bag failure by venting excess air pressure outside the air bag system. To relieve excess air pressure, the relief valve should be positioned between the air bag control valve and the air bag. In most high-pressure air bag systems, a relief valve is built into the control valve assembly. A rescue team using in-line relief valves should position the valves at least 25' away from the air bag to minimize risk to rescuers who may be required to disconnect, connect, and/or shut off an air bag during a rescue operation.

Lifting and Lowering Considerations Always pressurize the air bag system slowly. Once the air bag has made contact with the load, but before the load has begun to rise, stop the inflation process to assess the entire system, including the inflow air pressure, the regulator, the hose and hose fittings, the control valve, the air bag, the load, and the patient's condition. Use simple verbal commands in conjunction with practiced hand signals to communicate throughout the lifting process. Hand signals are a good way to indicate the speed and direction of the lift or deflation, especially when noise or distance affect the reliability of the verbal commands. The commands and hand signals should include up, down, hold, and emergency stop.

Make sure that the load is continuously supported by cribbing during both lifting and lowering processes. Air bag failure must always be considered a possibility, and protective measures must be in place to minimize any chance that a rescuer or the patient could be injured if the load falls. Use wood wedges to keep cribbing in constant contact with the load surface during both lifting and lowering processes. When the lifting process is completed, lower the load with the air bag so that the cribbing is fully supporting the load. The air bag is designed to lift the load, but it is not a stabilizing device. Whenever possible, multiple points of cribbing should be used to support a lifted load.

Low-Pressure Air Bags

Low-pressure air bag systems will often have the same basic components as high-pressure air bag systems (e.g., pressure regulator, relief valves, directional valves, small diameter hose, and fittings), or they may have components developed specifically for medium- or low-pressure air bag systems. The components designed specifically for medium- and low-pressure air bags are often larger and bulkier than the same components for high-pressure air bag systems.

Components of Low-Pressure Air Bag Systems One significant difference between low- and high-pressure air bag systems is that low-pressure systems require a high volume of air flow for inflation. This high volume of air flow is best handled by larger diameter air hoses, larger/multiple gang valves, and a high-volume/low-pressure air compressor. Low-pressure air bags are most often used in multiples of two or more and therefore require considerable air volume for inflation.

The air hose for low-pressure air bags can be of a larger diameter with a relatively thin wire-supported wall and quarter turn couplings. This hose can be bent and sometimes compressed to the point that air flow is restricted. It is possible with some of the larger diameter hoses to crimp the hose of an inflated air bag, disconnect the hose, and then place a quarter turn cap on the end of the hose.

Also of importance in the operation of low-pressure air bag systems is the ability to deflate the air bag using the vacuum side of a portable air compressor. The valves for the low-pressure air bag system, therefore, are often set up to allow for a vacuum deflation of the air bag.

A number of fabrics, such as aramid or canvas impregnated with neoprene, vinyl, or rubber compounds, are used to form the top and bottom of the air bag. Generally, multiple layers of these composite materials are used in the top and bottom air bag components. All of the components of the low-pressure air bag are cut to shape and cold-glued in place with epoxy. The side walls are usually single layers of a flexible material such as neoprene. The air inlet/discharge assembly is located in the side wall of the air bag, usually about halfway between the top and bottom.

Another notable difference between high- and low-pressure air bags is the shape and flexibility of the low-pressure air bag and its side walls (Figure 5.12). The top and bottom of the low-pressure air bag are very similar to layered belting material, but the side walls are built with maximum flexibility to allow for inflation and deflation. Low-pressure air bags inflate to a much greater height than do the high-pressure air bags and have a very definite, visible side wall. Some low-pressure air bags also have internal strapping that is used to add stability and control for the bag during high lifts.

Advantages of low-pressure air bags include the following:

1. Lifting heights range from 14" to 80", which provides good clearance for rescue operations.
2. The bags will lift thin-skinned vehicles such as combines and grain trailers without damaging or collapsing the vehicle walls.

FIGURE 5.12

A low-pressure air bag system can lift between 4,000 and 24,000 lb.

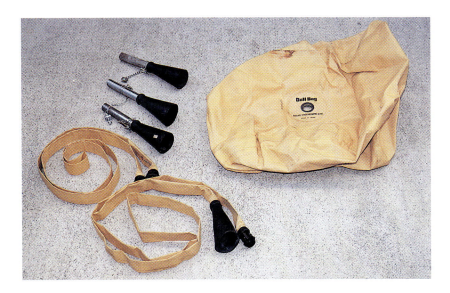

3. The wide lifting surface area of the bag provides good stability for the load and the bag.
4. Most damage to tops and side walls of the bags are repairable in the field with kits supplied by the manufacturer.
5. The bags are relatively lightweight for their lifting capacity. For example, a low-pressure air bag that weighs 95 lb can lift 34,000 lb.
6. The bags generally require little maintenance, except those bags made of natural materials such as virgin rubber.
7. The bags are flexible, which allows the bag to maintain more surface area contact with the load during the lift. This allows for potentially greater lifting power throughout the entire lift. High-pressure air bags lose lifting capacity as they reach full lifting height.

Disadvantages of low-pressure air bags include the following:

1. The wide surface areas of the bags require more storage space and a wider purchase point for placement during a rescue operation.
2. The hose lines are generally a larger diameter than those of high-pressure air bag systems. However, some manufacturers use the same hose and fittings for all air bags.
3. The bags cannot be stacked for greater lifting height.
4. Large volumes of air are required. For example, a 17-ton low-pressure air bag may require 287 cubic feet of air to fully inflate. As a result, the cycle time for inflation and deflation is longer for low-pressure air bags than for high-pressure air bags. In addition, using a small-diameter hose can considerably increase deflation time. It is not uncommon for low-pressure air bags to be repositioned during a rescue operation. A separate, high-volume air compressor may have to be used for multiple low-pressure air bag systems.

5. The thinner top, bottom, and side walls make the bag more vulnerable to punctures, tears, cuts, and other physical damage during rescue operations.

Stability Considerations The high lifting height of low-pressure air bags requires that rescuers pay close attention to vehicle or equipment stability throughout the lifting process. The rescuer must anticipate the potential for rolling (always ensure that wheel chocks are available for use or in place), sliding on inclined or slippery surfaces (use synthetic rope, wire rope, winches, webbing and/or chain to reduce the sliding potential), complete rollover (use wire rope and winches to control or prevent rollover and to help hold a vehicle at a given position), and load shifting during the lift (establish a wide safety zone to reduce injury from failure or movement of rescue equipment or uncontrolled movement of the vehicle).

The high lifting height of low-pressure air bags requires adequate cribbing to support the load during the lifting process. It may be necessary to use cribbing that is 2', 3', or 4' long to obtain a base wide enough to provide stability to the cribbing stack. All lifting operations must be performed in conjunction with a solid base of support such as cribbing.

Always estimate the location of the center of gravity of a load to determine the best placement of the air bags. A single air bag used to make a one-sided or rolling lift should, when possible, be positioned at right angles to the estimated center of gravity. Two air bags used to make a one-sided or rolling lift should be positioned with the estimated center of gravity between the two bags. If three air bags are used for this same lift, at least one air bag should be positioned at right angles to the estimated center of gravity and the other two bags positioned on either side of the estimated center of gravity.

Grain trailers may require that extra low-pressure air bags be placed directly under the load to prevent the load from deforming the side of the trailer.

On extremely slick surfaces, secure low-pressure air bags using synthetic ropes tied to the air bag shackles and a suitable anchor. A sheet of plywood may need to be placed under the air cushion with synthetic rope holding the plywood in place.

Safety Considerations Barrier protection should always be placed over air bags whenever they are not in full sight, or whenever there is a risk of puncture from antennas, glass, sharp metal edges, or hot surfaces. Because the side walls of low-pressure air bags may project out past the top and bottom of the bag during the lift, barrier protection should be placed over the top and side walls during all lifting operations.

HYDRAULIC SYSTEMS AND TOOLS

One type of rescue tool uses a closed fluid system to transform energy to work. This type of energy transmission is called **hydraulic power.** These tools include the following basic components: actuators to transform energy to work (such as cylinders attached to spreader arms, rams, and cutting tools); valves; fluid to transmit energy; fluid reservoirs; pumps to generate pressure and fluid movement; and hose lines and couplings.

Hydraulic systems operate by placing high pressure on a confined fluid. An engine or motor drives a hydraulic pump that forces oil from a reservoir through hydraulic lines to a fluid-powered cylinder or drive mechanism. The fluid-powered cylinder is the most common actuator used in rescue tools. Fluid-powered cylinders consist of a cylindrical body, a closure at each end, a movable piston, and a rod attached to the piston. Such cylinders can be found on both manual hydraulic tools and power hydraulic tools.

Hydraulic Cylinders

There are a number of different types of hydraulic cylinders used in rescue tools. The most common types are briefly described below.

Single-acting and double-acting cylinders are common in hydraulic systems. Single-acting cylinders are those in which fluid pressure is applied to the movable element in only one direction. Spring-return assemblies may be added to some single-acting cylinders to return the cylinder to the base after the pressure is released. Double-acting cylinders are those in which fluid pressure may be applied to either side of the movable element. Double-acting cylinders can be identified by the two hoses connected to the cylinder.

Ram cylinders are movable elements that have the same cross-sectional area as the piston rod.

Single rod cylinders are those in which the piston rod extends from only one end of the cylinder. Double rod cylinders are those with a single piston and single piston rods that extend from both ends of the cylinder.

Telescoping cylinders have multiple tubular rods that are contained within each other to provide a long working stroke with a short cylinder storage body.

Hydraulic Valves

Valves are mechanical devices consisting of a valve body and an internal moving part. The valve body contains internal passages that are either connected or disconnected by the internal moving part. The action of the internal moving part either changes the direction and rate of fluid flow or controls the maximum system pressure, acting as a relief valve.

A hydraulic system will have one or more valves. At a minimum, there must be a directional control valve in the hydraulic system for work to occur. Manual hydraulic pumps normally have directional control valves with two positions—open or shut—to allow the hydraulic fluid to flow toward or away from the pump. Powered hydraulic pumps normally have directional control valves with three positions—open left, open right, and neutral. This type of control valve (sometimes called a deadman valve) is held in a neutral position by spring tension until it is moved by the tool operator. The valve will return to the neutral position once the tool operator releases the valve lever. One variation of these two directional control valves is found on the Kinman rescue tool. The valve on the Kinman rescue tool is actually an electrical switch that controls the pump and the direction of the pump.

Another valve on a hydraulic system is often referred to as the dump valve. While this is not the technical name, it gives an indication of the valve's function. The dump valve, normally found only on powered pumps, redirects the hydraulic fluid from the pump directly into the fluid reservoir. The result is that pressure is taken off the hydraulic lines, which allows the rescuer to change tools or to start pump motors with little load on the pump.

Multiple-Tool Operations Some hydraulic systems have transfer valves that allow for more than one tool to be hooked up to the pump and ready for operation. The advantage here is that the rescuer can select a tool and then transfer hydraulic fluid power to that tool. A transfer valve permits sequential operation of different rescue tools without losing time connecting and disconnecting tools.

A manifold block may also be used in multiple-tool operations. A manifold block permits multiple tools to be hooked up to a single pump and reservoir, which potentially allows multiple-tool operation. Simultaneous tool operation off a single pump and reservoir reduces the performance of the tools that are operating. Consult the tool manufacturer for recommendations regarding multiple-tool operations.

Hydraulic Fluids

Hydraulic fluid is a caustic, toxic substance that is the lifeblood of a hydraulic tool system. Therefore, rescuers must understand how to select, use, and care for hydraulic fluids and tools in the safest manner possible. Hydraulic extrication equipment may produce up to 10,000 psi pressure if the equipment is operated at or close to maximum capacity. In addition, the hydraulic fluid may reach temperatures of up to 200°F while the equipment is operating. If the system fails, serious accidents and injuries will result. A ruptured hose can spray and burn a rescuer, patient, or bystander with hot fluid. Even pinhole leaks, because they are under so much pressure, can inject fluid into tissue. A detailed discussion of injuries associated with hydraulic fluids is presented in chapter 11.

This section discusses the basic factors involved in the selection and use of hydraulic fluids. The two types of hydraulic fluid discussed here are specially compounded petroleum oil fluid and one type of fire-resistant fluid. (More detailed information is provided in the Appendix.)

Hydraulic fluids serve four principal functions:

1. They transmit power; therefore, the fluid must be incompressible and flow easily.
2. They lubricate moving parts. The moving parts of the hydraulic system slide against each other on a film of fluid.
3. They seal clearances between parts. In many cases, the hydraulic fluid is the only seal between internal parts that minimizes leaks from the high-pressure side to the low-pressure side of moving parts.
4. They cool or dissipate heat. The activity of compressing, moving, changing direction, intensifying pressure, and restricting flow in a hydraulic system creates heat. The hydraulic fluid must be capable of maintaining its working characteristics and dissipating that heat in order to be effective.

In addition to these four primary functions, hydraulic fluids must also be formulated to prevent or resist the following: foaming under pressure; formation of rust, sludge, gum, and varnish; and pitting and corrosion of system parts. Hydraulic fluids should also have stability over a wide range of temperatures, and should be compatible with hydraulic system seals. Not all fluids meet all of these requirements to the same degree. Special compounds and formulas are developed by manufacturers to meet specific hydraulic system needs.

Selecting the Appropriate Hydraulic Fluid Manufacturers of hydraulic tools select hydraulic fluids that optimize the performance of their tools. Because there are significant differences between hydraulic fluids, extreme care must be taken not to mix different hydraulic fluids. Putting the wrong fluid into a hydraulic system may cause the seals to fail, or the hydraulic system to malfunction. All rescuers must be aware of the specific type of fluid that is used in each hydraulic rescue system and follow an established protocol for hydraulic system maintenance.

The hydraulic fluid supplier should provide a Material Safety Data Sheet for the fluid used in each rescue system. It is the responsibility of each rescue team to ensure that these sheets are obtained, read, and maintained.

Hydraulic Hoses and Couplings

Hydraulic hoses move the hydraulic fluid from the pump to the working tool and then return the hydraulic fluid back to the fluid reservoir. They are made of thermoplastic or a rubber-like material and strengthened with multiple layers of reinforced mesh. Hoses must be capable of handling the maximum working pressures of the pump, maximum surge pressures, and heat from the hydraulic fluid. The hose must also be resistant to chafing and other common external damage, be electrically nonconductive, and be compatible with the system's hydraulic fluid. Hydraulic hoses used in rescue systems have two pressure ratings: the working pressure and the bursting pressure. The safety factor built into the hose is the difference between the working pressure and the bursting pressure. The minimum acceptable safety factor for hydraulic system hoses used for rescue work is 2:1. The external jacket on the hose should list the rated bursting pressure for that hose.

The ends of the hose are coupled using a matched male and female coupler system. The couplers have check valves that keep the hydraulic system closed when the couplings are separated. Pushing the male and female couplers together opens the check valves and allows the hydraulic fluid to flow. The female coupler has a movable collar that must be pulled back to permit joining with the male coupler. This collar may have a pin-notch safety system that requires the pin and notch to be aligned before the collar can be retracted. This safety feature reduces the chances of accidental separation of the fittings such as when the hose is dragged along the ground. This safety feature also requires more manual dexterity on the part of the rescuer when operating the coupling.

There is no uniformity among manufacturers of hydraulic rescue tools regarding hydraulic hoses or hydraulic hose couplings. Thus, it is important to recognize and identify hoses for a specific hydraulic tool system so that valuable time is not lost at the scene of an incident trying to attach rescue tools to the wrong fittings and hoses (especially with multiple rescue systems present). It is even more important to identify specific hoses for specific rescue systems when hoses and couplings are compatible between two different systems, but the fluids used by each rescue system are not.

Operating Hydraulic Tools

Rescuers should always assume that the entire hydraulic system, including hoses, is under pressure. Hydraulic fluid is flammable; therefore, smoking, open flames, and sparks should not be allowed anywhere near the equipment. A charged fire hose or ABC-type fire extinguisher should be readily available during the operation of rescue equipment.

Experience operating hydraulic equipment should be required for all rescuers before they are allowed to operate equipment at an incident. An error in operation may move the equipment in the wrong direction, resulting in further injury to the patient.

Hydraulic Jack With Self-Contained Pump This hydraulic jack, one of the earliest hydraulic tools used in rescue work, combines a lifting piston with a manual hydraulic pump. The lifting capacity of the jacks used in rescue work range from 5 to 20 tons. The piston often has a screw-out capacity that allows limited adjustment of the piston before contacting and lifting the load. These jacks are normally used to make vertical lifts, but some are manufactured to allow horizontal applications.

Portable Manual Hydraulic Tools This group of hydraulic tools is most commonly known by its trademark name Porta-power spreader. The term portable or "Porta" evolved due to the ease of moving and placing hydraulic power after the development of a small manual hydraulic pump. Unlike the pump described above, the pump in the Porta-power spreader is separate from the working component. This allows the operator to use hydraulic power from a small manual pump by connecting a hose between the pump and a variety of working tools. These small manual pumps are generally designed to generate between 4,000 to 10,000 psi.

The three common types of tools that are attached to the manual hydraulic pump are spreaders, cutters, and rams (Figure 5.13). Because the power generated by the manual hydraulic pump may exceed the capacity rating of the working tool, it is important to check the capacity ratings on all tools, including hydraulic tools.

Advantages of using Porta-power spreading tools include the following:

1. They are light and portable.
2. One person can manipulate and control the tool.
3. They are widely used in many settings, so parts and service are usually readily available.
4. Ram tools have a number of adapters, which makes them versatile.
5. They are easily interchanged using the quick-connected type of couplers.

Disadvantages of using Porta-power spreading tools include the following:

1. The force generated by jaw-type spreading tools is limited to less than 2,000-lb capacity.
2. The closing cycle of most tools is generally passive. The closing force is supplied by gravity or spring(s).
3. Fittings often work loose in storage because of vehicle vibrations. This tends to cause a loss of hydraulic fluid, and oil covering tools and fittings, resulting in possible poor performance due to fluid loss, or time lost at the scene replacing hydraulic fluid.
4. Threaded fittings may become damaged during use or in storage, which makes special fittings and adapters unusable at a rescue scene.

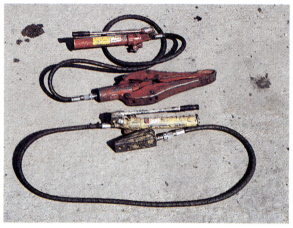

a.

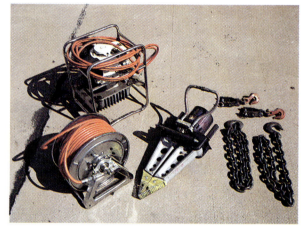

b.

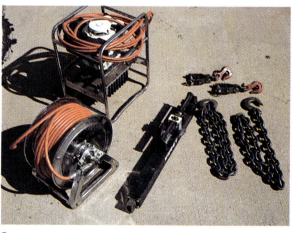

c.

FIGURE 5.13

a. to c. Commonly used manual hydraulic tools include Porta-power spreaders, hydraulic spreaders, and hydraulic rams.

5. Connecting points from the hydraulic hose to the working tool are often exposed to potential damage at incidents by bending metal or moving equipment components.

SUMMARY

An integral part of rescuer preparation is familiarity with and practice using a variety of extrication tools. These tools aid in the extrication process by cutting, lifting, spreading, disassembling, pushing, pulling, and stabilizing the heavy equipment found in agricultural-rural incidents. This chapter describes the components of several tool systems, explains the operating principles, and lists advantages and disadvantages of using specific types of tools.

Rescuers must have a basic understanding of the mechanics of extrication in order to stabilize vehicles and other heavy farm equipment, such as tractors and combines. Rescuers using rigging with pulleys and slings must be concerned with the angle created by the incoming and outgoing lines of a fixed pulley. The total load placed on the fixed pulley changes as the angle changes. A similar effect occurs in rigging a sling with two or more legs.

Manual effort tools cut, pull, lift, spread, and disassemble heavy equipment. Many manual effort tools increase available effort because they have extended handles or assemblies that provide leverage. Perhaps the most common manual effort pulling tool is the come-along.

Pneumatic hand tools perform a wide range of tasks in extrication. Of the several pneumatic tools used in agricultural-rural extrication, the one most commonly used is the pneumatic chisel. The pneumatic chisel cuts through plastic sheet metal and other materials.

Two types of air bags are commonly used in agricultural-rural rescue: high-pressure air bags and low-pressure air bags. One advantage to using high-pressure air bags is that they are capable of being stacked for greater lifting capacity. Low-pressure air bags are quite flexible, which allows the bag to maintain more surface area contact with the load during the lift. High-pressure air bags lose lifting capacity as they reach full lifting height.

Hydraulic systems and tools use a closed fluid system to transform energy to work. Rescuers should always assume that the entire hydraulic system, including hoses, is under pressure. Experience operating hydraulic equipment, such as hydraulic jacks and the Porta-power spreader, should be required for all rescuers before they are allowed to operate equipment at an incident.

TABLE 5.4 Rescue Tools Inventory

Power Spreader Unit

One pair goggles
One power unit
One 32' hydraulic hose
24 2-oz bottle oil additive
One 2-gallon UL listed gasoline safety can with hose/funnel attachment
One spare spark plug and necessary wrench
One quart hydraulic fluid
One spare power plant recoiler unit with rope
Two each clevis link/shackle unit with pins
Two 12'x 1/2" case-hardened steel chain with grab hooks at each end
One pair spreader unit training tips with pins
One spare pin for spreader unit
One spare pin for shackle unit
One cribbing and block set
(Store power plant, spreader unit, cutter unit, and hydraulic hoses preconnected.)

Rescue Air Bag System

One each air bag unit with complete accessory components
One 20'x 1" 7000-lb capacity nylon strap with ratchet
One each protective caps for bag nipples
One cribbing and block set
Two 36"x 36" open weave steel mesh base plates, OR
Two 6"x 36"x 3/4" plywood sheet base plates
Ten 45-cubic-feet compressed air cylinders (2,216 psi) or equivalent air source
(Store air source, regulator, control unit, and all hoses preconnected.)

Remote Controlled Hydraulic Jack Unit

Two hydraulic pumps
Two 10" hydraulic ram (10 tons)
One each: 5", 10", 18", and 30" extension tube
Two double male adapters
Two double female adapters
Five lock-on connections
Nine locking pins
One slip lock adjustable extension
Two serrated heads
Two 9° vee heads
Two wedge heads
Two rubber flex heads
Two flat bases
One plunger toe
One cylinder toe
One chain pull plate
Two 8'x 3/8" diameter chain with grab hook, one end only
One 10"x 3/8" diameter chain shortener
One clamp head (some units use a 2-piece head/toe attachment)
(NOTE: A 10-ton capacity unit is preferred over a 4-ton unit.)

Cribbing Blocks

40 2"x 4"x 18" hardwood cribbing blocks
40 4"x 4"x 18" hardwood cribbing blocks
20 4"x 4"x 48" hardwood cribbing blocks
10 4"x 18" wedge blocks
(Most cribbing blocks can be stored at the fire or rescue station.)

Forcible Entry Tools

One 6-lb flat-head axe with 36" fiberglass handle
One 6-lb pick-head axe with 36" fiberglass handle
Two Halligan-type entry bars
One pryaxe-type entry bar
One 8-lb sledge hammer
Two baling hooks (hay hooks)
One 66" pry bar
One 36" bolt cutter tool

Cutting Tools

Four sets of goggles, 1 set welder's goggles
Four hacksaws, 12" one-piece frame-type with shatterproof blades
12 spare shatterproof hacksaw blades
Two squirt cans with lightweight cutting oil
One pair tin snips
One air chisel (300 psi unit preferred)
Two air chisel double panel cutting chisel bits
Two air chisel flat chisel cutting bits, 8" to 11"
Four 45-cubic-feet air cylinders (2,216 psi) or equivalent

continued

TABLE 5.4 Rescue Tools Inventory, *continued*

One electric or pneumatic reciprocating saw
12 reciprocating saw blades, shatterproof type
One can-opener-type metal-cutting tool
Five pairs industrial-quality earmuff protective devices
One 24" chain saw with support accessories
One oxyacetylene cutting torch outfit with support accessories
One rotary power saw with support accessories

Pulling Tools

Two hand winch tools (come-along), 2-ton capacity
Two 9/32" or 3/8"x 12' alloy chain
Two 9/32" or 3/8"x 15' alloy chain
Two 9/32" or 3/8"x 10' alloy chain
(All chains have grab hooks at each end.)

Ropes and Rigging

Two 300' nylon kernmantle lifeline, 1/2" or 5/8"
Two 500' nylon kernmantle lifeline, 1/2" or 5/8"
One 100' nylon kernmantle accessory line, 3/8"
One 100' polypropylene, 1/2"
15 rated carabiners
Two full-body rescue harnesses with safety lines
Three rated pulley snatch block tools
Assorted quantity of 1" nylon webbing straps

Hand Tools

Two utility knives
One 12" adjustable wrench
One 8" adjustable wrench
One 1/2" drive socket wrench set, standard and metric
One 6"x 3/16" flat-bladed screwdriver
One 8"x 3/8" flat-bladed screwdriver
One Phillips screwdriver
One channel lock pliers
One 10" vise grips with wire cutter feature
Two 3-lb mallets
Two 12" pry bars
Two automatic spring-loaded center punch

One solid-type center punch
Two 1"x 12" long cold chisel
One finger ring cutter tool
Two 24" ripping-type crowbar
One 12'x 1" tape measure
One 3/8" chainbinder
Two stainless steel scissors with serrated blades
One carpenter-type leather tool pouch with waist belt

Safety/Control Tools

Two packages golf tees for temporary leak stoppages
12 30-minute road flares
Plastic barrier tape
One 5-gallon oil-absorbent material (quantity at fire or rescue station)
100 3/8"x 18" square industrial-type oil-absorbent pads
8 PVC fluorescent orange traffic cones
Two 3"x 60' duct tape
Two large 100% wool fire safety blankets
One 12'x 20' salvage cover
One 24" wide push broom
Three handlights
Three 10-lb ABC-type dry chemical fire extinguisher
Portable lights and generator for night extrications

Other Tools

Two 50'x 12 gauge extension cord with ground
One 8' folding ladder
One 8' fiberglass pike pole
One 36" closed hook pike pole
Three 7,000-lb capacity mechanical jack, handyman type
One 12-ton capacity hydraulic jack

CHAPTER 6

Tractors

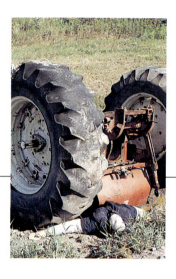

CHAPTER OUTLINE

Overview
Objectives
History of Tractor Design
   Rollover Protective Structure (ROPS)
   Four-Wheel Drive Tractors
Tractor Stability
   Center of Gravity
   Ballast
   Drawbar Pull
Rear Overturns and Side Rollovers
   Extrication Technique
   Rear Overturns Into Water
Collisions With Other Vehicles
Front-End Loaders
Summary

KEY TERMS

Articulated tractor: four-wheel drive tractor divided into two sections and steered by the articulation of the two sections.

Ballast: weight added to the tractor tires, usually in liquid form, to increase traction.

Center of gravity: the point in any body at which all of the body's weight is concentrated.

Drawbar pull: the force produced by the equipment pulled behind the tractor.

CHAPTER 6 Tractors

Field speed: speed of under 10 mph.

Front-end loader: hydraulically powered implement mounted to the front end of a tractor and equipped with a bucket for hauling a variety of materials.

Rollover protective structure (ROPS): a heavy steel frame mounted to the rear axle and the tractor frame designed to support the maximum weight of the tractor without breaking or collapsing.

OVERVIEW

The tractor is the one piece of farm equipment recognizable to everyone. Many farms have more than one tractor—oftentimes a newer model and one or two older models. When a new tractor is purchased for field work, an older model with fewer safety features may be relegated to upkeep or maintenance duties, such as mowing or clearing debris. When used as secondary tractors, these older models are frequently operated by less-experienced drivers (children) or by older individuals with slower reflexes. Consequently, these models are responsible for most fatal accidents.

Rescuers must be familiar with and recognize the potential dangers of the different types of tractors. This chapter describes the most common types of tractors found on farms and explains extrication techniques for rear overturns and side rollovers. Rescuers should know how to turn off equipment to prevent further injury to the patient during the rescue effort. Understanding how a tractor's center of gravity changes is also important in extricating patients from rear overturns and side rollovers.

As in all farm equipment rescues, both the rescue and medical teams should be outfitted with minimum protective gear, including helmets with face shields, goggles, boots, and heavy leather gloves.

OBJECTIVES

After reading this chapter, the rescuer should be able to:
- recognize the various types of tractors.
- estimate center of gravity for an overturned tractor.

continued

- recognize the symbols and safety signs found on tractors.
- describe the process by which an individual would be extricated from an overturned tractor.

HISTORY OF TRACTOR DESIGN

The first tractor, called the Froelich, was developed in 1892. The Froelich was powered by an internal combustion engine and looked more like a steam railroad engine than a tractor (Figure 6.1). In 1906, the Hart-Parr company introduced the first vehicle actually called a "tractor." This vehicle was also powered by an internal combustion engine, but was small enough to be used for tillage operations (Figure 6.2). These early tractors had wide front axles, large steel rear wheels, and smaller steel front wheels. The operator sat in a small, high, open seat between the rear wheels; this area carried most of the weight of the tractor. These tractors were at high risk for rear overturns when pulling equipment if the equipment became stuck in the ground. The additional pull was often enough to throw the tractor off balance. The engine and front end were simply not heavy enough to provide the needed stability.

During the 1920s, the "row crop" or tricycle chassis design was introduced. These tractors had narrow front axles with small wheels, high ground clearance, and large rear wheels on a wide axle (Figure 6.3). This design allowed the tractor to be driven between crop rows without

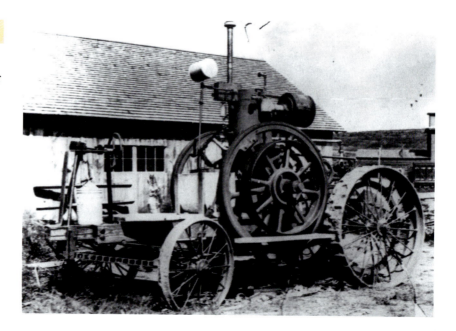

FIGURE 6.1

The Froelich was built in 1892 by the Waterloo Tractor Engine Company.

Photo courtesy of American Society of Agricultural Engineers, St. Joseph, Michigan

CHAPTER 6 Tractors 97

FIGURE 6.2

In 1906, the Hart-Parr Company introduced the first vehicle called a "tractor."

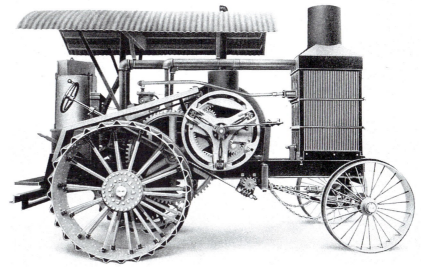

Photo courtesy of Floyd Co. (Iowa) Historical Society

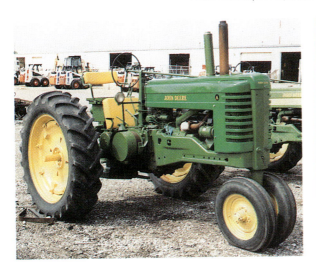
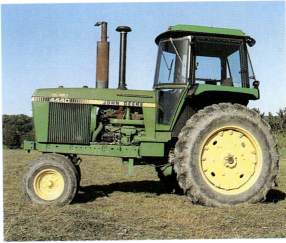

FIGURE 6.3

Two styles of row crop, or tricycle chassis, tractors.

damaging the plants. However, the narrow chassis was also unstable, and the number of side rollovers increased. A comparable situation exists with three-wheel all-terrain vehicles.

By 1940, rubber tires replaced steel wheels, enabling faster movement through the field and on the road. Operators took advantage of "road gears" to drive their tractors on rural roads, thus creating another hazard: collisions between tractors and motor vehicles.

Narrow front-end designs were phased out of tractor design in the 1960s, but many of these older models are still used as secondary tractors. They are often used to mow along ditches, waterways, canals or dams, or to clear driveways and feedlots of snow or mud. Because these tractors are still widely used, they are often involved in side rollovers.

Rollover Protective Structure (ROPS)

In 1966, an important safety feature was added to tractors: the **rollover protective structure (ROPS)**. This heavy steel frame is mounted to the rear axle and the tractor frame. The ROPS is designed to support the maximum weight of the tractor without breaking or collapsing, and must be certified to Occupational Safety and Health Administration (OSHA) standards. Tractor cabs without ROPS may crush like the passenger compartment of an automobile (Figure 6.4). The ROPS may be an open frame of two or four posts, with or without a sunshade. It may also be incorporated into a cab as an integral part of the cab framework. All tractors with ROPS are required to be equipped with seat belts (Figure 6.5).

The ROPS protects the operator in two ways. First, it limits side rollovers and rear overturns to 90 degrees in most situations. This prevents the severe crushing injuries that could result from a complete rear overturn, especially if the operator is wearing a seat belt. Second, the ROPS provides a survival zone for the operator because it is designed to support the maximum force generated by the tractor's weight during a rear overturn. ROPS are not indestructible, however. A high-speed highway collision with a loaded truck, a collision with a moving train, or an overturn from a bridge may cause the ROPS to collapse.

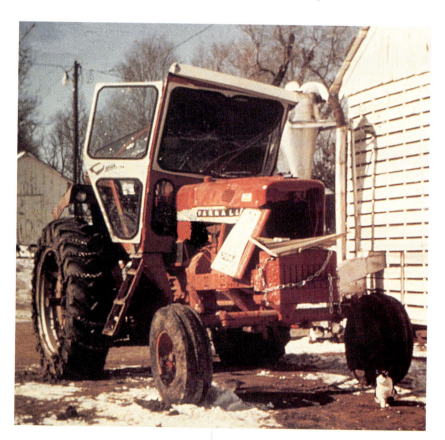

FIGURE 6.4

A tractor cab without a ROPS will deform in an overturn or rollover.

CHAPTER 6　Tractors　　99

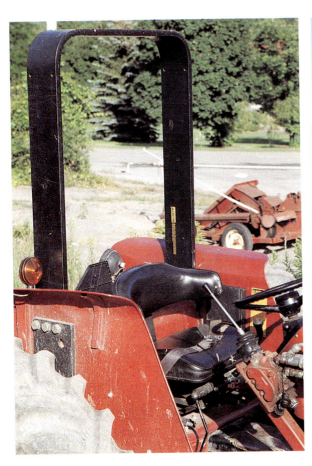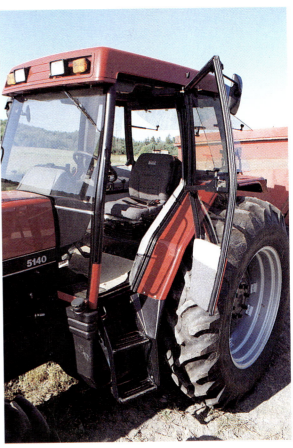

FIGURE 6.5　All ROPS-equipped tractors are required to have seat belts.

Four-Wheel Drive Tractors

Four-wheel drive tractors became common in the mid-1970s. These tractors may weigh up to 60,000 lb and have added traction due to the four-wheel drive and large tires. Many models will have two or three tires in both the front and the rear. These tractors are very stable on slopes and will normally slide, rather than overturn, when operating at **field speed** (under 10 mph). The front tires of four-wheel drive tractors carry 60% to 70% of the total weight, which helps to prevent rear overturns.

Some four-wheel drive tractors are **articulated** models, which means that they have two sections connected by a vertical hinge (Figure 6.6). The cab is usually mounted on the front section and can be reached by steps near the hinge joint. The driving axles of both sections are rigidly mounted, so paired, double-acting hydraulic cylinders are used for steering. One cylinder extends (pushes) as the other retracts (pulls), articulating the hinge joint.

FIGURE 6.6

A four-wheel drive articulated tractor has two sections connected by a vertical hinge.

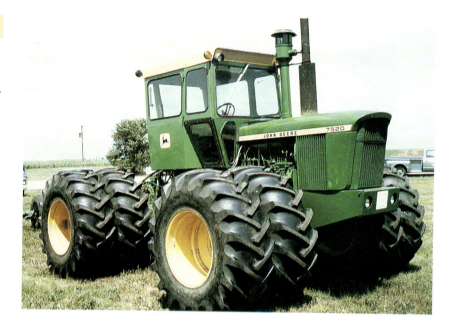

FIGURE 6.7

Another type of four-wheel drive tractor is capable of turning the axles in either the same or opposite directions.

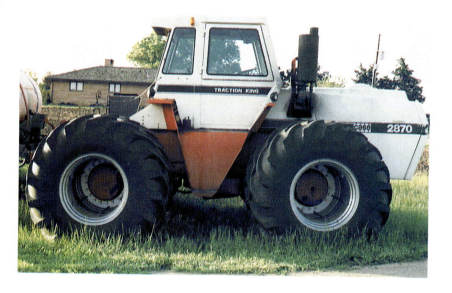

Another type of four-wheel drive tractor has a rigid, one-section frame with steerable front and rear axles (Figure 6.7). Both axles are equipped with universal joints similar to those used in front-wheel drive automobiles. This type of tractor has two primary steering modes—independent and coordinated. In independent mode, the steering wheel controls the front axle, and a rocker switch or lever controls the rear axle. As a result, front and rear wheel position is determined by the operator. In coordinated mode, the steering wheel controls both axles at the same time. A selector switch determines whether both axles turn in the same direction (crab steering) or in opposite directions (coordinated steering). Crab steering is used primarily on hillsides in which the tractor moves across a slope with all four wheels turned slightly uphill. Coordinated steering is used to reduce turning radius.

The design of the newest four-wheel drive tractors combines a standard articulated tractor frame with a rigid front axle that turns 5 to 10 degrees in the horizontal plane. The pivoting front axle allows fine steering control for working in row crops. The front axle is pivoted by hydraulic cylinders separate from those moving the hinge joint. As the operator turns the steering wheel, the axle moves. Once the axle reaches its limit, continued steering input causes the hinge joint to articulate, producing a variable ratio system.

Most side rollovers of four-wheel drive tractors occur during transport on roads rather than in fields. Higher travel speeds (15 to 20 mph), along with rapid steering rates, can cause inattentive or inexperienced operators to easily lose control. Small movement of the steering wheel will result in large directional changes; when the operator reacts, he or she usually over corrects, setting up a severe oscillation. If the tractor is towing equipment, the equipment may begin to oscillate or may even touch one set of rear tires and roll up onto the tractor. The operator may not be able to keep the tractor on the road, and a side rollover may occur.

Side rollovers may also be caused by mechanical failure. Each axle on a four-wheel drive tractor is driven by a separate drive shaft equipped with two universal joints. When either joint fails, the shaft flails about inside the tractor frame and damages the hydraulic steering hoses, brake lines, engine crankcase, and/or transmission case. Unbalanced steering force is created when one or both hydraulic hoses to a single steering cylinder are broken. The hinge will articulate to its limit, producing a hard left or right turn. The operator will be unable to correct this problem, and a side rollover may result if the tractor leaves the road.

When the hydraulic hoses to both steering cylinders are broken, the operator loses all steering control. The hinge joint of an articulated tractor may move either partially or completely to the left or the right. Leaving the road at transport speed without steering control may result in a side rollover.

Most four-wheel drive tractor service brakes consist of a large disk brake assembly mounted on the front or rear drive shaft. The system uses a hydraulic power assist, so broken brake lines or a broken drive shaft will make it impossible to stop the tractor with the brakes.

FIGURE 6.8

The two-wheel drive tractor with a powered front axle (front-wheel assist) gained popularity in the 1980s.

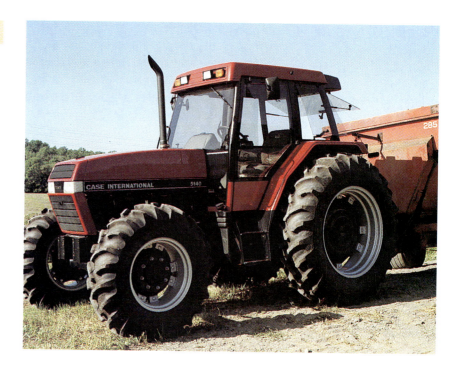

In the 1980s, two-wheel drive tractors equipped with a powered front axle (front-wheel assist) became popular (Figure 6.8). The increased weight of the front drive axle and larger front tires give these tractors added stability and should decrease the frequency of rear overturns.

TRACTOR STABILITY

Understanding stability and how a tractor's center of gravity changes is important because many rescue operations in agricultural-rural settings involve an upset and/or unstable tractor, such as a rear overturn or a side rollover. These rescue operations involve lifting and/or supporting the tractor and attached equipment. Side rollovers and rear overturns occur on both level surfaces and on slopes.

Rescuers must be able to evaluate the stability or potential instability of the tractor and any attached equipment on different types of surfaces to prevent additional or more serious injuries to the patient and potential injuries to the rescuers. Rescuers must also understand how the type of tractor, the distribution of weight, and the addition of liquid ballast and/or mounted or attached equipment affect the stability of an overturned tractor.

The following sections briefly define and discuss center of gravity, and how additional equipment and liquid ballast affect the center of gravity as it relates to overturned vehicles.

Center of Gravity

Center of gravity is defined as the point in any body at which all of the body's weight is concentrated. In a tractor, the center of gravity is determined by the distribution of weight. Weight is considered a vector, which means that it has both magnitude and direction. The magnitude is described in pounds, and the direction is toward the center of the earth. Rescuers have an unconscious awareness of their own and their patient's center of gravity. They use this awareness every time they lift and move a patient. However, rescuers are less likely to have such an awareness of a tractor's center of gravity. Therefore, lifting and moving a tractor requires estimating the location of the center of gravity and understanding how it shifts.

The center of gravity in an upright, two-wheel drive tractor, without additional ballast or mounted equipment, is approximately 24" to 36" in front of the rear axle, 30" to 50" above the ground, and within 1" of either side of the longitudinal center line (Figure 6.9). Liquid or cast iron ballast, mounted equipment, or towed equipment will change the location of the center of gravity, moving it toward the added weight. Equipment, tanks, or weights mounted on the front of the tractor will shift the center of gravity forward. Rear-mounted or towed equipment, or rear wheel ballast will shift the center of gravity to the rear. Mounted equipment that changes position in relation to the tractor will move the center of gravity up or down. For example, a front-end loader mounted on a tractor will shift the center of gravity upward. If the bucket of the loader is full of grain, the upward shift is increased even more.

FIGURE 6.9

The center of gravity in an upright, two-wheel drive tractor, without additional ballast or mounted equipment, is located just in front of the rear wheels.

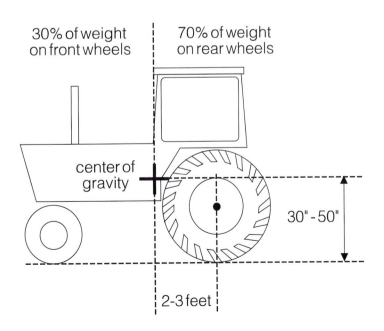

Ballast

Liquid **ballast**, usually water or calcium chloride solution, is usually carried inside the rear tires to increase traction. One large tractor tire can hold over 500 lb of liquid ballast. Ballast will lower the center of gravity, and move it toward the added weight. Liquid ballast flows, which means it remains in the lowest part of the tire when the tractor operates at field speed, is stopped, or is overturned. Lifting the tractor after a side rollover or rear overturn will change the tire position, causing the liquid to flow to a different low point. A shift in this much weight during extrication can significantly shift the center of gravity, resulting in unexpected tractor movement.

Drawbar Pull

Another force affecting tractor stability is **drawbar pull**. This is the force produced by the equipment pulled behind the tractor. The magnitude is determined by the amount of resistance of the implement, and the direction is opposite the direction of motion of the tractor. A wheeled trailer without any attached equipment or with raised equipment has much less resistance than a large plow, tandem disc, or field cultivator being pulled through the soil. Drawbar pull causes a dynamic change in the distribution of weight by reducing the front weight and increasing the rear weight.

Similarly, increasing the height of the drawbar changes the distribution of weight. If the drawbar hitch is raised above the rear axle, all of the front end weight will be transferred to the rear, and the tractor will overturn (Figure 6.10). Loads carried by a tractor's three-point lift can cause enough weight transfer for a rear overturn.

Once a tractor has overturned or rolled over, there may be some tension in the drawbar due to the weight and position of the implement, and this tension must be considered when lifting the tractor.

To prevent unwanted tractor movement after a side rollover or rear overturn, rescuers must determine how the shape of the stability footprint has changed, and then estimate how the center of gravity line may have shifted. The tractor will tip or roll when the center of gravity line is outside the periphery of the stability footprint.

Evaluating the shift in the weight distribution will also make extrication easier and possibly faster, as lifting a 4,000-lb front end is much easier than lifting a 10,000-lb rear end. Lifting away from the center of gravity may also provide a mechanical advantage through the lever effect. This may be offset by reduced lift or movement where the patient is trapped.

REAR OVERTURNS AND SIDE ROLLOVERS

Approximately 85% of tractor upsets are side rollovers, 14% are rear overturns, and 1% are front overturns. Even though rear overturns do

FIGURE 6.10

Increasing the height of the drawbar changes the distribution of weight. A drawbar hitch higher than the pivot point will cause the tractor to overturn.

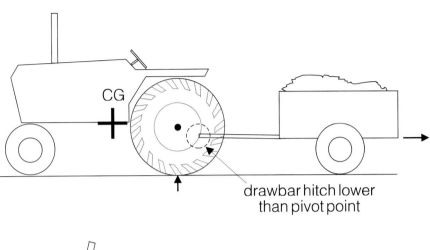

drawbar hitch lower than pivot point

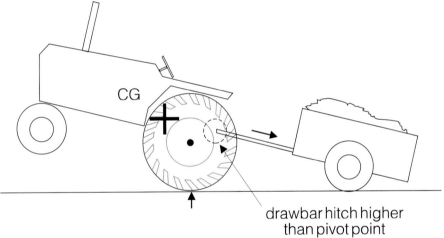

drawbar hitch higher than pivot point

not occur as often as rollovers, they are responsible for nearly half of all tractor-related fatalities. In a side rollover, the operator often jumps or is thrown free, but in a rear overturn, there is often no escape. A rear overturn occurs in 1.5 seconds, while average reaction time in an adult is three quarters of a second. Therefore, by the time the operator reacts, the overturn cannot be stopped.

Most overturn fatalities occur with tractors that are not equipped with ROPS. As the tractor comes to rest, the seat becomes the focal point that supports most of the tractor's weight. Unless the tractor is equipped with ROPS, the trapped operator will be crushed under the weight of the tractor. If the operator is trapped in the cab of the tractor, automobile extrication techniques may be used.

Extrication Technique

Extricating a patient from a rear overturn is a step-by-step process that must be followed to ensure the safety of both the patient and the rescuers. The extrication process for an overturn is described below.

Securing the Scene. Securing the scene includes establishing a safety zone, moving bystanders to a safe area, and ensuring that the tractor is turned off and stabilized.

1. **Establish a safety zone.** The first step in any rescue operation is to establish a safety zone. As you approach the scene, look for potential hazards, such as downed power lines, fire, or a hazardous materials spill. Approach slowly so you can see how the tractor is situated, and if there is potential for movement, or if the tractor is on an incline.

   The safety zone should encompass an area of at least 50' from the tractor in all directions. The safety zone should be expanded if there is spilled gasoline or agricultural chemicals, if there is the possibility of fire, or if there is a possibility that the tractor may move unexpectedly. If the tractor is on an incline, the area of the slope below the tractor should be considered a "no entry" zone. Plastic barrier tape and light stakes should be used to outline the safety zone.

2. **Escort bystanders out of the safety zone.** In many rescue operations, rescuers are called only after family and friends are unable to extricate the patient themselves. Escort neighbors, co-workers, family members, and other bystanders out of the safety zone as soon as it is marked. One member of the rescue team should be assigned to communicate with the patient's family and friends throughout the rescue operation. Law enforcement personnel at the scene are often assigned this role. But regardless of who is assigned the role, remember that it is a crucial part of the rescue operation.

3. **Turn off the engine.** Even if the engine does

FIGURE 6.11
a. Gasoline-powered tractors can be identified by the spark plugs and distributor in the engine.
b. Disconnect the high-voltage wire between the coil and distributor to shut off the engine.

a.
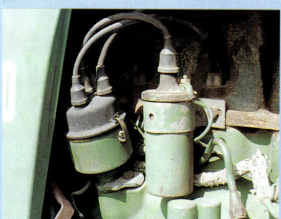

b.
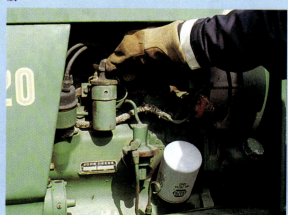

not appear to be running, make sure that the engine is shut off. Overturned gasoline engines will usually stop running because the carburetor float will not operate properly unless it is in a vertical position. Fuel-injected, propane, or diesel engines use a pressurized fuel supply and may continue to run even if the engine is upside down.

Gasoline-powered tractors are easily identified by the spark plugs and distributor in the engine (Figure 6.11a). These tractors also have an ignition switch on the control panel near the steering wheel. To shut off the engine, turn off the switch and remove the key. Disconnect the high-voltage wire located between the coil and the distributor (Figure 6.11b). Older models equipped with magnetos can be shut off by removing all spark plug wires.

Diesel-powered tractors may also have a shut-off key or fuel shut-off knob on the control panel. This key or knob may be red or orange and marked with an international symbol (Figure 6.12a). On some tractors, the fuel shut-off knob will have to be pushed or pulled into the off position, and the key will have to be removed to disable the starting circuit. On others, simply turning the key will turn off the fuel and shut off the engine. Smaller diesel tractors may have a separate lever that is not readily identifiable as a fuel shut-off (Figure 6.12b). All shut-off controls must be locked in the off position with a small vise grip clamped to the cable at the fuel pump or at the control panel (Figure 6.13).

If these procedures do not work, a diesel engine can be stopped by manually operating the fuel shut-off lever on the fuel injection pump (Figure 6.14). As a last resort, a carbon dioxide fire extinguisher can be discharged into the engine's air intake or air cleaner. The discharge from the fire extinguisher will prevent air from reaching the engine and the engine will stop. A stream of cool water or carbon dioxide can be applied to the injection pump to shrink the case, which will in turn, jam the pump.

4. **Secure the tractor.** The tractor must be secured so it does not move in unwanted direc-

FIGURE 6.12
a. Secure the tractor by turning off the fuel shut-off key and knob on the panel of a diesel-powered tractor. The knob is colored either red or orange and is marked with an international symbol.
b. A separate lever in a smaller diesel tractor operates as the fuel shut-off.

a.
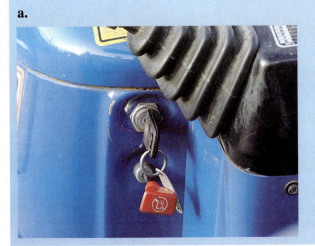
b.
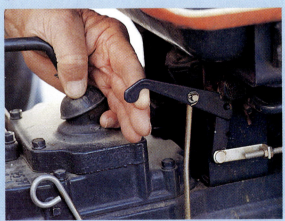

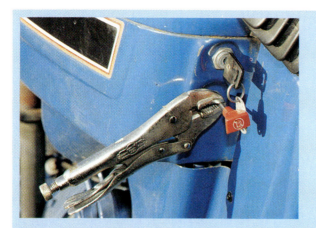

FIGURE 6.13

Lock the fuel shut-off knob in place with a small vise grip.

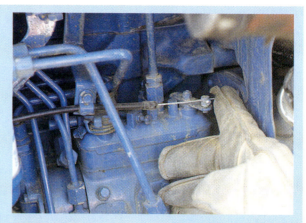

FIGURE 6.14

A diesel engine can be stopped by manually operating the fuel shut-off lever on the fuel injection pump.

tions during the extrication process. Chock any wheels touching the ground. Use cribbing under the tractor frame to prevent unwanted movement. Make sure to crib both sections of an articulated tractor.

If the tractor is on a slope, first fasten chains or cable to the axle housing or tractor frame as these parts support the entire weight of the tractor. Then, anchor the chains securely to a large tree or to a vehicle heavier than the tractor. Make sure the anchor vehicle's transmission is in park, the parking brake is set, and the wheels are chocked. Drape tarps over the chains so they will drop to the ground rather than whip about if they break.

With some rear overturns, the tractor may turn over no more than 120° to 130° (Figure 6.15a). In this type of overturn, it is important to chock the rear tires—both in front and in back. The tractor must then be anchored to a heavier vehicle with three restraint lines, one connected to the rear axle, the second (tow line) to the front tractor frame, and the third to the front axle (Figures 6.15b, c). The tow line prevents lateral movement, the top restraint line prevents the tractor from overturning, and the bottom line prevents the tractor from moving.

If the rear tires are not chocked, the tractor could roll back onto the patient and/or rescuers. The tractor might also "bounce" back onto all four tires as the load is lifted from the patient. Chocking the rear tires will also prevent the tractor from pivoting as the tractor is lifted.

In this type of overturn, the tractor is also likely to be left in gear. If the tractor tire lug climbs the chock, the engine may try to start if it comes under compression. During extrication, the tractor may be either left in gear or taken out of gear, if the proper restraints are used.

Do not use any type of rope to anchor an overturned tractor. Synthetic rope may stretch too much to provide adequate support, and it may become a source of stored energy if it breaks. Natural fiber rope deteriorates easily; therefore, it is not considered safe, especially if the condition of the fiber is not known. Patient assessment cannot begin until the tractor is secured.

CHAPTER 6   Tractors

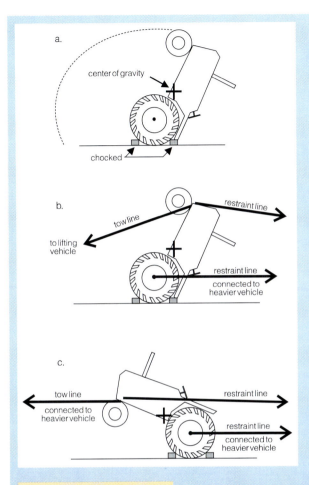

FIGURE 6.15

a. Some tractors may overturn no more than 120 to 130°.
b. and c. Anchor the tractor with one restraint line to the front of the tractor and another restraint line to the tractor frame.

Accessing the Patient. Accessing the patient may be difficult if the tractor has overturned into a ditch or roadbed, or if it is located in a field far from the road. Tilled fields or wet soil may require use of a four-wheel drive vehicle to access the scene.

The extrication method used to access the patient will depend on how much of the patient is pinned, the soil condition, and the tractor size. Possible extrication methods include digging, lifting, a combination of digging and lifting, gaining window access, and straightening or cutting a deformed cab. No matter which technique is used, only trained, knowledgeable rescuers should plan strategies and tactics. Rescuers must also ensure that they are wearing appropriate protective clothing, such as leather gloves, goggles, and a helmet with a face shield during the extrication process.

On rear overturns of non-ROPS open tractors, the patient's entire body may be trapped beneath the weight of the tractor (Figure 6.16). Side rollovers usually do not pin the entire body. If the tractor is equipped with a ROPS, the patient is usually in an area known as the survival zone, regardless of whether the tractor has overturned or rolled over.

1. **Dig around the tractor.** This is a possibility only if the ground is soft or sandy, and the tractor is securely anchored and blocked. As you dig, block and crib to support the tractor. Do not dig on the downhill side of the slope.
2. **Gain access through a door or window.** Few ROPS-equipped cabs have two doors, so if the door cannot be opened because it is lying on the ground, window access is required. All ROPS-equipped cabs have an emergency exit window. These emergency exit windows are usually hinged along the top or side, and have an adjustable linkage that locks in the open position and provides a positive seal when closed (Figure 6.17a). Quick-release pins allow the operator to remove the linkage and open the window completely when necessary. If the patient is conscious and has motor control, he or she should be able to release the emergency window with the help of rescuers.

Some windows are mounted by cap screws that are accessible from outside the cab (Figure 6.17b). If the patient seems unconscious or immobile and cannot release the emergency exit window, first see if the window can be removed by releasing the cap

FIGURE 6.16

A rear overturn of a non-ROPS, open tractor may entrap the victim's entire body.

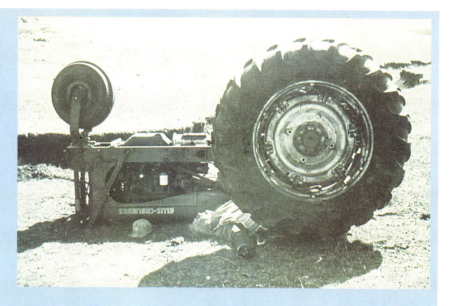

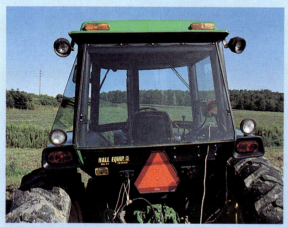
a.

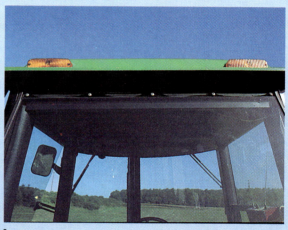
b.

FIGURE 6.17

a. An emergency exit window in a ROPS-equipped tractor cab is hinged on the top or side and can be locked into an open position.
b. Rescuers can gain access through a window by releasing the cap screws at the top of the window.

screws. If not, tell the patient that you are about to break the glass.

Select the window farthest from the patient. Apply duct or masking tape in a lattice pattern to the window and shatter it with a window punch. All window glass in modern tractors is tempered glass, so you can even tape and break the windshield if necessary. Tractor cab windows are much larger than automobile windows, so once they are removed, access to the patient is fairly easy. Place a blanket on the frame if shards of glass remain on the frame. This protection will permit access to the patient without injury to the rescuer, and will enable the rescuer to safely remove the patient. When removing the patient, use a short back board between the window frame and the patient to ensure that the remaining slivers of glass do not cause further injury to the patient.

3. **Straighten or cut a deformed ROPS cab.** This method may be necessary if the force of the overturn was unusually high, such as in a collision with a loaded truck or train, or a tip-over fall from a considerable height. Hand-held and power spreader units will be ineffective for two reasons. First, these units must be able to deform the material against which they press to prevent the tips from slipping. The high-strength, thick-walled ROPS will not deform and may break the tips of the spreader unit. Second, the distance between the ROPS posts usually exceeds the maximum width of conventional spreader tools.

In this situation, heavy-duty hydraulic rams can be used to displace the ROPS frame. Place the bottom of the ram against a firm surface on another part of the ROPS frame. Direct the ram against the narrowest part of the framework and push the parts away from each other. Do not place the ram on the ground in an attempt to displace the frame; the entire tractor may move as you begin to push.

Hydraulic lifting units with a lifting capacity of 5 to 12 tons may also be used to raise part of a tractor and free a patient. You will need 2' to 3' of solid wood blocking to enable the jack to reach an axle or other solid part of the tractor. The tractor part against which the unit pushes must be able to bear the entire weight of the tractor. The axle on both sides should be blocked before and during the lift to prevent the tractor from rocking onto the patient. Lift only as high as necessary to release the patient.

4. **Use automobile extrication techniques.** A cab with a non-ROPS frame may deform extensively during a rear overturn. Bystanders may want to try straightening the cab and extricating the patient using a front-end loader. **This is a dangerous technique and should not be attempted.** If the loader is positioned above the cab, rescuers must work beneath it. Front-end loaders are lowered either by gravity or by hydraulic systems. In either case, if the loader drops, rescuers may be trapped or injured.

Because non-ROPS cab frames are lightly constructed, automobile extrication techniques can be used. *Always try to open the doors manually before using tools to pry them open.* If the doors cannot be opened, try entering through the rear window. The rear window is usually made of tempered safety glass that will break into small rounded pieces when tapped. Tell the patient of your intention to break the glass. If the patient is conscious, he or she should use a blanket, jacket, or other material to shield the face. To permit access to the patient without injury to the rescuer, cover the frame and any remaining shards of glass with a protective blanket. When removing the patient, use a short back board between the window frame and the patient to ensure that the remaining slivers of glass do not cause further injury.

Lifting the Tractor. If other methods for accessing the patient are unsuccessful, consider lifting the tractor with air bags or with a wrecker. Air bags are very effective and can be easily inflated. Using a wrecker requires more care as it is a more dangerous way to lift the tractor.

High-pressure air bags are useful for agricultural-rural rescue operations because they can be inflated without a power compressor unit. As a result, they are especially suitable for use in off-road or difficult terrain rescue operations. High-pressure air bags come with their own hoses and regulators and can be attached to any self-contained breathing apparatus (SCBA) air cylinder. They are also considerably smaller than low-pressure air bags and are thus able to fit in tight areas.

1. **Use high-pressure air bags to lift the tractor.** This method for lifting a tractor is very effective, especially with side rollovers. Although they work best against a flat surface, air bags can be used on contoured or plowed ground and against the curves of the tractor, as long as they are positioned to avoid sharp objects or projectiles. Their broad support surface is effective even on soft soil.

   Place the air bag(s) as close to the patient as possible. Lift against the tractor frame, rather than against sheet metal (which may deform) or tires (which may cause unwanted movement). As the air bags lift the tractor, insert cribbing (2"x4" or 4"x4" wood or wedge blocks) on each side of the patient to support the tractor's weight. For every 1" of lift, 1" of cribbing is needed. Wedged cribbing is useful in this type of rescue operation, because the wedge can be inserted as the weight is lifted, providing constant support. Lift the tractor only as high as needed to release the patient. Lifting is a continuous motion; once the lift has begun, it must be continued until the patient is extricated. The medical team must be ready to begin care as soon as the patient is extricated.

   Ideally, an air bag should be placed on either side of the patient, and cribbing inserted between the bags and the patient as the bags are inflated simultaneously. Assign one rescuer to each air bag to monitor the rate of inflation. The rescuer at the controls should begin inflating both air bags at the same time, and should regularly check to ensure equal lifting movement from both bags.

   If the tractor must be lifted higher than possible using a single air bag, consider using cribbing with a single air bag, or try stacking two air bags. When using only one air bag, you can inflate the bag, crib to support the tractor weight, deflate the bag completely, place additional cribbing under the bag, and then reinflate the air bag. Two air bags can be stacked, with the smaller bag on top of the larger bag (Figure 6.18). Inflate the smaller bag to the maximum pressure first, then inflate the larger bag. Keep the pressure in the larger bag lower than the pressure in the smaller bag. The larger bag will cradle

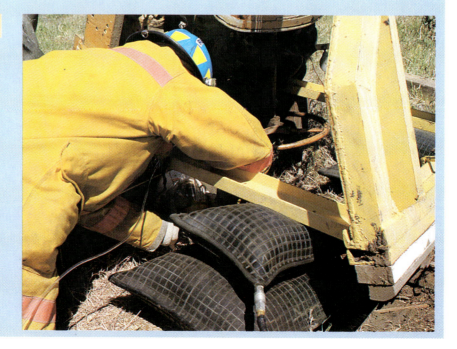

FIGURE 6.18

Lift the tractor with two stacked air bags positioned as close as possible to the patient's body.

around and conform to the shape of the smaller bag, as long as the larger bag contains less air pressure.

2. **Use a heavy-duty wrecker or other machine to lift the tractor.** This method may be necessary if the tractor is on a steep slope, or if bystanders have begun their own rescue operation. Use caution if attempting this technique. Make sure the wrecker operator knows what is expected and is aware of proper rescue techniques. If possible, a trained rescuer should be with the wrecker operator at all times, providing instruction.

Standard wreckers, designed for towing 3,000- to 4,000-lb automobiles, do not have enough weight or lift capacity to lift an overturned tractor that weighs 70,000 lb. If a heavy-duty wrecker is available, and if the tractor is on a steep slope, securely fasten the chain or cable to the tractor axle on the side opposite the wrecker. Drape tarps over the chains that will carry the tension so that if the chains break, they will drop to the ground. Chock all wheels securely to ensure that the tractor will not slip sideways. Chock the rear wheels with a wedge or block as an added

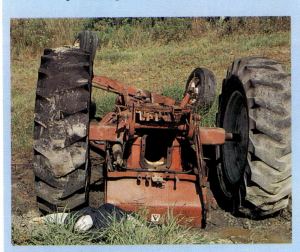
a.

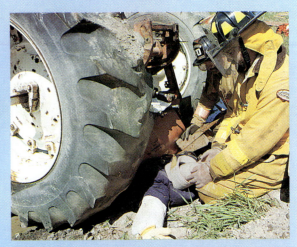
b.

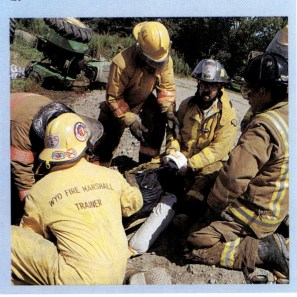
c.

FIGURE 6.19

a. Upon arrival at the incident, assess the situation for possible hazards to rescuers.
b. Protect the cervical spine and maintain an adequate airway throughout extrication.
c. Secure the patient on a back board before transport to a medical facility.

precaution. Place cribbing under the tractor as it is lifted. Do not use concrete blocks as cribbing or support because they might break.

3. **Conduct a primary assessment.** As soon as you reach the patient, begin the primary assessment. Once the patient has been extricated, recheck the patient's airway, breathing, circulation, and disability (ABCD). In all overturn and rollover incidents, protect the patient's cervical spine as you establish and maintain an adequate airway (Figure 6.19).

Assess breathing effort and lung sounds. If the patient is breathing, administer high-flow oxygen via a nonrebreathing mask. If the patient's respirations are under 10 or over 30 breaths per minute, assist ventilations with a bag-valve-mask device. If the patient is not breathing, use a pocket mask to initiate rescue breathing. *If within your scope of practice and if according to local protocols,* insert the appropriate airway. Nasal airways should be considered if the patient still has a gag reflex or a possible injury to the cervical spine. Oropharyngeal airways should only be used if injury to the spine has been ruled out.

4. **Control external bleeding.** Patients involved in tractor upsets, particularly rear overturns, are likely to experience severe bleeding, and possibly hypovolemic shock. If possible, apply direct pressure to control the bleeding using universal precautions; use indirect pressure at the arterial pressure points if direct pressure is not possible. Monitor the patient for signs and symptoms of hypovolemic shock.

Table 6.1 illustrates some of the most common injuries associated with tractor overturns.

TABLE 6.1   Common Injuries Involving Tractors

Mechanism of Injury	Result	Typical Injuries
Tractor overturn—open tractor without ROPS	Major crush injuries	**Chest injuries** (mechanical asphyxia, flail chest, pneumothorax, hemothorax, subcutaneous/mediastinal emphysema); **Abdominal injuries** (laceration of liver and spleen, rupture of hollow organs, penetrating wounds); **Spinal injuries** (fractures and dislocations); **Pelvic injuries** (fracture with associated internal bleeding, ruptured bladder, lacerated rectum); **Head injuries** (fractured skull, usually depressed, severe concussion, decreased level of consciousness)
Tractor overturn—closed cab without ROPS	Laceration and shearing from torn metal in addition to crush injuries	
Tractor overturn—ROPS-equipped cab	Major trauma if operator is ejected; deceleration injuries if operator not using seat belt	Minor cuts and bruises from broken glass and loose objects in cab

Rear Overturns Into Water

While rear overturns into water are rare, a tractor may overturn into a ditch or roll off a bridge into a stream. In most rural areas, if the operator is trapped in the cab under water, the rescue team will often arrive too late to do anything except recover the body. A first responder could try to reach the operator with a length of pipe, hose, or hollow tube that could be used as a snorkel and enable the operator to continue breathing. This type of situation is basically an underwater rescue, and, depending on the water depth, a specialized diving team may be needed. Rescuers should not place themselves at risk for possible drowning; therefore, personal flotation devices (PFDs) and helmets designed for water rescue should always be worn when working in and around water.

COLLISIONS WITH OTHER VEHICLES

Tractors involved in on-road collisions with other vehicles will not usually sustain extensive damage because of their size and heavy construction. If the other vehicle is an automobile, it may suffer more damage; if it is a large truck, damage to both tractor and truck will be similar. Tractors are occasionally involved in collisions with trains because many railroad crossings in rural areas are not marked or gated. A slow-moving tractor will be unable to escape a fast-moving train, but the operator may be able to jump clear. If the operator does not escape, the collision will usually be fatal.

FRONT-END LOADERS

Handling heavy materials is the principal function of a **front-end loader**, which gets its name because it is mounted on the front end of a tractor (Figure 6.20). Most front-end loaders have single-acting hy-

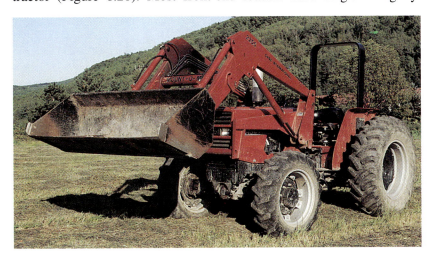

FIGURE 6.20

The hydraulic system of a front-end loader may fail, causing injury to a patient or rescuers.

draulic systems; that is, the hydraulic system is used in one direction—only to raise the loader. Normally, gravity is sufficient to lower the loader. Double-acting systems exert force in either direction and can be identified by the two hoses connected to the cylinder (Figure 6.21). Front-end loaders usually have one cylinder on each side of the frame to lift and another pair to tilt the bucket.

The addition of a front-end loader to a tractor raises and moves the tractor's center of gravity forward, especially if the loader is in a raised position. A loader that is raised too high could cause a tractor to roll over (Figure 6.22). If a front-end loader is attached to a tractor, a counterbalancing weight, such as another piece of equipment at the rear of the tractor, will also likely be added. The rear tires may be filled with liquid ballast, or weights may be added to the rear axle hubs as counterweights. The counterweight will also affect the center of gravity (Figure 6.23).

Most accidents with front-end loaders result from failure of the hydraulic system. The loader bucket falls, trapping or crushing a person working underneath it. In this situation, the initial steps for rescue are slightly different than those for a rear overturn or side rollover. After rescuers secure the scene, they should chock the wheels and crib under the loader *before* turning off and securing the power. The fact that the front-end loader has collapsed indicates that the hydraulic system failed, perhaps due to a leaking cylinder, ruptured hose, or collapsed support. However, if there is any pressure left in the system, it will be lost when the power is turned off. Chocking first protects the patient from further injury and increased pressure due to further settling of the loader bucket or frame.

FIGURE 6.21

Double-acting systems exert force in either direction and can be identified by the two hoses connected to the cylinder.

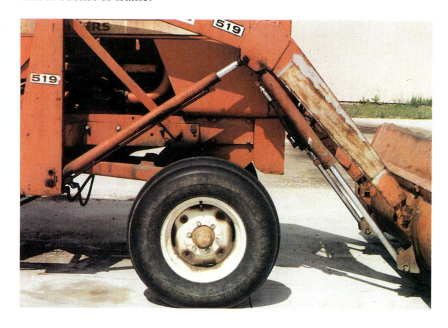

FIGURE 6.22 The addition of a front-end loader moves the tractor's center of gravity forward. A front-end loader raised too high could cause the tractor to roll over.

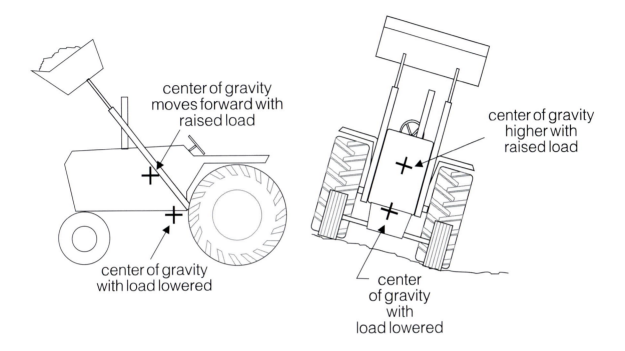

FIGURE 6.23 Adding a counterweight to the rear of a tractor equipped with a front-end loader changes the tractor's center of gravity.

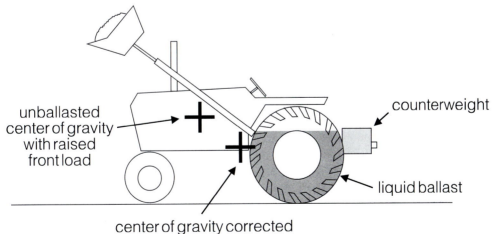

FIGURE 6.24

If the ground is soft, rescuers can dig under the front-end loader to access the patient. Block and crib the bucket before digging to avoid additional injury to the patient or to the rescuers.

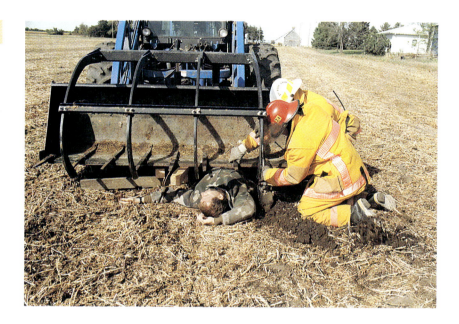

Rescuers should not attempt to locate or repair damage to the hydraulic system in order to lift the loader bucket. Attempting to release pressure by operating unfamiliar controls can be extremely dangerous for both the patient and the rescuers.

If the ground is soft, it may be possible to dig under the loader to free the patient (Figure 6.24). Continue to support the loader with blocking or cribbing throughout the extrication process. High-pressure air bags or heavy-duty hydraulic jacks may also be used to lift the loader. Place the lifting equipment against the frame of the loader and lift only enough to free the patient.

SUMMARY

Rescuers must be familiar with and recognize the potential dangers associated with different types of tractors. The first tractors looked and operated much like steam railroad engines. As tractor design evolved, the lighter, small front-end models were replaced with designs that included ROPS and four-wheel drive.

Before attempting to extricate a patient from a rear overturn, rescuers must understand tractor stability and how a tractor's center of gravity changes. Attaching equipment or adding ballast will change a tractor's center of gravity.

Extricating a patient from a rear overturn or side rollover incident involves a standardized process in which rescuer and patient safety is of primary importance.

CHAPTER 6   Tractors

Major crush injuries to the chest, abdomen, spine, pelvis, and head are common as a result of tractor overturns. Rescuers must always protect the cervical spine of a patient who has been injured in an overturn. Patients involved in tractor upsets, particularly rear overturns, are likely to experience severe bleeding. Therefore, rescuers must render care using universal precautions.

Extrication from a rear overturn may be complicated by the introduction of a front-end loader. Oftentimes, bystanders will attempt extrication with a front-end loader before the rescue team arrives. Therefore, rescuers must also understand the operation of and potential hazards associated with front-end loaders.

CHAPTER 7

Combines

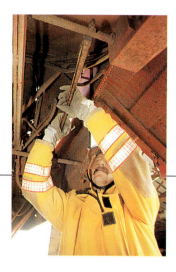

CHAPTER OUTLINE

Overview
Objectives
History of Combine Design
Overturns
   Extrication Technique
Entanglements
Drive Belts or Chains
   Extrication Technique
Grain Tank Augers
   Extrication Technique
Snapping Rolls
   Extrication Technique
Straw Walkers
   Extrication Technique
Header Collapse
Summary

KEY TERMS

Flighting: large, fluted blades on a turning shaft that moves grain or some other product from one point to another.

Header: part of the combine that cuts the grain.

Snapping rolls: paired rollers that are part of the row unit of a combine.

Straw walkers: part of the combine that separates threshed grain from the straw, consisting of several longitudinal sections that move in an alternating rise and fall motion.

CHAPTER 7 Combines

OVERVIEW

The combine received its name because it combines several operations, such as cutting, harvesting, and threshing in a single machine. Combines have several units, including a cutting unit, a threshing unit, a separating unit, a cleaning unit, and a grain-handling unit (Figure 7.1). The many moving parts of a combine mean there is constant danger of an accident. In addition, fires on combines may be caused by a combination of oil and chaff or debris in the engine compartment.

Rescuers must be familiar with and recognize the potential dangers of the different units of a combine. This chapter describes the most common injuries that result from entanglement in a combine and explains extrication techniques for these incidents. Rescuers should know how to turn off the different units to prevent further injury to the patient during the rescue effort. Understanding how a combine's center of gravity changes is also important in extricating patients from an overturn.

As in all farm equipment rescues, both the rescue and medical teams should be outfitted with minimum protective gear, including helmets with face shields, goggles, boots, and heavy leather gloves.

OBJECTIVES

After reading this chapter, the rescuer should be able to:

- recognize the various parts and safety features of a combine.
- describe extrication principles for incidents involving entanglement in various parts of a combine.
- describe extrication principles for incidents involving a collapsed combine header.

HISTORY OF COMBINE DESIGN

Combines were developed from two earlier machines: the reaper and the threshing machine. Cyrus McCormick invented his horse-drawn reaper in 1831, and reapers were first used in 1833. Reapers cut and bound the grain into bundles. The stationary threshing machine was introduced in 1837 to meet the increased cleaning needs produced by the reapers.

FIGURE 7.1

a. The combine is a familiar sight in many rural areas.
b. Several moving units of a combine pose potential threats to the safety of the operator.

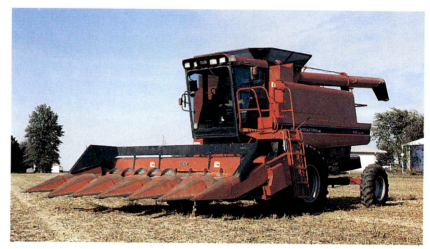

a.

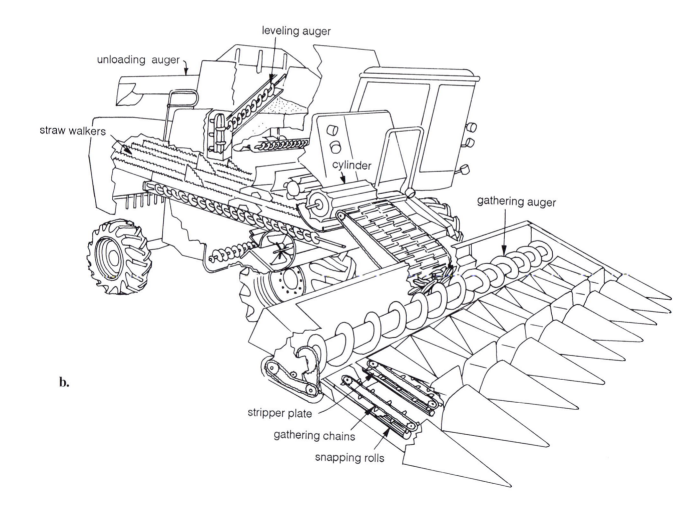

b.

CHAPTER 7   Combines

The bundles of grain were then transported by horse and wagon from the field to the threshing machine. Threshing machines were first powered by steam engines and then early tractors, using long, flat drive belts.

The first combine was built in 1837, but was not put into general use until 1854. The early machines were pulled by teams of horses, and the cutting and separating mechanisms were engine powered. The first self-propelled unit was not developed until 1935. These early machines had unshielded drive systems and very few safety features, resulting in many injuries and fatalities.

Most newer combines include several safety features, such as anti-skid ladders, locking parking brakes, handrails, safety shields, safety stands, locking brake pedals, and safety alert symbols and signs. Separate parking brakes, support stands, and shielded drive mechanisms, when used properly, also protect the operator inspecting or servicing the combine. Some combines have a sensor that disengages the header drive and separation unit if the operator's weight is removed from the seat. However, many operators remove the safety shields for repair or adjustment, then do not replace them. As a result, exposed parts can catch shirtsleeves, pant cuffs, belts, or sweatshirt tie strings, as well as fingers, hands, and feet.

The speed of the moving parts is also a factor; an arm can be pulled in faster than a hand can let go. Since combines are harvest machines, many operators, in their haste to get the crop in while weather and other conditions are good, tend to be hurried and careless around them, increasing the chances of an accident.

OVERTURNS

Because combines have a wide track width and a relatively low center of gravity when the grain tank is empty, they rarely overturn. A combine that runs off the road will usually slide down the embankment without tipping over. An overturn will not usually occur unless the grain tank is filled or the operator loses control next to a very steep, deep embankment. However, because combine cabs do not have rollover protective structures (ROPS), injuries that result from an overturn may be serious.

Extrication techniques are very similar to those used for a non-ROPS tractor overturn, described in chapter 6.

Extrication Technique

Securing the Scene.

1. **Establish a safety zone.** As you approach the scene, look for potential hazards, such as downed power lines, fire, or a hazardous materials spill. Approach slowly so you can see how the combine is situated, and if there is potential for movement.

    The safety zone should encompass an area of at least 50' from the combine in all directions. The safety zone should be expanded if there is spilled gasoline or agricultural chemicals, if there is the possibility of fire, or if there is a possibility that the combine may move unexpectedly. If the combine is on an incline, the area of the slope below the combine should be considered a "no entry" zone. Plastic barrier tape and light stakes should be used to outline the safety zone.

2. **Escort bystanders out of the safety zone.** In many rescue operations, rescuers are called only after family and friends are unable to extricate the patient themselves. Escort neighbors, co-workers, family members, and other bystanders out of the safety zone as soon as it is marked. Remember, however, to keep family members informed throughout the rescue operation.

3. **Turn off the engine, whether it is running or not.** Combines, like tractors, may have gasoline, fuel-injected, or diesel engines. Follow the same guidelines as outlined for tractors to shut off and secure the engine. Combines also have a control lever or switch for activating the header and another lever or switch for engaging the auger when unloading grain from the grain tank (Figure 7.2). These levers or switches must be turned to the off position once the power to the combine is shut off.

4. **Secure the combine.** The combine must be secured so there is no unwanted movement during extrication. Chock any wheels touch-

FIGURE 7.2 **a. and b.** Combines have separate levers or switches that control the header and unloading auger.

a.
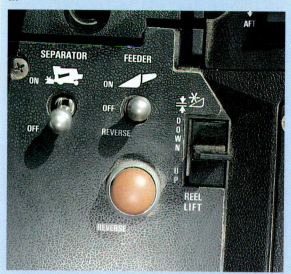

b.
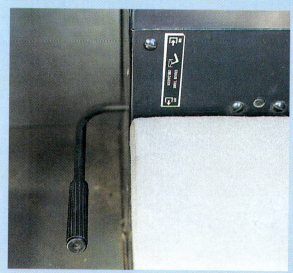

ing the ground. Use cribbing under the frame to prevent unwanted movement.

If the combine is on a slope, first fasten chains or cable to the axle housing or frame as these parts support the entire weight of the combine. Then, anchor the chains securely to a vehicle heavier than the combine, such as a fire or rescue vehicle. Make sure the anchor vehicle's transmission is in park, the parking brake is set, and the wheels are chocked. Drape tarps over the chains so they will drop to the ground rather than whip about if they break.

Do not use any type of rope to anchor an overturned combine. Synthetic rope may stretch too much to provide adequate support, and it may become a source of stored energy if it breaks. Natural fiber rope deteriorates easily; therefore, it is not usually considered safe, especially if the condition of the fiber is not known.

Accessing the Patient. Accessing the patient may be difficult if the combine has overturned into a ditch or roadbed, or if it is located in a field far from the road. Possible extrication methods include gaining window access and lifting the combine with air bags. No matter which technique is used, only trained, knowledgeable rescuers should plan strategies and tactics. Rescuers must also ensure that they are wearing appropriate protective clothing, such as leather gloves, goggles, and a helmet with a face shield during the extrication process.

Combine cabs have non-ROPS frames and may deform extensively during an overturn. Cabs on older machines are not as strong as those on newer models. Automobile extrication techniques can be used to free an operator trapped in the cab. *Always try to open the doors manually before using tools to pry them open.*

1. **Gain access through a door or window.** If the doors cannot be opened, the next entry to consider is through a rear or side window. Access to the rear window may be difficult because on most models the grain tank is behind the cab. A side window may permit easier access.

   Combine windows are usually made of tempered safety glass that will break into small, rounded pieces when tapped. Notify the patient of your intent to break the glass. If the patient is conscious, he or she should use a blanket, jacket, or other material to shield the face. Place a blanket on the frame to cover any remaining shards of glass. This protection will permit access to the patient without injury to the rescuer, and will enable the rescuer to safely remove the patient. When removing the patient, use a short back board between the window frame and the patient to ensure that the remaining slivers of glass do not cause further injury to the patient.

2. **Use high-pressure air bags to lift the combine, if the patient is trapped under the combine.** Use a direct vertical lift, rather than a rolling lift, to raise the combine. Place high-pressure air bags as close to the patient as possible. Lift against the combine frame, rather than against sheet metal (which may deform) or tires (which may cause unwanted movement). As the air bags lift the combine, insert wedged cribbing (2"x4" or 4"x4" wood blocks) on each side of the patient to support the combine's weight. For every 1" of lift, 1" of cribbing is needed. Wedged cribbing is useful in this type of rescue operation, because the wedge can be inserted as the weight is lifted, providing constant support. Lift the combine only as high as needed to release the patient. Lifting is a continuous motion; once the lift is begun, it must be continued until the patient is extricated. The medical team must be ready to begin care as soon as the patient is extricated.

   Ideally, an air bag should be placed on either side of the patient, and cribbing inserted between the bags and the patient as the bags are inflated simultaneously. Assign one rescuer to each air bag to monitor the rate of inflation. The rescuer at the controls should begin inflating both air bags at the same time, and should regularly check to ensure equal lifting movement from both bags.

If the combine must be lifted higher than possible using a single air bag, consider using cribbing with a single air bag, or try stacking two air bags. When using only one air bag, you can inflate the bag, crib to support the combine's weight, deflate the bag completely, place additional cribbing under the bag, and then reinflate the air bag. Two air bags can be stacked, with the smaller bag on top of the larger bag. Inflate the smaller bag to the maximum pressure first, then inflate the larger bag. Keep the pressure in the larger bag lower than the pressure in the smaller bag. The larger bag will cradle around and conform to the shape of the smaller bag, as long as the larger bag contains less air pressure.

3. **Conduct a primary assessment.** As soon as you reach the patient, begin the primary assessment. Once the patient has been extricated, recheck the patient's airway, breathing, circulation, and disability (ABCD). In all overturn incidents, protect the patient's cervical spine as you establish and maintain an adequate airway.

Assess breathing effort and lung sounds. If the patient is breathing, administer high-flow oxygen via a nonrebreathing mask. If the patient's respirations are under 10 or over 30 breaths per minute, assist ventilation with a bag-valve-mask device. If the patient is not breathing, use a pocket mask or bag-valve-mask device to initiate ventilation. *If within your scope of practice and if according to local protocols,* insert the appropriate airway. Nasal airways should be considered if the patient still has a gag reflex or a possible injury to the cervical spine. Oropharyngeal airways should only be used if injury to the spine has been ruled out.

4. **Control external bleeding.** Patients involved in combine overturns are likely to experience severe bleeding and possible hypovolemic shock. If possible, apply direct pressure to control the bleeding using universal precautions; use indirect pressure at the arterial pressure points if direct pressure is not possible. Monitor the patient for signs and symptoms of hypovolemic shock. Begin fluid replacement, *if within your scope of practice.*

ENTANGLEMENTS

Most combine accidents involve entanglement in parts of the equipment, such as in the drive belts or chains (Figure 7.3). Clothing, fingers, hands, or legs may be caught, resulting in burns, severe cuts, crush injuries, and amputations (Figure 7.4). Less frequent, but more severe injuries, occur when the operator becomes entangled in the grain tank auger or the snapping rolls of the header or pinned under the header.

DRIVE BELTS OR CHAINS

Pinch points occur in all types of equipment. Although each machine is different, basic extrication principles apply. In every entanglement, there will be stored energy in the system. Cutting chains or belts may result in explosive release of this energy and could cause further injury to the patient.

CHAPTER 7 Combines

FIGURE 7.3

Exposed drive belts or chains are sources of potential injury. (Shield removed for viewing purposes.)

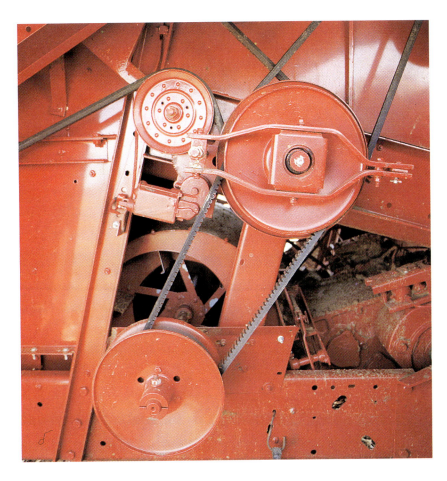

FIGURE 7.4

Soft tissue damage to a hand caught in a combine drive belt.

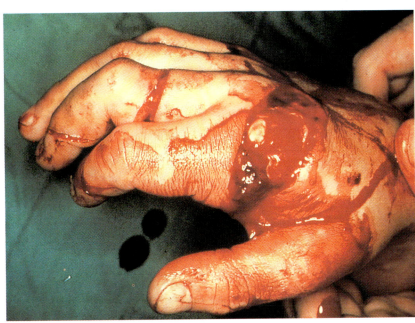

Extrication Technique

1. **Establish a safety zone.**
2. **Escort bystanders out of the safety zone.**
3. **Turn off and secure the power source.**
4. **Use a hacksaw to cut the drive belt.** Most rubber belts for farm machinery contain numerous strands of tough steel and cannot be cut with a knife. Support the ends of the drive belt on both sides of the cut point.
5. **Use a bolt cutter or separate the master link to release chains.** If cutting the drive chain with a bolt cutter, cut the side plates, not the pins or rollers because they are made of hard steel (Figure 7.5a). The master link is similar to those found on a bicycle chain. Usually a pair of pliers or a screwdriver can be used to open the link and remove it from the chain (Figure 7.5b).
6. **Call a farm equipment mechanic.** If the patient is entangled, disassembly of the equipment may be required. However, disassembly should only be undertaken with the supervision of a farm equipment mechanic or an individual knowledgeable about this type of equipment.
7. **Conduct a primary assessment.** Conduct a primary assessment as described earlier in the chapter.
8. **Control external bleeding.** Begin fluid replacement, *if within your scope of practice, and if according to local protocols.* Use universal precautions any time you may be exposed to bodily fluids.

FIGURE 7.5

a. Cut the drive chain with a bolt cutter, or
b. Use a screwdriver to separate the master link.

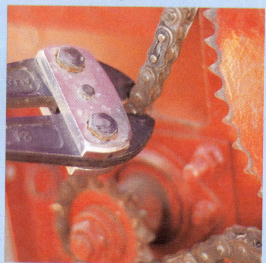

a.

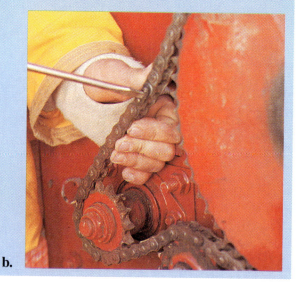

b.

GRAIN TANK AUGERS

Large combines have two exposed augers—a leveling auger at the top and an unloading auger on the bottom (Figure 7.6). Augers apply the screw theory to move material from one point to another. The grain tank

CHAPTER 7 Combines

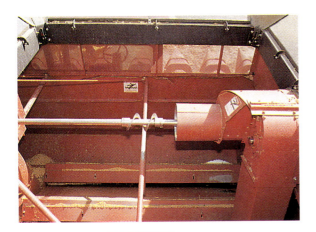

FIGURE 7.6

A large combine has a leveling auger at the top of the grain tank and an unloading auger on the bottom.

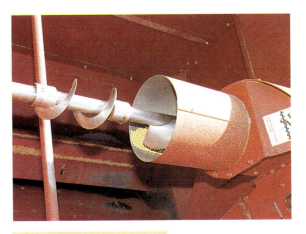

FIGURE 7.7

Large, fluted blades (flighting) move the grain forward.

auger in a combine has large, fluted blades called **flighting** that catch the grain and move it forward (Figure 7.7). The grain tank itself has sloping sides and a sloping bottom, which makes footing treacherous. Therefore, leather boots with nonskid soles should be part of the rescuer's protective gear, along with leather gloves, goggles, a helmet with a face shield, and protective clothing appropriate for the weather and type of rescue situation. A back board may be placed across the bottom of the tank to provide a working surface for rescuers.

Injuries usually occur when the operator enters the grain tank while the combine is running, and then he or she loses footing and slips into the unloading auger mechanism. The feet are caught by the exposed, rotating auger flighting and may be entangled or amputated.

Extrication Technique

1. **Establish a safety zone.**
2. **Escort bystanders out of the safety zone.**
3. **Turn off and secure the power source.** First shut off the power to the combine, and then shut off the grain tank auger using the appropriate lever on the control panel.
4. **Cut the drive belt with a hacksaw.** Unloading augers are usually driven by a V-belt connected to a pulley at the bottom of the auger. A hacksaw should be used unless someone at the scene understands the equipment and can disconnect the main and unloading auger drives. On most combines, the drive belt or chain must be disconnected (cut) before the auger can be reversed (Figure 7.8a). If the

auger is driven directly with a hydraulic motor, remove the hydraulic hoses.

5. **Rotate the auger backwards with a pipe wrench.** If the patient is minimally entangled, simply reversing the rotation of the auger will free the patient (Figure 7.8b). The pipe wrench can be applied at either end of the auger—whichever end is free. Before extricating the patient, ensure that he or she is supported with a long spine board or safety harness. The appropriate support device will depend on the patient's weight and condition, as well as the desired removal technique.

6. **Conduct a primary assessment.** Conduct a primary assessment as described earlier in this chapter.

7. **Control external bleeding.** Begin fluid replacement, *if within your scope of practice, and if according to local protocols.* Use universal precautions any time you may be exposed to bodily fluids.

FIGURE 7.8
a. Cut the drive belt with a hacksaw before reversing the auger.
b. Rotate the auger backwards using a pipe wrench.

a.
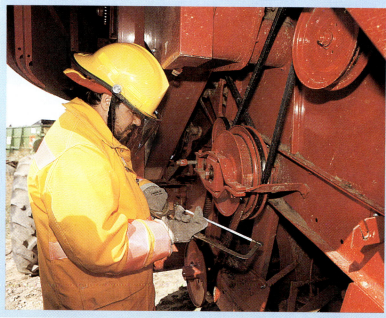

b.
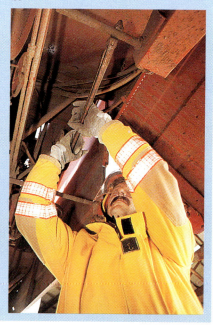

SNAPPING ROLLS

Snapping rolls are paired rollers found on the row unit of a combine. The row unit consists of the "snouts" or points, the gathering chains, stripper plates, and snapping rolls. The gathering chains have steel fingers, called "flights," which support the stalks and move them into the mechanism (Figure 7.9a).

The corn ears are "snapped" from the stalks by a pair of long, closely spaced rolls. Although the rolls may have different designs, they all have raised spirals or longitudinal fluting that rotate toward each other

CHAPTER 7 Combines

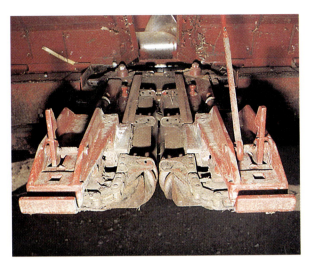 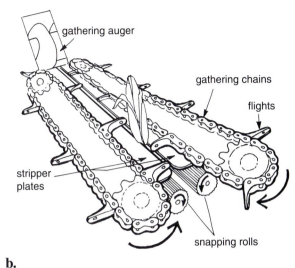

a.   b.

FIGURE 7.9

a. Entanglement in the moving snapping rolls on a combine header can result in serious injury. (Shield removed for viewing purposes.)
b. Parts of the row unit containing the snapping rolls.

(Figure 7.9b). Snapping rolls pull the ear against stripper plates to snap it from the stalk. The rolls are set in heavy metal housings built as an integral part of the machine.

Occasionally, the snapping rolls may get clogged. Incidents occur when an operator tries to dislodge a plug of stalks or other debris by pulling or kicking at the plug while the machine is still running. Once the plug is free, the speed of the rolls carries the extremity into the machine.

Extrication can be quite difficult, not only because the rolls are covered by the metal housing, but also because in most cases, it is nearly impossible to reverse the direction of the roll. The power reverse on newer models should not be engaged, as it may cause additional injury to the patient. As part of the response to this type of accident, a farm equipment mechanic and a physician trained in field amputation should be dispatched to the scene as quickly as possible. The mechanic may be able to assist in the extrication, and the physician may need to perform a field amputation to free the patient.

Extrication Technique

1. Establish a safety zone.
2. Escort bystanders out of the safety zone.
3. Turn off and secure the power source.
4. **Dismantle the row unit according to instructions given by a farm equipment mechanic or an individual knowledgeable about the equipment.** This is the safest way to extricate the patient, if the patient's condition allows the time necessary for disassem-

bly. If the patient's condition is deteriorating, the options are field amputation by a trained physician, or an attempt to pry the rollers apart with high-pressure air bags or a spreader tool.

The prying method may be possible on older (pre-1970) machines, but it will not work with newer models. To pry the rolls apart, begin at the widest section, toward the front. Watch for flying bits of metal while prying the rolls apart. Use wedge blocks to maintain any separation, and to hold the rolls apart while you reposition the spreader tool. Do not use cable to pull the rollers apart as cables may slip or break without warning.

5. **Conduct a primary assessment.** Conduct a primary assessment as described earlier in the chapter.

6. **Control external bleeding.** Entanglement in snapping rolls commonly results in traumatic amputation of the extremity. As long as the pressure is maintained, there will be little bleeding, but as the extrication proceeds and the pressure is released, bleeding may be severe. Rescuers must be ready to control the bleeding using universal precautions, treat the patient for hypovolemic shock, and recover any amputated parts. These wounds will be very dirty and contaminated with dust, dirt, and chaff.

STRAW WALKERS

Straw walkers are the part of the combine that separates threshed grain from the straw. The straw rack of the combine has several longitudinal sections that move in an alternating rise and fall motion (Figure 7.10).

A large fan forces air up through the straw walkers and out the discharge opening at the rear of the combine. Grain kernels (which are heavier than dust, chaff, and straw) fall through the spaces between walker sections and are moved on a conveyor to the grain tank. The dust, chaff, and straw are lifted by the movement of the straw walker and carried by the air stream to the discharge opening. Horizontal rotating beaters spread the chaff and straw leaving the combine. Some combines are equipped with straw choppers rather than beaters. These choppers use flails or swinging knives to pulverize the straw.

Operators typically do not enter the discharge opening when the main drive is running, since dust, chaff, and straw are being forcefully ejected. However, an operator may enter the discharge opening to inspect the mechanism when the main drive is not running. Other individuals, such as children playing, may enter the discharge area, and not be visible to the operator. They will be injured if the main drive is engaged.

Once the main drive is engaged, individuals inside the discharge opening will lose their footing and then either slip between the two walker sections or be severely cut by the edges of the walker sections. The extremities may become entangled in the drive system, which is similar to a crankshaft, or fractured by the alternating movement of the adjacent sections. Extensive entanglement may necessitate disassembly by a farm equipment mechanic or an individual knowledgeable about the equipment.

CHAPTER 7 Combines

FIGURE 7.10

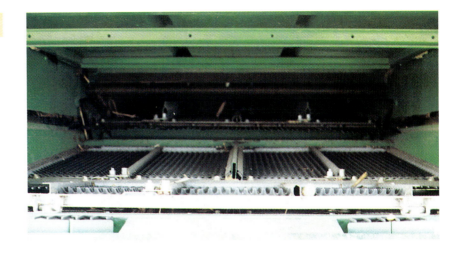

The straw walker of a combine has several sections that "walk" in an alternating rise and fall motion to separate grain from the straw.

Because of the large quantities of dust, chaff, and straw associated with these types of incidents, a member of the rescue team should be assigned to a charged hose throughout the extrication process. Because extrication involves cutting metal, there is a possibility of fire. Therefore, a rescuer with a charged hose should stand near the extrication team.

Extrication Technique

1. **Establish a safety zone.**
2. **Escort bystanders out of the safety zone.**
3. **Turn off and secure the power source.**
4. **Cut the drive belts or chains with a hacksaw.** If a hacksaw will not cut the belts or chains, use a manual or power cutter. As you begin cutting, make sure that the patient is supported on a long spine board and protected with goggles and/or a helmet with a face shield.
5. **Drape tarps or a heavy blanket on top of the straw walkers.** This will provide further protection for the patient and will help provide secure footing for the rescuers. Plywood or sheets of light metal may be used, if available. Supplemental lighting may also be necessary.
6. **For entanglement between the sections of the straw walker, separate the sections with either a manual or power spreader.** As the sections are separated, insert wedge blocks to stabilize the opening.
7. **For entanglement in the drive system, cut the crankshaft with shears or an extrication saw.** Try cutting with shears first. Powered cutting equipment should be used as a last resort since this type of equipment produces a large number of sparks.
8. **Conduct a primary assessment.** Conduct a primary assessment as described earlier in the chapter.
9. **Control external bleeding.** Use universal precautions any time you may be exposed to bodily fluids.

HEADER COLLAPSE

The **header** is the cutting unit of a combine, and can weigh from 2,000 to 5,000 lb (Figure 7.11). The header is so named because it cuts the grain just below the "head." Headers are adjustable for the height of the cut. Today's large combines use hydraulic cylinders to raise and lower the header. If the hydraulic cylinder fails while the header is raised, it may fall and crush an individual working below it. Safety stands and hydraulic cylinder locks, when they are used, help prevent these accidents (Figure 7.12).

Rescuers should follow the extrication technique for a collapsed front-end loader described in chapter 6. Digging under the header to free the patient may be possible if the ground is soft, or use high-pressure air bags placed closely to the patient. In either case, continue to support the header with blocking or cribbing throughout the extrication process (Figure 7.13).

Table 7.1 illustrates some of the most common injuries from incidents involving combines.

TABLE 7.1   Common Injuries Involving Combines

Mechanism of Injury	Result	Typical Injuries
Entanglement in snapping rolls	Fractures; amputations	**Traumatic amputation** of fingers, toes, hands, arms, legs **Fractures**
Header collapse	Crush injuries	**Chest injuries** (mechanical asphyxia, flail chest, pneumothorax, hemothorax, subcutaneous/mediastinal emphysema); **Abdominal trauma** (laceration of liver and spleen, rupture of hollow organs, penetrating wounds); **Spinal injuries** (fractures and dislocations); **Pelvic injuries** (fracture with associated internal bleeding, ruptured bladder, lacerated rectum); **Head injuries** (fractured skull, usually depressed, severe concussion, decreased level of consciousness)
Entanglement in straw walkers/choppers	Fractures; lacerations	**Fractures; lacerations**

CHAPTER 7 Combines 135

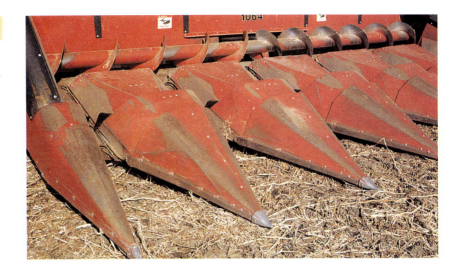

FIGURE 7.11

The header is the cutting unit of a combine. Different headers are used to harvest corn, soybeans, and other grain crops.

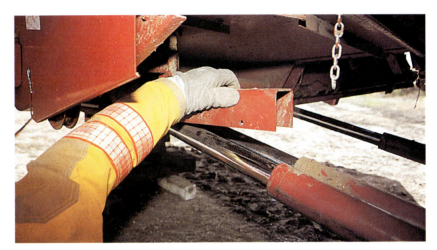

a.

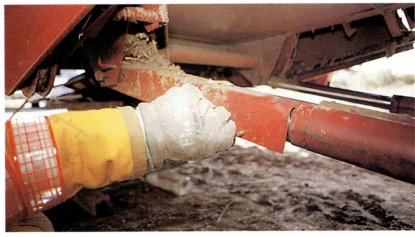

b.

FIGURE 7.12

a. The hydraulic cylinder lock in the up position.
b. The lock is secured to prevent downward movement of the header.

FIGURE 7.13

a. During extrication, place high-pressure air bags as close to the patient as possible.
b. As the air bags are inflated, support the header with blocking and cribbing.

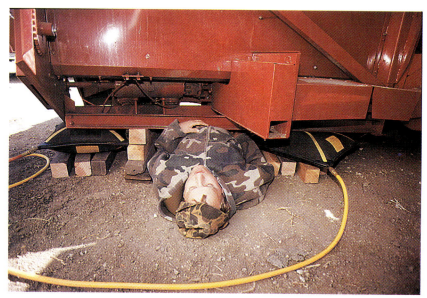

a.

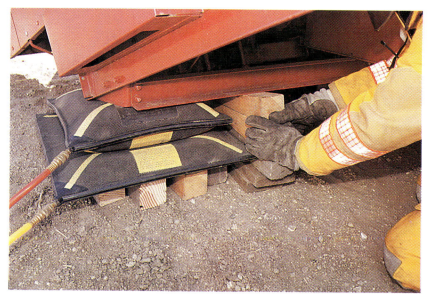

b.

SUMMARY

The combine is a harvesting machine composed of several units: a cutting unit; a threshing unit; a separating unit; a cleaning unit; and a grain-handling unit. Each of these units is a potential source of serious injury if the operator becomes entangled. Rescuers must be able to identify each of the units of the combine so that appropriate precautions may be taken before proceeding with a rescue.

The extrication technique for combines is essentially the same as that for a tractor. However, disentangling patients from specific combine units requires that rescuers recognize and understand how these units operate. Common injuries include traumatic amputations, fractures, and severe crushing injuries.

CHAPTER 8

Agricultural Equipment

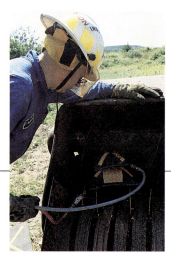

CHAPTER OUTLINE

Overview
Objectives
Power Take-Offs
   PTO Entanglement
      Extrication Technique
   Minor Entanglement
   Severe Entanglement
   Disassembling the PTO
   Disentangling the Extremities
      or Body
Augers
   Portable Auger
      Entanglement
      Extrication Technique
   Minor Entanglement
   Open Auger Entanglement
      Extrication Technique

Balers
   Conventional Balers
      Extrication Technique
   Large Round Balers
      Extrication Technique
Cotton Pickers
Tandem Disc
Ensilage Cutters
   Extrication Technique
Irrigation Systems
Mixing Wagons
   Extrication Technique
Tub Grinders
Sugar Beet Harvesters/
   Potato Diggers
Manure Spreaders
Summary

KEY TERMS

Auger: implement that applies the screw theory to move material from one point to another.

CHAPTER 8 Agricultural Equipment

Implement input shaft: shaft that connects the implement to the intermediate shaft.

Intermediate shaft: shaft that transfers the tractor power to the attached implement.

Power take-off (PTO): a shaft or shafts that transmit power from a mechanism to an accompanying machine.

Primary driveline: transfers power from the engine or tractor to a gearbox.

Secondary driveline: connects the gearbox with the equipment.

Torque: force that produces rotation or torsion.

Tractor output shaft: shaft that delivers power from the engine and protrudes from the rear of the tractor.

Universal joint: joints at the ends of the PTO drivelines that connect the tractor to the implement, and allow the driveline to change angles.

Windrow: crop that has been cut and raked into a row.

OVERVIEW

Agricultural equipment is pulled by, attached to, or powered by a tractor, portable engine, or electric motor. Some agricultural equipment may also be component parts of several kinds of machines. As many as 35 different machines may be used during any single growing season or on any single farm. Each piece of equipment has the potential to cause serious injury.

Many types of agricultural equipment are not self-powered; they draw power from a tractor or portable engine. A power take-off (PTO) is usually used to transfer power from a tractor to trailing equipment (such as a baler) or to stationary implements (such as a feed grinder). Portable engines may also use PTOs to supply power to implements such as portable augers and irrigation systems. The complexity of some of this machinery may mean that a qualified farm equipment mechanic should be dispatched to the scene as soon as the rescue team is sent; the mechanic may be able to help in the extrication operation.

Rescuers must be familiar with these different agricultural implements and must be able to recognize their potential dangers. Several types of equipment use hydraulic systems, so rescuers

continued

should recognize the special hazards associated with hydraulic fluid leaks. Rescuers should also be aware of potential electrical hazards from contact between overhead power lines and high-standing farm equipment. Selecting the appropriate tools and techniques is vital to the safety of the rescuers, the success of the rescue operation, and possibly even to the life of the patient.

This chapter describes the most common pieces of agricultural equipment and outlines general extrication techniques. Although the chapter does not cover every possible situation, the techniques described may be applied to other situations. Because many rescue operations in agricultural-rural settings involve severe trauma or serious medical conditions, basic life support and medical assistance must be provided throughout the extrication process.

OBJECTIVES

After reading this chapter, the rescuer should be able to:

- recognize various types of agricultural equipment.
- identify potential hazards in dealing with agricultural equipment.
- determine appropriate extrication techniques based on the type of equipment and general extrication and safety principles.

POWER TAKE-OFFS

A **power take-off** or **PTO** refers to a shaft or shafts that transmit power to the mechanism of an accompanying machine (Figure 8.1). With it, a single engine supplies both pulling power and remote operation power. PTO-driven equipment may be stationary, pulled behind, or mounted on a tractor, and include mowers, balers, grain augers, self-unloading wagons, choppers, or feed mills.

The first PTOs were introduced in the 1920s. Early manufacturers developed a protective, inverted-U shield to cover the rotating drive; however, many operators remove these shields, increasing their risk of entanglement.

PTOs revolve at two standard speeds. Older, less-powerful tractors are usually equipped with a six-spline shaft that turns at 540 revolutions per minute (rpm); larger, high-horsepower tractors will have a 21-spline shaft that rotates at 1,000 rpm. Some tractors are able to accommodate both speeds by using separate or interchangeable shafts (Figure 8.2). An

CHAPTER 8   Agricultural Equipment   141

FIGURE 8.1

A power take-off (PTO) enables the tractor engine to transmit power to another machine.

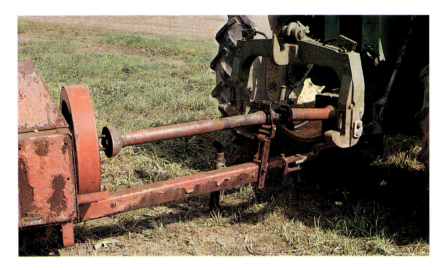

FIGURE 8.2

Newer tractors have both 6-spline and 21-spline shafts. (Note: Master safety shield removed for viewing purposes.)

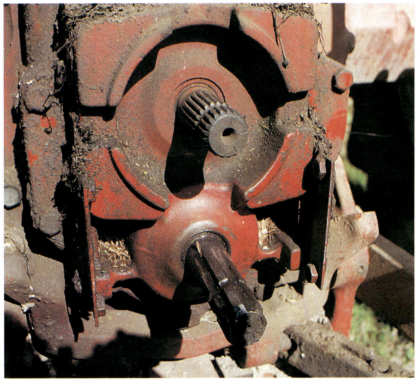

operator standing behind the tractor and looking forward, will see that the shafts of all PTOs rotate clockwise.

The PTO driveline connects the tractor to the attached implement. At one end of the driveline is a **universal joint** with internal splines that match and connect to the tractor output shaft.

An **intermediate shaft** connects the first universal joint to a second universal joint; this shaft transfers the tractor power to the attached implement. The simplest form of intermediate shaft is a single square shaft that telescopes into a hollow square tube. Newer shafts may have different shapes or designs to prevent misalignment of the joint. Some PTO drivelines may be quite complicated, with multiple intermediate shafts that may or may not telescope, or be supported by bearings.

The **tractor output shaft** delivers power from the engine and protrudes from the rear of the tractor. The output shaft is splined so it can be connected to the PTO driveline. The output shaft is protected by a fixed master safety shield (Figure 8.3). On older tractors, a simple pin or bolt inserted through the universal joint and the output shaft is used to lock the components together. On newer models, a spring-loaded pin or a sliding collar is used to lock the joint and shaft together (Figure 8.4).

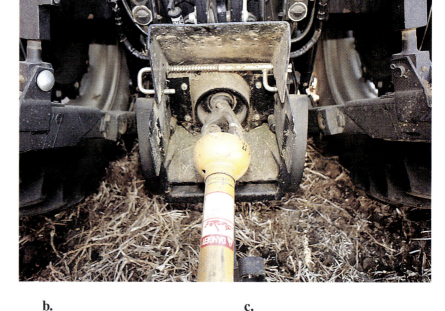

FIGURE 8.3

The tractor output shaft is protected by a fixed master safety shield. The shaft is splined to connect the PTO driveline to the output shaft. (Note: Top portion of safety shield raised for viewing purposes.)

FIGURE 8.4

An operator can lock the shaft and driveline together by using **(a)** a simple pin or bolt, **(b)** a spring-loaded pin, or **(c)** a sliding collar.

a.

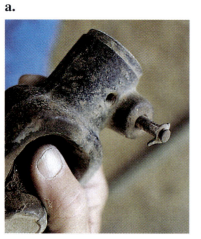

b.

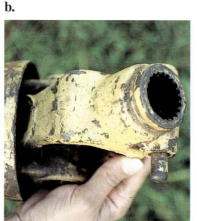

c.

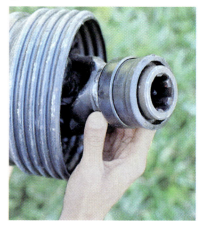

At the far end of the intermediate shaft is another universal joint that connects to the **input shaft** of the implement. Modern PTO drivelines are completely shielded with a master shield on the tractor, free-rotating shields surrounding the intermediate shaft, and a shield for each universal joint (Figure 8.5). However, on older tractors and equipment, these shields may be missing, damaged, or provide only partial protection. Remember that damaged or deformed shields provide no protection.

Sometimes two or more PTO drivelines are needed to operate an implement (Figure 8.6). In this situation, the **primary driveline** transfers power from the engine or tractor to a gearbox, and a **secondary driveline** connects the gearbox with the equipment. The secondary driveline may rotate at a different speed than the primary driveline, depending on the gear ratio. If the speed of the secondary driveline is slower than that of the primary driveline, the force or **torque** produced is greater. However, if the speed of the secondary driveline is faster than that of the primary driveline, the torque produced is lower.

PTO Entanglement

Incidents involving PTOs usually occur when an individual wearing loose clothing gets too close to an unshielded shaft or joint. An open shirtsleeve, baggy pant cuff, tie strings from sweatshirts, loose belts, or sweaters can easily become caught by and entangled in the rotating shaft. Depending on the speed of the rotating shaft and the type of clothing, the PTO may rip the clothing away or entangle both the clothing and the operator before he or she can turn off the machine or remove the caught piece of clothing (Figure 8.7).

Becoming entangled in a PTO occurs very quickly. A PTO driveline operating at 540 rpm makes nine complete rotations every second. If the

FIGURE 8.5

All PTO drivelines should be completely shielded to prevent injury to the operator. However, shields are sometimes removed by the operator.

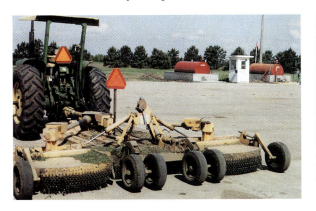

FIGURE 8.6

Two or more PTO drivelines are needed to operate some types of farm equipment.

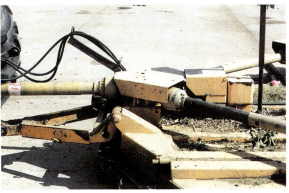

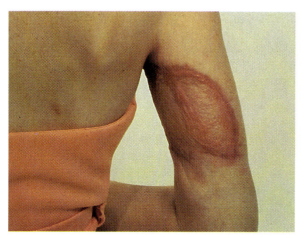
a.

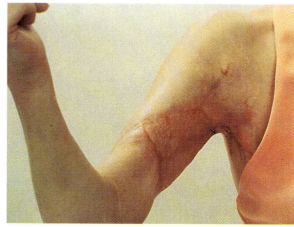
b.

FIGURE 8.7

a. and b. Loose clothing is easily caught in the rotating PTO and can entangle the operator.

driveline is 4" in circumference, this means that 36" of shirtsleeve, or an entire arm, can wrap around the driveline in just 1 second. Only half a second is needed to entangle an entire arm or leg at 1,000 rpm.

Most PTO entanglements take place at the connecting points between the PTO and the tractor or between the PTO and the attached implement. While these areas should be protected by safety shields, operators often remove shields or fail to replace damaged shields. Entanglements also occur at the point where the intermediate shaft of the PTO telescopes.

Extrication Technique

Several extrication techniques may be used for PTO entanglements, depending on the degree and the site of the entanglement. Therefore, several options will be presented. However, for all incidents involving a PTO, the first steps, securing the scene and accessing the patient, are the same.

Securing the Scene. Securing the scene includes establishing a safety zone, escorting bystanders to a safe area, and turning off the power and stabilizing the equipment.

1. **Establish a safety zone.** Approach the scene slowly from the front so the patient can see you. Do not let the patient turn his or her head. As you approach, look for any potential hazards. Do not permit any open flames, including smoking, around the site.

   The safety zone should encompass an area of at least 50' from the equipment in all directions. The safety zone should be expanded if there is spilled gasoline or agricultural chemicals, if there is the possibility of fire, or if the equipment may move unexpectedly. Plastic barrier tape and light stakes should be used to outline the safety zone.

2. **Escort bystanders out of the safety zone.** Escort neighbors, co-workers, family members, and other bystanders out of the safety zone as soon as it is marked. One member of the rescue team should be assigned to com-

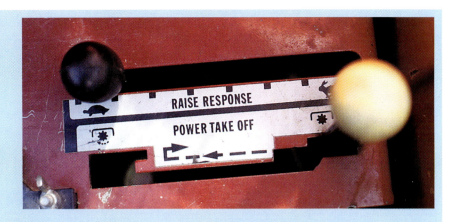

FIGURE 8.8

Some PTOs have a second clutch to permit independent shifting. The clutch should be marked with an international symbol or decal.

municate with the patient's family and friends throughout the rescue operation. Law enforcement personnel at the scene are often assigned this role. Regardless of who is assigned this role, it is important to remember that communication with the family is a crucial part of the operation.

3. **Shut off and secure the power source.** This is usually the tractor engine or the portable power supply. Review the procedures for turning off tractor engines discussed in chapter 6. On some tractor models, the engine may start if the PTO is rotated, so it is very important that the power source be prevented from starting.

4. **Secure the equipment so it will not move, and then disengage the PTO.** Support the PTO with cribbing and chock the equipment to ensure a stable working area before beginning disentanglement. Most tractors will have international symbols or decals to identify the function of each control. All tractor PTO systems have a reduction gear set and a clutch; newer systems may also have a PTO brake inside the transmission. On older, smaller tractors, power to the PTO is interrupted when the main drive clutch, controlled by the operator's foot, is depressed as the operator shifts gears. After ensuring that the tractor engine will not restart, move the PTO shift lever into neutral.

A second type of system uses the main drive clutch to shift the PTO in and out of gear, but also has a second clutch that permits independent shifting. This is usually referred to as "live" power. The unit should have an international symbol or decal that identifies this control (Figure 8.8).

On some newer tractors, there may be two PTO levers. The main lever can be shifted only if the transmission clutch is disengaged or the engine is shut off. The rotation of the output shaft is controlled by a second clutch, operated by a hand lever. This hand lever may have a latch that is controlled by a thumb button on the handle. The latch must be released before the clutch can be disengaged. There may also be a brake that is activated if the lever is pushed past the disengaged position. Tractors with very high horsepower may use a hydraulically operated clutch pack and a system of constant mesh gears. With these tractors, the only PTO control will be a lever on the unit.

Accessing the Patient. When the incident commander or operation leader signals that it is safe, rescuers should immediately begin assessing the patient.

1. **Conduct a primary assessment.** As soon as you reach the patient, you should prepare to begin the primary assessment. Check the patient's airway, breathing, circulation, and disability (ABCD). Checking the airway and

breathing is particularly important, especially if clothing is wrapped tightly around the body, or if there is upper body entanglement (Figure 8.9).

2. **Control external bleeding.** Patients entangled in PTOs are likely to sustain injuries in which the bones in the extremities are crushed or severely fractured. Attempt to control external bleeding as close to the point of entanglement as possible. If possible, apply direct pressure to control the bleeding; use indirect pressure at the arterial pressure points if direct pressure is not possible. Remember to use universal precautions whenever you may be exposed to bodily fluids. Monitor the patient for signs and symptoms of hypovolemic shock.

Table 8.1 summarizes some of the most common injuries that result from incidents involving a PTO.

TABLE 8.1 Common Injuries Involving PTOs

Mechanism of Injury	Result	Typical Injuries
Entanglement in power take-off	Clothing entanglement produces extensive soft tissue and severe deceleration injuries.	**Head injuries** (closed and open skull fractures); **Spinal injuries** (severe fractures and dislocations); **Chest injuries** (flail chest, sucking chest wounds, pneumothorax, hemothorax, tension pneumothorax, pulmonary contusion, myocardial contusion)
Entanglement in secondary drive	Strangulation; hand fractures; avulsion of fingers and soft tissue; degloving of extremities; hair entanglement may result in scalping.	**Abdominal injuries** (blunt trauma, internal bleeding, possible extensive evisceration); **Pelvic injuries** (fractures with internal bleeding, ruptured bladder, ruptured rectum, degloving or avulsion of external male genitalia); **Extremity injuries** (open fractures and dislocations; closed fractures with extensive comminution; soft tissue wrapped around PTO drive shaft; complete avulsion of hands, feet, lower arms, and legs; extensive degloving of large areas of skin)

Minor Entanglement

Several tactics may be used to disentangle a patient, depending on the site and the degree of entanglement. Listed below are several options for disentangling a patient, from cutting clothing in a minor entanglement to disassembling the PTO in cases of severe entanglement of the extremities.

If only clothing is wrapped around the shaft, the patient can usually be freed by cutting the entangled clothing with a sharp knife.

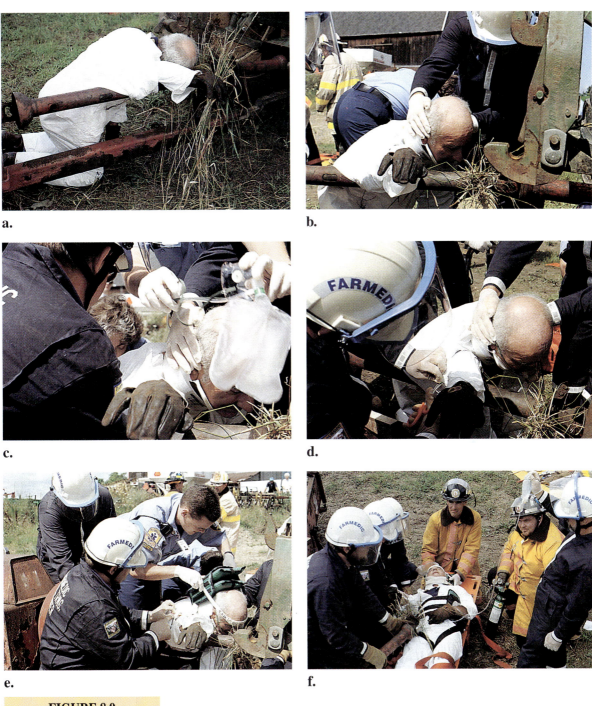

FIGURE 8.9

If the patient's upper body is entangled (**a**), first check the patient's ABCDs (**b, c**), then attempt to control external bleeding (**d, e**). If the patient's extremity cannot be disentangled from the PTO at the scene, disassemble and transport the PTO with the patient. Place the patient on a back board to stabilize the spine and provide additional support (**f**).

If the entanglement is not severe, or if clothing is caught around the locking pin or sliding collar, rotate the PTO counterclockwise to free the patient. Remember to follow the steps described above for turning off the power, securing the implement, and disengaging the PTO before attempting to reverse rotation. Universal standards require that the PTO operate in a clockwise direction as you face the rear of the tractor. This means that the shaft must be turned counterclockwise to free the patient. Insert a crowbar in the universal joint between the PTO and the power source and turn counterclockwise, or use a large pipe wrench on the solid portion of the shaft and slowly rotate the PTO shaft counterclockwise (Figure 8.10).

Severe Entanglement

If the entanglement is more severe, attempt to separate the ends of the intermediate shaft using the telescoping connection. Depress the locking pin on the front universal joint to release it from the tractor output shaft. If the locking pin is stuck or rusted, tap it gently. The intermedi-

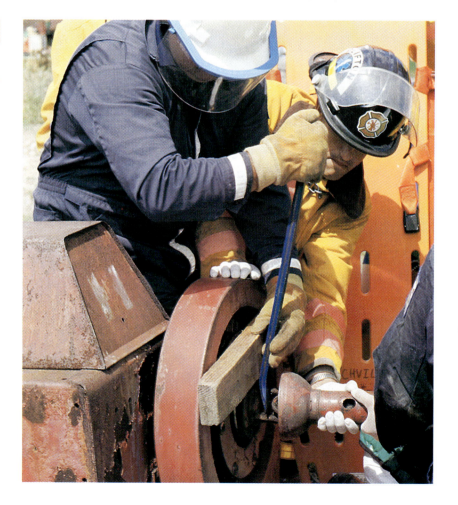

FIGURE 8.10

To free a patient minimally entangled, insert a crowbar in the universal joint and slowly turn the shaft counterclockwise.

ate shaft may be connected to the implement with a C-ring, a large nut, or a shear pin driven through the shaft. Use a snap-ring tool to enlarge the circle of the C-ring and then release it. An appropriately sized wrench can be used to loosen a nut connection, and a hammer and punch should be used to force the shear pin through the shaft. Newer PTO drivelines will have locking pins or collars and splines at both the tractor end and the implement end.

On older tractors, the locking pin and internal/external spline may be rusted and difficult to remove. Place the tip of a crowbar against the front of the tractor output shaft housing and gently apply force against the tractor. Once the PTO is free of the tractor, move the patient and the shaft to allow room to slide the solid shaft out of the hollow shaft, separating them and freeing the patient.

If the PTO cannot be disengaged from the tractor output shaft, try the same procedure at the **implement input shaft**. Disassemble the slip clutch or remove the shear pin to free the PTO.

Disassembling the PTO

If there is no other way to remove the intermediate shaft from the power source or the attached implement, it may have to be disassembled or separated by cutting or shearing. A farm equipment mechanic should be consulted or at the scene before any equipment is disassembled.

Cutting the intermediate shaft and moving the tractor are last resort efforts. If you must cut, cut only the hollow section of the telescoping shaft as far from the patient as possible, using hydraulic shears or a hacksaw. Support both the shaft and the patient securely. Do not use an acetylene torch because the heat of the cutter may cause further injury to the patient. While cutting, remember that the shaft may be under load, and that energy will be released proportional to the size of the shaft. If there is torque in the system, cutting the shaft will cause additional rotation and could cause further injury to the patient or injure the rescuers. Insert a crowbar or pry bar to prevent unwanted rotation. If the two parts will not separate, transport the patient while still entangled in the shaft.

On some tractors, it is possible to remove the driveline shaft from inside the differential housing. If the shaft is removed from the housing, a large amount of fluid may come out with the shaft. If the fluid is hot, it may burn the patient and/or the rescue team.

Disentangling the Extremities or Body

Entanglement of the foot or entire leg can occur if the operator steps onto the drawbar of the tractor. A loose shoelace or pant leg can be caught by the rotating intermediate shaft, wrapping the foot or leg around the shaft two or three times (Figure 8.11). Common injuries include total amputation at the ankle; degloving injuries in which the calf becomes wrapped around the shaft; and deboning injuries in which the

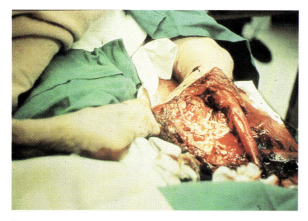 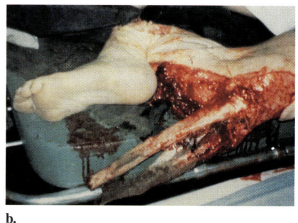

a. b.

FIGURE 8.11

a. and b. An extremity can be wrapped two or three times around the PTO shaft, resulting in amputation, degloving injuries, or deboning injuries.

tibia and fibula are pulled downward and separated from soft tissues. Complete knee dislocations or disarticulations may also occur.

This type of entanglement usually occurs at the forward universal joint where the PTO connects to the tractor. The patient's clothing or tissue usually wraps around the joint, covering the locking pin. In this situation, rescuers will not be able to release the PTO from the tractor. The PTO must be disconnected from the implement end and reverse rotation must be used to unwrap the patient.

If the body becomes entangled, place a long back board or scoop stretcher under the patient, and lift until the patient's body is level with the PTO. This will enable rescuers to work on the PTO without causing further injury to the patient. The patient's body should be supported in this position by cribbing or other members of the rescue team to prevent additional movement. Use a half back board or self-conforming short spine board to stabilize the spine and provide additional lifting support.

AUGERS

The **auger** is an ancient tool that was first applied to agriculture in the late 1940s. Most people are familiar with augers as drills or boring tools. In agriculture, augers apply the screw theory to move material from one point to another and are used as part of complex materials handling systems. Today, augers are found in self-unloading wagons, grain bins, combine grain tanks, feed mixers, and silos. They are used not only on farms, but in grain elevators, food processing plants, and any industry where loose material must be moved.

Portable augers are used to move large quantities of grain, feed, or fertilizer quickly and easily (Figure 8.12). Open augers are often found in grain bins, silos, self-unloading wagons, and combine grain tanks (Figure 8.13). These large open augers are used to level or sweep grain from the center of a structure to the outer edge. Accidents with open augers can occur if an individual slips and falls or tries to kick loose

CHAPTER 8　　Agricultural Equipment　　151

FIGURE 8.12

Portable augers can move large quantities of grain, feed, or fertilizer quickly and easily.

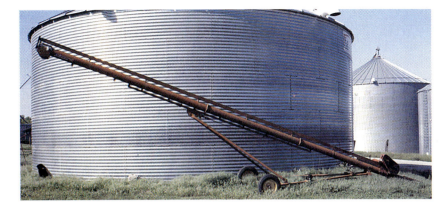

FIGURE 8.13

Open augers, such as this one in a feed mixer, are found in a variety of implements or in storage structures.

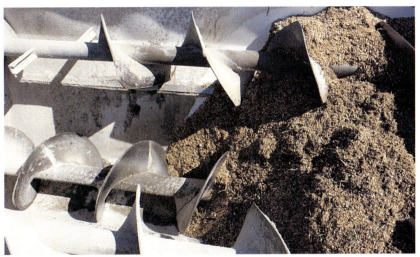

matted grain and loses his or her balance. Per hour of use, the auger is the most dangerous piece of farm equipment.

Portable Auger Entanglement

Portable augers may be 10' to 60' long, and when loaded with grain, they may weigh several thousand pounds. The portable auger has an outer tube to contain the grain, a central shaft wrapped by a spiral of flat spring steel (the **flighting**), a drive mechanism to rotate the central shaft, and a wheeled undercarriage that supports and allows the auger to be moved. At the joining of the undercarriage and the auger, a crank and rachet assembly is used to raise or lower the auger (Figure 8.14a). Rescuers must ensure that this crank and rachet assembly is secured to prevent collapse of the auger.

Material is moved by screw action from the inlet source to the discharge opening of the tube. Usually a rubber V-belt or chain drive connected to an external drive shaft is used to rotate the center shaft (Figure 8.14b). The external drive shaft is connected to a right-angle gearbox that draws power from an electric motor, a small internal combustion engine, or a PTO.

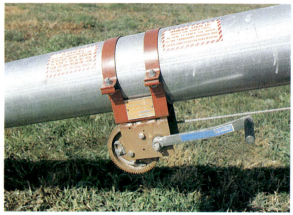
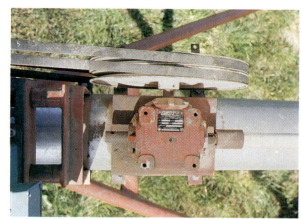

FIGURE 8.14
a. A crank and rachet assembly is used to raise or lower the auger.
b. A rubber V-belt or chain drive connected to an external drive shaft rotates the center shaft. (Note: Safety shield removed for viewing purposes.)

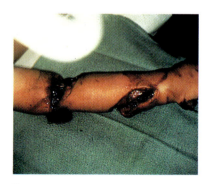
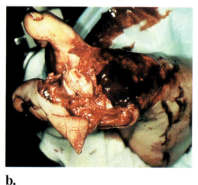
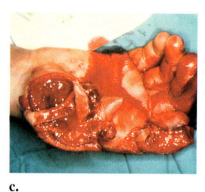

FIGURE 8.15
Most incidents with portable augers involve the hands or feet. The resulting injuries include severe soft tissue lacerations and amputation.

Most incidents with portable augers involve entanglement of the hands or feet, and occur when a piece of loose clothing, glove, tie string, or shoelace is caught in the flighting, or when an operator attempts to free a grain clump and the arm or leg is drawn into the auger (Figure 8.15). Electrical injuries may occur when elevated augers come into contact with overhead power lines.

CHAPTER 8 Agricultural Equipment

Extrication Technique

Securing the Scene.

1. **Establish a safety zone.** As you approach the scene, watch for overhead power lines. If there is potential contact, do not proceed with the rescue. Immediately request that the local utility company turn off the power and provide scene safety assistance. The safety zone should encompass an area of 50' from the equipment in all directions. Plastic barrier tape and light stakes should be used to outline the safety zone.
2. **Escort bystanders out of the safety zone.** Move all bystanders to a safe distance, and provide psychological support to family members, neighbors, and co-workers. Reassure them that you will free the patient without further injury, although extrication may take some time. Remember it is important to keep the family informed throughout the rescue operation.
3. **Shut off power to the auger drive.** Shut off all electric motor switches and disconnect any extension or power cables. Shut off small gasoline engines by grounding the ignition with a shut-off switch or by short-circuiting the spark plug to the cylinder head. Hold a screwdriver blade firmly against the cylinder head, and then touch the screwdriver shaft to the spark plug terminal (Figure 8.16). After the engine stops turning, disconnect the spark plug wire. If the auger is driven by a tractor, shut off the engine and secure the tractor, disengage the PTO, and block the tractor wheels to prevent unwanted movement. Torque may be stored in the system, and if released, could cause additional injury to the patient, or even restart the small combustion engine that powers the auger.
4. **Secure the auger to prevent unwanted movement.** Chock the auger wheels and drive a stake or a long bolt through the draw-

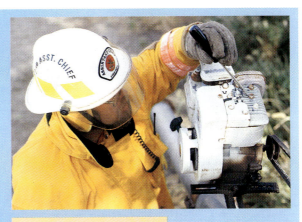

FIGURE 8.16

One way to shut off power to the auger drive is to hold a screwdriver blade against the cylinder head, and then touch the screwdriver shaft to the spark plug terminal. Disconnect the spark plug wire after the engine stops turning.

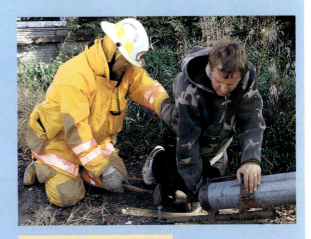

FIGURE 8.17

Chock the auger wheels and drive a stake or long bolt through the drawbar pin hole at the inlet end to prevent the auger from moving during extrication.

bar pin hole located at the inlet end (Figure 8.17). Portable augers are unstable in the raised position, and can easily overturn if there are strong winds or if the ground is sloping. Grain in the upper or discharge section of the tube can overbalance the auger; the stake will prevent this from occurring.

Accessing the Patient. When the incident commander or operation leader signals that it is safe, rescuers should immediately begin assessing the patient.

1. **Conduct a primary assessment.** As soon as you reach the patient, begin the primary assessment. Check the patient's airway, breathing, circulation, and disability (ABCD). In all auger incidents, protect the patient's cervical spine as you establish and maintain an adequate airway.

   Assess breathing effort and lung sounds. If the patient is breathing, administer high-flow oxygen via a nonrebreathing mask. If the patient's respirations are under 10 or over 30 breaths per minute, assist ventilation with a bag-valve-mask device. If the patient is not breathing, use a pocket mask to initiate ventilation. *If within your scope of practice and if according to local protocol*, insert the appropriate airway. Nasal airways should be considered if the patient still has a gag reflex or a possible injury to the cervical spine. Oropharyngeal airways should be used only if injury to the spine has been ruled out (Figure 8.18).

2. **Control external bleeding.** Severe lacerations and/or amputation may have caused considerable blood loss. Be prepared to initiate treatment for hypovolemic shock, because severe blood loss and resultant shock is common in auger accidents. Remember to use universal precautions whenever you may be exposed to bodily fluids.

   Direct pressure to control bleeding is impossible until the rescue team exposes the extremity; therefore, use indirect pressure against the axillary or brachial artery for arm entanglement, or against the femoral or popliteal artery for leg entanglements until you can apply direct pressure.

Table 8.2 illustrates some of the most common injuries that result from entanglement in a portable auger.

TABLE 8.2 Common Injuries Involving Portable Augers

Mechanism of Injury	Result	Typical Injuries
Entanglement in portable augers	Amputation or deep lacerations from auger flighting; electrical burns if auger contacts overhead power lines; crush and shear injuries if auger collapses	**Head injuries** (concussion and/or fracture if auger collapses); **Spinal injuries;** **Chest injuries;** **Abdominal injuries** (evisceration if victim is small and auger is large); **Pelvic injuries** (if victim is small); **Extremity injuries** (amputation of fingers, toes, feet, arms, legs, hands; spaced, deep lacerations; spiral fractures; localized crush injuries); **Electrical injuries**

Minor Entanglement

If there is minimal entanglement, reverse the rotation of the auger flighting to remove the extremity. Insert a crowbar or pry bar in the universal joint and turn the shaft backwards. Or, use a pipe wrench to rotate the shaft backwards. Use extreme caution to prevent additional rotation of the trapped extremity when you rotate the flighting. If the

CHAPTER 8 Agricultural Equipment

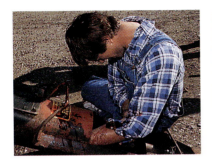

a.

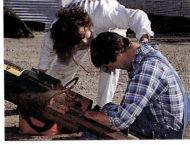

b.

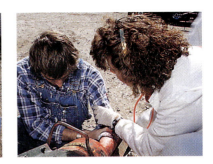

c.

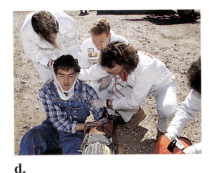

d.

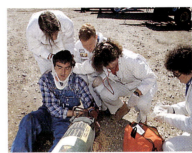

e.

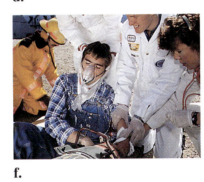

f.

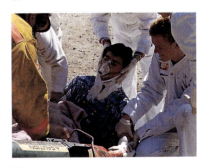

g.

FIGURE 8.18

As soon as you reach the patient (**a**), check the ABCDs (**b, c**). In all auger incidents, protect the patient's cervical spine (**d, e**). If the patient is breathing, administer high-flow oxygen via a nonrebreathing mask (**f, g**).

trapped extremity rotates with the flighting, stop immediately. Even with minor entanglements, the tissue and clothing may be so tightly compressed between the tube and the flighting that reverse rotation will not work.

Use a heavy-duty air chisel to cut open the auger tubing if you cannot reverse the rotation. If the patient is conscious, explain what you are doing. An air chisel creates high levels of noise and vibration, and you do not want to alarm the patient. If an air chisel is not available, a hand chisel may be used, although extrication will take much longer. Shield the patient with a heavy fire-retardant blanket, protect the eyes with safety goggles, and protect the head with a helmet and face shield. All members of the medical team should wear heavy-duty leather gloves, eye protection, and minimum protective gear. Members of the rescue team should wear full bunker gear.

Begin the cut about 90 degrees from where the extremity enters the auger. Cut the auger tubing slowly and carefully lengthwise, well past the full length of the extremity to permit adequate clearance. If bones are fractured, the soft tissue will stretch, increasing the distance of entanglement. The extremity may be wrapped around the center shaft, but this will not be apparent until the auger tubing is open. Continue cutting in a smooth arc toward the trapped extremity. Finish the cut back toward the auger inlet, always remembering to stay well away from the entangled extremity.

Pry or pull the cut section of tubing away to expose the injury. The edges of the cut will be sharp and jagged, but the metal will probably be light enough that you can lift it by hand. If you must use a crowbar, do so carefully to avoid placing any pressure against the trapped extremity. Insert the very tip of the crowbar between the tubing and the cut section and lift, using the edge of the uncut tube as the fulcrum for lifting. If the tubing will not bend, make a complete, U-shaped cut back to the inlet.

Once the extremity is released, locate any amputated or avulsed tissue and prepare for transport. Amputated or avulsed tissue may be caught between the "steps" of the flighting. Auger injuries will usually be grossly contaminated by grain, dust, mold, and other debris. Rinse all parts with normal saline solution or sterile water to decontaminate; wrap the parts in dry, sterile dressings; seal in a plastic bag (do NOT put water, saline solution, or ice in the bag), and keep cool during transport according to local protocols. As the extremity is freed and pressure released, bleeding will increase. Apply direct pressure to control bleeding using universal precautions and treat the patient for shock.

In most portable auger entanglements, the patient will be conscious during both the entanglement and the extrication. The entanglement is not as instantaneous as with a PTO, so the patient fully realizes what is happening, and may be experiencing an autonomic stress reaction. An autonomic stress reaction commonly occurs in association with emotional situations such as fear, bad news, or good news. The patient needs constant reassurance and emotional support throughout the extrication process and during transport.

Open Auger Entanglement

Large-diameter, open augers such as a sweep auger or unloading auger can be found in many agricultural-rural settings, such as in combine grain tanks, silos, and feed mixers. Grain bins and silos are equipped with sweep augers that consist only of open flighting (Figure 8.19). Sweep augers operate on top of the grain or silage to move it to the unloading auger inlet at the center of the structure, and to keep the surface of the material level.

CHAPTER 8 Agricultural Equipment   157

FIGURE 8.19

Grain bins and silos are equipped with sweep augers that consist only of open flighting. The auger rotates around the grain bin or silo to keep the material level.

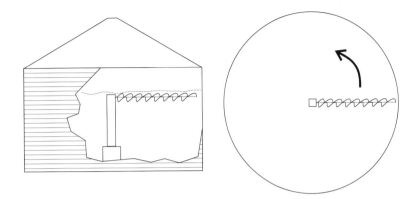

FIGURE 8.20

When the bones fracture after being wrapped around the auger, the tissue may then wrap tightly around the flighting and shaft. Wrapping continues until the extremity is avulsed or until the auger stops.

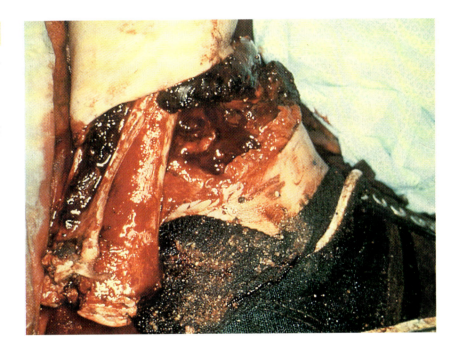

Entanglement in a sweep auger usually occurs when the grain bin or silo is almost completely empty. An individual enters the grain bin to clean while the auger is still operating. Because there is little grain to provide resistance, the auger is spinning faster and sweeping around the silo faster as well. The individual may be caught unaware.

Typically, one or both legs become wrapped around the auger. When the bones fracture, the tissue may wrap tightly around the flighting and shaft, similar to a PTO entanglement (Figure 8.20). Wrapping continues until the extremity is avulsed or until the increased load stops the auger.

Extrication Technique

Entanglement in this type of auger is totally different from entanglement in a portable auger. Grain bins and silos are confined spaces. Always assume that the atmosphere within a grain bin, silo, or other confined space is hazardous until proven otherwise. Wear a self-contained breathing apparatus (SCBA), a safety harness, and a safety line when working in them.

Securing the Scene.
1. **Establish a safety zone.** The safety zone should encompass an area of 50' from the grain bin or silo in all directions. Plastic barrier tape and light stakes should be used to outline the safety zone.
2. **Escort bystanders out of the safety zone.** Move all bystanders to a safe distance, and under no circumstances allow family members, friends, neighbors, or co-workers into the bin or silo. However, remember to keep family members informed throughout the rescue operation.
3. **Shut off and secure the power to the auger before entering the grain bin.** Shut off all electric motors, and if possible, pull all circuit breakers.
4. **Enter the scene as if it were a confined space/hazardous atmosphere rescue.** Because sweep auger entanglement usually occurs when the silo or grain bin is almost empty, the risk of a hazardous atmosphere is lessened. However, rescuers should wear a self-contained breathing apparatus (SCBA) until the area is well ventilated, and the atmosphere is safe for breathing. Rescuers should always wear a safety harness and a safety line when entering a confined space. (See chapter 9 for a complete discussion.)

Disentangling the Patient.
1. **Extricate the patient by reversing the rotation of the auger.** Use a pipe wrench to grasp the auger at one end of the center shaft and turn backwards slowly.
2. **Support the patient on a long spine board to minimize movement.** These patients, if still alive, will have sustained injuries to multiple systems. Spinal injury and head and chest trauma are common. Follow the steps for assessing the patient and controlling bleeding as described for portable auger entanglements. Remember to use universal precautions in all rescue operations.

BALERS

Balers are used to compress hay or other crops into a compact form for easier handling and storage. The small round baler was developed in 1892 and is still used on many smaller farms. It forms hay into round bales weighing 50 lb to 150 lb. The conventional baler forms rectangular bales that weigh between 50 lb and 150 lb. The large round baler was introduced in 1971 and has become very common, in many places replacing the small round and conventional balers (Figure 8.21). A fully formed bale may weigh 800 lb to 1,500 lb, and may be 6' long and 6' in diameter.

Most incidents with conventional balers involve the tying mechanism. If the twine does not feed properly, a hurried operator may try to correct the situation without turning off the machine. As a result, the operator's hand could become entangled in the mechanism (Figure

CHAPTER 8 Agricultural Equipment

8.22). The most common incident with large round balers involves entanglement in the pick-up mechanism as the operator tries to unclog the rollers. If this is attempted while the baler is operating, the roller may catch and pull the operator as well as the hay into the baling chamber when the clog is loosened (Figure 8.23).

Whenever working on an incident involving a baler, clear any loose hay surrounding the baler and tractor to reduce the risk of fire.

FIGURE 8.21 Three popular styles of balers are the closed throat round baler **(a)**, conventional baler **(b)**, and the open throat round baler **(c)**.

a.
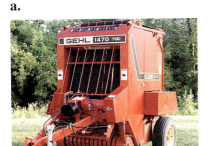

b.
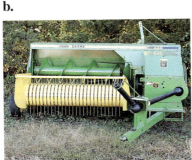

c.
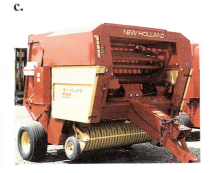

FIGURE 8.22 An operator's hand and arm may become caught in the baler **(a)**, resulting in severe lacerations and amputation **(b)**.

a.
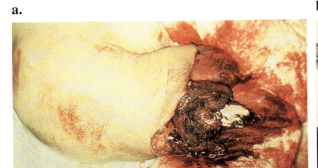

b.
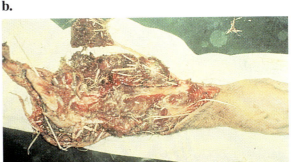

FIGURE 8.23 Injuries to the feet can occur when an operator tries to kick loose clogs in the rollers and becomes entrapped. Heat from the rollers caused extensive tissue damage.

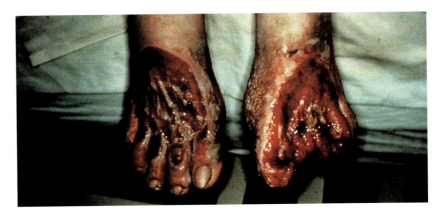

Conventional Balers

In conventional balers, the pick-up mechanism is a drum with spring steel tines or teeth that lift the hay from the **windrow** (row of cut and raked hay) to feed the auger that transports it to the bale chamber. A spring-loaded set of packer fingers holds the hay against the pick-up teeth. Once the hay reaches the chamber, the feeder plunger pushes it to the rear and compacts it into a bale. A feeder plunger head passes the bale chamber opening, and a knife cuts the hay. The bale is then tied with either wire or twine. The twine wraps around the bale and is cut as the bale is ejected. The entire tying operation takes only 3 seconds. Smaller balers may be self-powered or operated by a PTO attached to a tractor.

Types of Entanglement Entanglement in the tying mechanism occurs when the twine does not feed properly, and the operator tries to correct the problem without stopping the baler. Fingers and hands can quickly become entangled in the knotting mechanism, resulting in pinches, lacerations, or hand fractures.

Other mechanisms of injury include entanglement in the PTO, impalement on the pick-up assembly, or entanglement in the feed auger or the compression chamber. Extrication techniques for entanglement in the PTO were discussed earlier in this chapter. Impalement injuries occur when the operator slips to the ground and cannot get out of the way fast enough. The operator may then be caught by the tines of the pick-up mechanism and sustain extensive lacerations and possibly severe puncture wounds.

Entanglement in the compression chamber can be fatal. In this chamber, the hay is shaped to form the rectangular bale. As the shaping process begins, a large knife cuts the hay entering the chamber, and may amputate body parts as well. If the equipment is still running, the operator may also be caught in the compression process as the feeder plunger enters the chamber to squeeze the hay into shape. Disassembling the baler will be necessary to recover body parts. A farm equipment mechanic will be needed to supervise the disassembly process.

Extrication Technique

Extrication from a conventional baler may require disassembly of the equipment; therefore, a farm equipment mechanic should be called to assist with the rescue operation.

Securing the Scene.
1. **Establish a safety zone.**
2. **Escort bystanders out of the safety zone.**
3. **Shut off and secure the power source.** Chock the wheels of the tractor and the baler to prevent unwanted movement. Disconnect the PTO from the tractor to permit reverse movement of most moving components on a conventional baler.

Disentangling the Patient.

1. **With entanglement in the tying mechanism, disassemble the knotting mechanism.** A farm equipment mechanic can disassemble a knotter quickly. If a mechanic is not available, check the baler tool box or twine box to find an operator's manual. Disassembling the tying mechanism is time consuming, but it is not difficult, and close examination of the knotter will make disassembly procedures apparent.
2. **With entanglement in the pick-up mechanism, insert a wedge block between the pick-up assembly and the spring-loaded bar.** This will release the pressure on the patient. Insert the wedge block near the frame of the pick-up assembly, and then chock and crib. Move the wedge block closer to the patient, if necessary, to continue raising the bar, cribbing as you proceed.
3. **With impalement injuries, cut the tines with bolt cutters.** The tines are made of spring steel and are approximately 1/8" in diameter. Do not remove the tines from the patient, as this may cause severe hemorrhaging. Stabilize the tines and provide rapid transport to the emergency department (Figure 8.24).

Table 8.3 illustrates some of the most common injuries that result from entanglements in conventional balers.

TABLE 8.3   Common Injuries Involving Conventional Balers

Mechanism of Injury	Result	Typical Injuries
Entanglement in rectangular baler	Crush injuries Hands and fingers caught in knotting mechanism	High incidence of fatality Severe lacerations; possible amputation
Entanglement in small round baler		

Large Round Balers

The large round baler has a pick-up assembly similar to that of the conventional baler. However, early models have two large steel rollers instead of a spring-loaded bar that compress and feed the hay into the bale chamber. In principle, these rollers operate like those of a wringer washing machine, which presses or squeezes water out of clothing.

The rollers of a large round baler range from 3" to 12" in diameter, and may have either a smooth surface or a textured rubber covering. The rollers may allow for no clearance (closed throat) or as much as 18" (open throat) of clearance between them. Large, heavy springs on the rollers provide the tension needed to compress the hay. The same mechanism is used in hay swathers or hay crimpers. Within the bale chamber, a series of springs and belts shapes the bale.

Types of Entanglement Entanglements occur when the operator tries to remove clogged material while the baler is running. As the plug is freed, and the material drawn into the baler, the operator's hands and

FIGURE 8.24 With impalement injuries (**a**), ensure the wheels of the tractor and the baler are chocked (**b, c**) and support the baler with cribbing (**d**). Do not remove the tines from the patient (**e**). Stablize the tines (**f**) and provide rapid transport after the patient is freed from the machine.

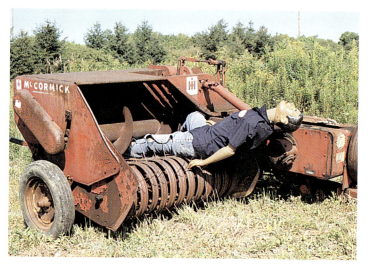
a.

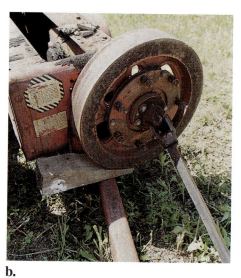
b.

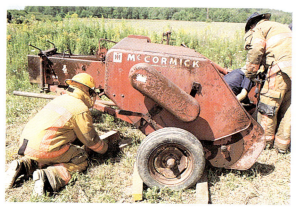
c.

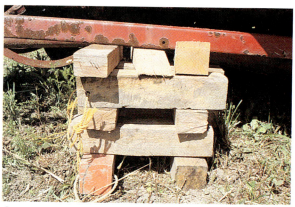
d.

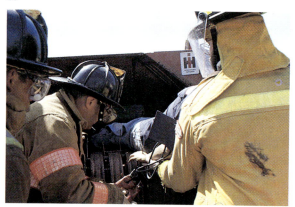
e.

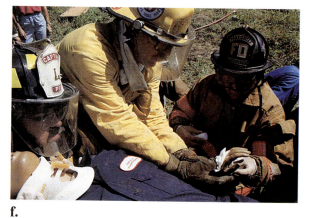
f.

CHAPTER 8   Agricultural Equipment

FIGURE 8.25

Entanglement in a large round baler can occur as the operator tries to remove clogged material from the rollers. As the plug is freed, the operator's hands and feet, or hands and arms may be pulled in along with the straw.

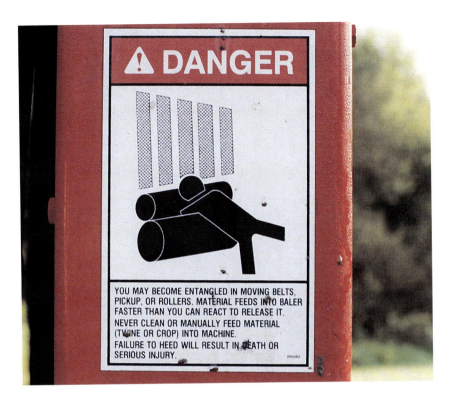

arms, or feet and legs, may also be pulled between the rollers (Figure 8.25). Commonly, the extremity is pulled in until the rollers reach their maximum limit of separation. Large round balers do not have slip clutches, so the rollers will continue to turn until the power is shut off or the tractor runs out of fuel.

Machines running at high speed or those with little clearance between the rollers may avulse the extremity entirely. If the patient is braced against the baler frame to prevent being drawn in further, hyperextension of the head and a collapsed trachea may result.

Entanglement in large round balers usually results in fatal crushing injuries. Advanced life support personnel and a farm equipment mechanic should be dispatched to the scene in all cases.

Extrication Technique

Securing the Scene.

1. **Establish a safety zone.**
2. **Escort bystanders out of the safety zone.**
3. **Shut off and secure all power.** Chock the wheels of both the tractor and the baler to prevent any unwanted movement. Leave the PTO engaged, if the tractor can be prevented from starting. Place two pry bars through the PTO universal joint and secure them with rope to the baler tongue or to the tractor drawbar to prevent rotation of the PTO in either direction.

Disentangling the Patient.

1. **Expose the ends of the rollers by removing the sheet metal shielding.** Block the bottom roller from both the front and the back to prevent it from turning. It may be possible to jam the drive pulley or sprocket at the end of the roll with a large alignment punch or small crowbar.
2. **Insert a long pry bar between the roller shafts.** Using the baler frame as the fulcrum, push the top roller up and insert wedge blocks to maintain the spacing.
3. **Insert a small 6"x 6" high-pressure air bag between the rollers.** Center the bag precisely to prevent the rollers from turning. As the bag inflates, it will increase the separation enough to either remove the extremity or to allow placement of a larger bag. Use wedge blocks to maintain the opening as the air bag inflates.
4. **If wedge blocks or air bags cannot be used, use a 3" wide piece of cargo strapping.** Pass the strapping around the top (movable) roller. Place a large high-pressure air bag on the top of the baler frame above the top roller and fasten the strap over it. Inflate the bag, and the strap will pull up the top roller. As the space between the rollers increases, block with wedges to protect both the patient and the rescuers. Once there is 2" to 3" of space, the extremity can be extricated.
5. **Disassemble the baler as a last resort.** As a last resort, disassembly of the baler may be required to extricate the patient. For this reason, a farm equipment mechanic should be summoned to the scene immediately if the initial scene survey indicates severe entrapment. The mechanic can begin disassembly while the rescue team begins extrication. The rescue team should not attempt this disassembly, unless someone is familiar with the specific equipment.
6. **With entrapment in the bale chamber, cut into the chamber.** In some instances, an operator is pulled completely through the rollers into the bale chamber. If not crushed by the rollers, these individuals will probably suffocate in the chamber before extrication is complete. To access an individual trapped in the bale chamber, rescuers will have to work their way into the chamber by cutting the several long, flat belts that form the bale. The belts are mounted on a spring-loaded arm that moves to accommodate the growing bale. Loosen the spring or secure the arm with a chain, strap, or come-along. This will reduce the pressure on the bale, giving rescuers access to the bale. Use a knife or saw to cut the belts. The design of the bale chamber may mean that the belts will need to be cut several times. As you enter the chamber, remove the hay to access the patient. *Do not reverse the baler to "back" the patient out.*

Table 8.4 illustrates common injuries that result from entanglement in a large round baler.

TABLE 8.4   Common Injuries Involving Large Round Balers

Mechanism of Injury	Result	Typical Injuries
Entanglement in compression rollers of large round baler	Crush injuries	High incidence of fatality
Entanglement in open throat round baler	Crush injuries	Incidence of fatality limited—very few since switch to open throat baler

CHAPTER 8 Agricultural Equipment

COTTON PICKERS

While the cotton picker looks much like a combine, the mechanism for removing the crop from the plant is quite different. A corn combine uses rotating spiral "snapping rolls" to snap the ears off the stalks; the cotton picker uses vertical rotating drums with spindles to remove the cotton bolls. As the drums rotate, the spindles contact the bolls, remove them from the plants, and move them into a cleaning conveyor. After dirt, dust, and trash are separated from the bolls, the bolls are blown into a storage basket mounted on the picker. On some models, a hydraulic ram compresses the cotton in the basket to allow for more capacity.

Entanglement usually occurs in the gathering mechanism. If material clogs the spindles and drums, the drum drive may slip. The operator may try to remove the clog while the picker is running. The drum begins to rotate as soon as the clog is removed, and the operator is drawn into the mechanism. The sharp metal spindles penetrate the extremity and occasionally bore into underlying bone.

Extrication requires the assistance of a farm equipment mechanic; therefore, a mechanic should be dispatched to the scene when the rescue team is summoned. This type of incident should be treated as an impalement, rather than an entanglement. The patient should not be removed from the equipment. A farm equipment mechanic should be called at the same time as the rescue team to supervise the disassembly of the gathering unit. Once the drum is removed, the spindles can be removed from the drum.

Treat the spindles as any impaled object. Do not move or attempt to remove them unless there is upper airway obstruction. Apply direct pressure to stop bleeding using universal precautions, but avoid exerting any force on the spindle itself or on any tissue adjacent to its cutting edge. Use a bulky dressing to stabilize the spindles and provide prompt transport to the emergency department.

TANDEM DISC

The tandem disc is a rolling cutter, which cuts and moves soil and trash in a rolling action (Figure 8.26). Each section has several disc blades,

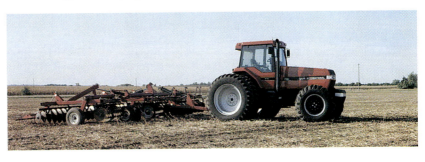

FIGURE 8.26

The tandem disc is a rolling cutter that cuts and moves soil and trash in a rolling action.

FIGURE 8.27

Ensilage cutters used to harvest and process crops are either self-propelled or pulled behind a tractor and powered by a PTO.

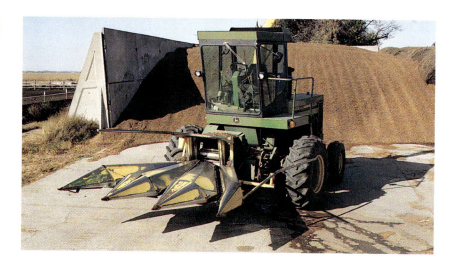

each with its own bearings spaced a fixed distance apart on a common shaft. The tandem disc usually consists of four or more sections. Discs are usually pulled behind the tractor. Although the blades are sharp, few incidents involve discs. However, rescuers should be able to recognize this piece of equipment. A disc connected to an overturned tractor drawbar will alter the tractor's center of gravity, moving it down and closer to the rear.

ENSILAGE CUTTERS

An ensilage cutter is used to harvest and process crops such as corn, sorghum, or hay for storage in a silo (Figure 8.27). Ensilage cutters are either self-propelled or pulled behind a tractor and powered by a PTO. The main parts of the ensilage cutter are the shearing and gathering unit, the feed rolls, the chopping cylinder, the blower, and the discharge chute.

The shearing and gathering unit for row crops looks much like the snapping roll combine header (Figure 8.28a). This unit is usually operated low to the ground, so that it cuts the entire plant off just above ground level, but it may be raised to allow for cleaning or maintenance. There are three types of cutting mechanisms: a short sickle bar with large sections; a horizontally turning star wheel; or a set of two overlapping horizontal cutting discs. Gathering chains, with steel flighting, carry the cut plants to the horizontal feed rolls (Figure 8.28b).

The feed rolls direct the stalks into the rotating chopping cylinder, which is equipped with very sharp knives (Figure 8.28c, d). There the stalks are cut into small pieces, approximately 1/4" to 3/8" long (Figure 8.28e). A series of paddles then throws or "blows" the cut silage through the discharge chute. The chute deposits the material into a wagon pulled behind the unit, or into a truck driven alongside it.

CHAPTER 8 Agricultural Equipment

FIGURE 8.28

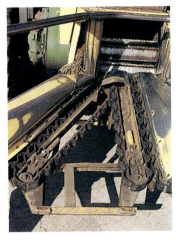

a. The shearing and gathering unit looks much like the snapping roll combine header.
b. Gathering chains, with steel or rubber flighting, carry the cut plants to the horizontal feed rolls.
c. The feed rolls direct the stalks into the rotating chopper cylinder.
d. A view of the shear bar shows how closely the bar bypasses the plate, chopping the stalks into small pieces.
e. The ensilage chopper will process crops or human flesh in much the same way.
f. Injuries may also occur at the cutting mechanism at the very front of the row unit. During operation, the cutting mechanism moves in a scissoring fashion.
(Note: Safety shields removed for viewing purposes.)

a.

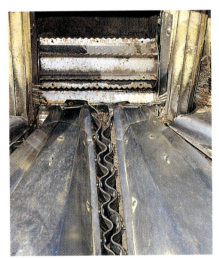

b.

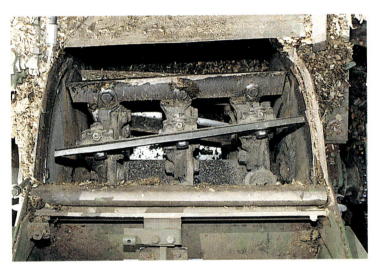

c.

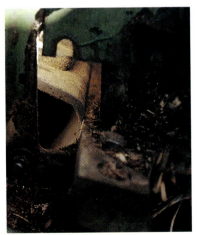

d.

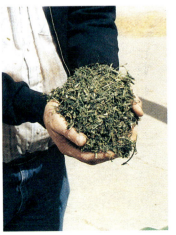

e.

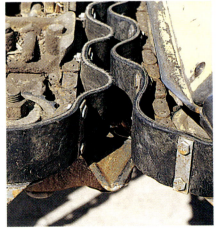

f.

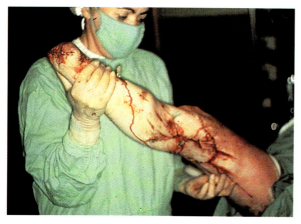
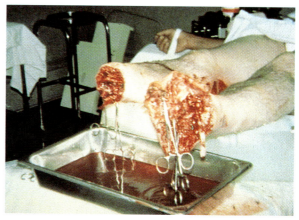

FIGURE 8.29

a. and b. Injuries from the cutting mechanism can result in severe lacerations or amputation of the foot, just above the ankle.

Most incidents involving ensilage cutters occur at the row units. These row units are much more lightweight than those used for corn harvesting. An individual walking too close to the cutter, or wearing loose pants or untied shoes may become entangled in the gathering belts or chains.

Another potential for injuries involves the cutting mechanism, located at the very front of the row unit (Figure 8.28f). These cutters are very sharp and can cleanly amputate a foot, usually just above the ankle (Figure 8.29).

Carelessness in working around the PTO may also result in entanglement. Use the techniques described earlier in this chapter to extricate a patient entangled in the PTO. Injuries may also result if the operator raises the gathering unit to clean under it, but does not adequately secure or support the unit, and the unit falls. These are similar to a combine header collapse, and rescuers should use the extrication techniques presented in chapter 7.

Extrication Technique

Securing the Scene.

1. **Establish a safety zone.**
2. **Escort bystanders out of the safety zone.**
3. **Shut off and secure the power source.** If the cutter is powered by a tractor, shut off and secure the tractor. If the cutter has its own engine, it will be easily identifiable, and the techniques used for securing the tractor engine may be used for the cutter engine.

Disentangling the Patient.

1. **If entanglement involves the row units, insert wedge blocks or high-pressure air bags.** Position the blocks or air bags above the site of entanglement (Figure 8.30).
2. **If entanglement involves the gathering chains or belts, use bolt cutters to cut the belts and release the extremity.**
3. **If entanglement results in amputation, in-**

sert wedge blocks, hydraulic spreader, or high-pressure air bags above the site of the amputation. This will enable rescuers to separate the units and retrieve the amputated part. Since the cut is clean and since there is little "mashing" of tissue, there is more potential for bleeding. A pressure dressing should be applied to the stump, and universal precautions followed.

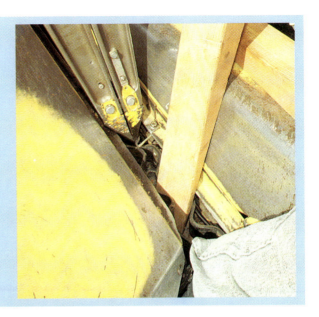

FIGURE 8.30

For entanglement at the row unit, insert wedge blocks or a high-pressure air bag. Place the blocks or air bags above the site of entanglement to force separation of the row unit.

IRRIGATION SYSTEMS

The long pipes of a center pivot irrigation system are a familiar sight in fields, and are supported by a series of triangular, wheeled frames (Figure 8.31a). They are driven by an electric motor or internal combustion engine. The electrical power is typically a three-phase system. There is also a backup ground to the grounding conduction on the electric drive system. These systems have a number of moving parts, including chains and sprockets, V-belts, pulleys, and PTOs for aligning the towers (Figure 8.31b, c).

Individuals may become caught and entangled in these moving parts. Even though the PTO moves slowly, there is still potential for dismemberment or death. Children who use the system as a playground or jungle gym may fall, or be struck by a moving part, caught up in the PTO, or electrocuted if the machine begins running unexpectedly.

The greatest danger from center pivot irrigation systems is electrocution, as some operators try to perform maintenance tasks without turning off the electrical power. Center pivot irrigation systems also act as lightning rods during electrical storms.

Rescuers are usually not trained or equipped to manage electrical hazards. When there are downed power lines or below-ground electrical feeds at the scene, call the utility company first to shut off the power. Remember to establish a safety zone, even larger than 50' in all directions, until the utility company arrives. Because there is no way to tell which way an electrical feed will travel, always assume that any downed power line or any piece of equipment in contact with a power line is energized.

FIGURE 8.31

a. A center pivot irrigation system.
b. A center pivot irrigation system is powered by a PTO that rotates at 54 rpm. Despite its slow rotation, a PTO can entangle an arm in about 10 seconds. Note how tightly the cornstalk is wrapped around the PTO on the right.
c. A well-shielded PTO on a center pivot irrigation system.

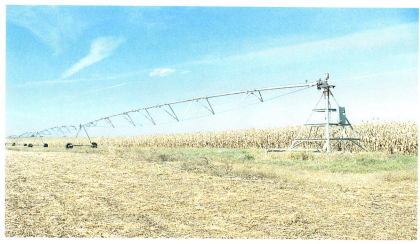
a.

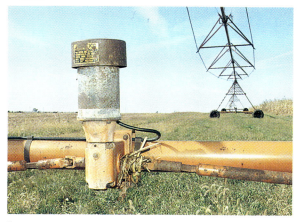
b.

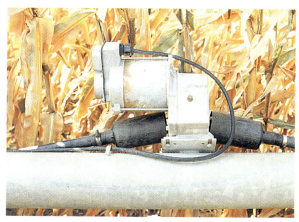
c.

The ground around an electrical incident involving an irrigation system may be wet or muddy. Ordinary fire-fighting gloves and boots do not provide adequate protection against electrocution. Electricity will pass through the body along the path of least resistance and may affect the body organs through which it passes. Injury and illness resulting from electrical shock vary greatly. Burns may be the most obvious injury, though not always readily apparent. Assessment of the patient should be as thorough as possible prior to transport. The extrication technique for entanglement in a PTO is presented earlier in this chapter.

MIXING WAGONS

Mixing wagons are used to blend components such as ground corn, ground alfalfa, and soybean meal into a feed ration. The wagon is a

CHAPTER 8 Agricultural Equipment

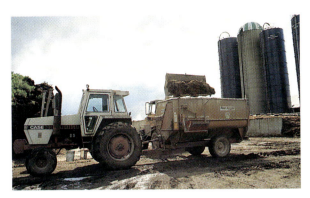

a.

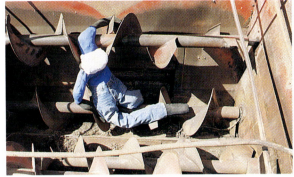

b.

FIGURE 8.32

a. The mixing wagon contains horizontal open augers that stir and blend feed.

b. An operator can become entangled, or trapped between the augers and the wagon side.

strongly constructed box with horizontal open augers that stir and blend the feed (Figure 8.32a). There is very little clearance between individual augers and between the augers and the box walls. Mixing wagons are usually powered by a tractor through a PTO.

Incidents occur when an operator loses balance and falls into the wagon while trying to loosen or kick free clogged material. Because the augers do not have a protective sheathing, the operator can easily become entangled, or trapped between the augers and the wagon side (Figure 8.32b). One or both legs may become entangled, resulting in multiple lacerations and fractures. If the operator falls in head first, the resulting injuries are usually immediately fatal.

Extrication Technique

Securing the Scene.

1. **Establish a safety zone.**
2. **Escort bystanders out of the safety zone.**
3. **Shut off and secure the power source.** Chock the wheels on both the tractor and the wagon to prevent any unwanted movement. Disengage the PTO.

Accessing the Patient.

1. **Lay a heavy rescue blanket, folded several times, on the grain.** This will protect rescuers from the sharp edges of the exposed auger flighting. The grain may have to be removed by bucket and by hand to uncover the patient. The wagon's unload mode cannot be used, as this would start the augers moving and result in further injury to the patient. It may be possible to cut through the side of the wagon at the end farthest from the patient, to empty the grain.

2. **Dismantle the auger housing.** At the end of the auger farthest from the patient, begin dismantling the housing by slowly and carefully unbolting the shaft bearing support. *Do not attempt to reverse the auger to release the patient.* A farm equipment mechanic may need to be called to assist in this operation. If the patient is caught between the side of the wagon and an auger, a hydraulic spreader tool can be used between the auger and the wagon side to provide sufficient clearance to remove the extremity. Or, once the auger is released, lift the shaft by hand or with a hoist only enough to free the patient. If the patient

is caught between two augers, both augers may require disassembly to complete the extrication.
3. **If the auger cannot be dismantled, cut through the auger shaft.** Cut at the end farthest from the patient, where the shaft meets the bearing support. An extrication saw or hydraulic shears will be able to cut through the shaft. Remember that using an extrication saw will produce heat and sparks. Make sure both the patient and the rescuers are wearing appropriate protective gear. Again, if the patient is caught between two augers, you may have to cut through both augers to release the extremity. Ensure that a charged hose is at the site in the event of a fire.

TUB GRINDERS

Tub grinders are specialized tools used primarily at large feedlots, at commercial units, and at sanitary landfills (Figure 8.33a). At feedlots and commercial units, they are used to chop large quantities of hay, including the stems and leaves, into small bits for feeding. At landfills, they are used to grind and compact solid waste. Tub grinders are extremely dangerous tools.

A standard tub grinder is a large, horizontal drum lined with flat metal pieces, or vanes. As the drum rotates, the vanes catch and move the hay into a horizontal hammer mill. The mill is also a rotating drum, lined with dozens of swinging hammers that chops the hay into bits. An open auger moves the hay into a belt elevator that carries it to a truck or feed wagon (Figure 8.33b).

Tub grinders are powered by large diesel engines that can exceed 500 hp. Most can chop a 1,500-lb round hay bale into small pieces in just a few minutes. They can be mounted on a semitrailer for transport from one job site to another, but when in operation, they are stationary.

An individual who climbs to the top of a tub grinder to watch, or who tries to unclog the grinder while it is running may lose his or her

FIGURE 8.33

a. Tub grinders can chop large quantities of hay into small bits for feeding.
b. The open auger on a standard-size tub grinder moves feed into a belt elevator that carries it to a truck or feed wagon.

a.
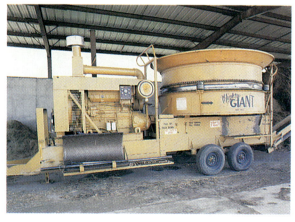

b.
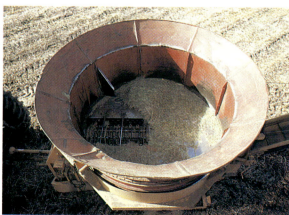

balance and fall in. In less time than a bystander can turn off the engine, the individual may be totally ground up, or suffer severe lower extremity amputation.

If summoned to an incident involving a tub grinder, immediately request on-scene support from a qualified physician. If the patient is alive and severely entangled, on-scene amputation may be the most expeditious method of extrication. Tub grinders may be on a platform, and the top of the grinder may be 10' to 12' above the ground. When the rescue team arrives, they must secure the scene, shut off and secure the engine, and chock the wheels of the grinder so it does not move. Because of the height of the grinder, this should be treated as a high-angle rescue, with two teams—one inside to extricate the patient, the other outside to lift and lower the patient to transport.

SUGAR BEET HARVESTERS/POTATO DIGGERS

Sugar beet harvesters lift the beets from the ground and then transport them on an open chain belt to a holding bin or transport vehicle. Potato diggers operate in the same way (Figure 8.34). Compression-type injuries where a body part, usually the foot, is trapped between rolls are most common. Incidents involving these machines are usually not fatal.

Extrication usually involves opening the machine part so that the body part can be released. Air bags and/or wedges can be inserted in an attempt to separate the rolls. If this is unsuccessful, the equipment will need to be disassembled.

FIGURE 8.34

Sugar beet harvesters (**a**) and potato diggers (**b**) lift the crops from the ground and then move them to a transport vehicle via an open chain belt.

MANURE SPREADERS

Manure spreaders are used to transport livestock manure, usually mixed with bedding (straw) to fields, and then to spread it on the ground as fertilizer. Modern machines are powered with a PTO. The manure is

a.

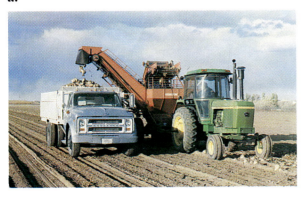

b.

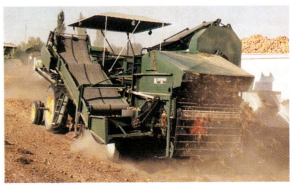

moved by either a movable floor or chain-driven bars to the rear of the box, where rotary beaters break up and disperse the material. Self-unloading wagons and gravity-flow wagons operate using the same principles. Potential injuries from this machine include driveline entanglement and being caught or ejected by the beater/spreader mechanism. Beaters/spreaders can be shafts with long steel teeth or drums with serrated, spiral metal flighting (Figure 8.35).

Injuries usually include extensive soft tissue trauma and possible closed and open fractures (Figure 8.36). The nature of the material handled by manure spreaders creates optimal conditions for massive bacterial infection of any open wounds. All open wounds should be rinsed with sterile saline solution or sterile water before bandages or dressings are applied. Entanglement in the beater/spreader mechanism is usually fatal, unless the PTO is shut off immediately.

Table 8.5 illustrates some of the most common injuries that result from incidents involving miscellaneous agricultural equipment.

FIGURE 8.35

Manure spreaders are equipped with beaters/spreaders that have long steel teeth or drums with serrated, spiral metal flighting.

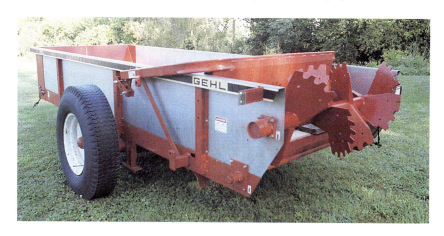

FIGURE 8.36

a. and b. Injuries usually include extensive soft tissue trauma and possible closed or open fractures.

a.

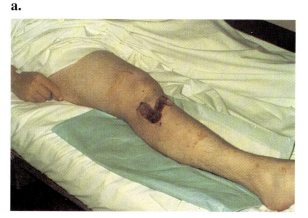

b.

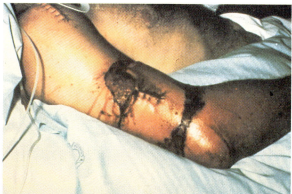

TABLE 8.5 Common Injuries Involving Other Equipment

Mechanism of Injury	Result	Typical Injuries
Falls into tub grinder	Massive blunt trauma to body	High incidence of fatality
Entanglement in ensilage cutter	Amputation of extremities	Traumatic amputation Open fractures
Entanglement in potato digger	Shear injuries	Traumatic amputation Fractures
Entanglement in sugar beet harvester	Shear injuries	Traumatic amputation Fractures
Entanglement in cotton picker	Amputation; puncture wounds	Traumatic amputation Fractures
Entanglement in drive belts and chains of any equipment	Local compression injuries	Traumatic amputation Fractures Degloving injuries

SUMMARY

The use of heavy equipment on farms has greatly increased the possibility of incidents resulting in injuries. Rescuers must be able to identify the type of equipment involved, and know the potential for injury, so that appropriate precautions may be taken before proceeding safely with a rescue.

Augers, a basic tool, are used in several ways: as a part of another implement (such as the open augers found in mixing wagons), or as a free-standing unit (such as a grain auger used to load a silo). Other agricultural implements include various kinds of PTOs, balers, blowers, choppers, cutters, grinders, loaders, mixers, pickers, and shredders. Irrigation systems are a primary source of electrical injuries.

Newer equipment is usually marked with standard safety symbols, which must be obeyed for a safe rescue. However, since many agricultural implements have a long life, incidents often involve older equipment that does not have safety features or markings. Rescuers must be aware of the potential dangers involved with this equipment as well.

CHAPTER 9

Grain and Silage Storage Facility Rescues

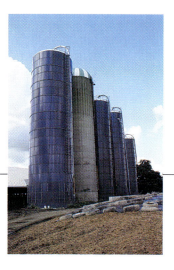

CHAPTER OUTLINE

Overview
Objectives
Special Considerations
Preincident Planning
Hazards in Confined Spaces
   Atmospheric Hazards
   Physical Hazards
   Psychological Hazards

Flowing Grain Entrapment
   Extrication Technique
Silos
   Extrication Technique
   Silo Fires
Liquid Manure Storage
Summary

KEY TERMS

Confined space: any space not intended for continuous occupancy, with limited or no ventilation, and limited entrance and exit.

IDLH: immediately dangerous to life and health.

Lockout: a process by which all power sources are shut off and secured.

Lower explosive limit (LEL): the point at which a gas mixes with just the proper amount of oxygen to burn.

CHAPTER 9 Grain and Silage Storage Facility Rescues

Maillard reaction: chemical reaction responsible for silo fires.

Silo gas: nitrogen dioxide that tends to collect at the surface of silage and flows down the silo chute to low areas around the base of the silo. The gas may appear yellow or reddish-brown.

Venturi effect: increased volume of air created by a pressurized air stream.

OVERVIEW

Grain and silage storage facility rescues are classified as confined space situations. Working in these tight quarters is difficult, unnatural, and dangerous. Suffocation, entrapment, exposure to harmful gases, and fires are just some of the hazards associated with confined space rescue operations. Confined spaces are one of the most hazardous environments rescuers encounter.

This chapter defines and describes confined spaces in agricultural-rural settings and illustrates the atmospheric, physical, and psychological hazards commonly associated with confined spaces. The chapter also explains how to manage potentially hazardous conditions in grain and silage storage facility rescues.

OBJECTIVES

After reading this chapter, the rescuer should be able to:

- describe a confined space situation in an agricultural-rural setting.
- list conditions that determine whether a confined space is safe to enter.
- describe a plan for conducting a confined space rescue.
- describe the atmospheric, physical, and psychological hazards in a confined space rescue.
- describe a safe ventilation system and when and how to use one.
- discuss how to prevent physical injuries and hazards during a grain or silage storage facility rescue.
- discuss how to avoid potential psychological anxieties by training and experience.

SPECIAL CONSIDERATIONS

A **confined space** is defined as any space not intended for continuous occupancy, with limited or no ventilation, and limited entrance and exit. In agricultural-rural areas, confined spaces include grain bins, storage tanks, silos, manure pits, and well pits. Many of these areas are not small in size, but they do have limited ventilation and limited entrance and exit. For example, a large grain elevator is considered a confined space. Even though many people could comfortably fit within its walls, a grain elevator or large fruit/vegetable storage facility is not intended for continuous occupancy. It has little, if any, natural ventilation and is difficult to enter or exit. The contents of a grain elevator also have the potential for engulfing the rescuer or the patient.

A major risk associated with grain and silage storage facility rescues is that the space or the surface area may look safe. Even experienced rescuers can develop tunnel vision. They may commit themselves to the dangers of the confined space without using protective gear, thus making themselves potential victims. The situation may be compounded when other rescuers attempt to save team members and become victims themselves. As many as 40% to 60% of confined space fatalities are would-be rescuers. Confined space entry and patient stabilization must be attempted only with the proper equipment, after the appropriate training, and after the environment has been made as safe as possible.

Never enter any confined space unless it has been determined absolutely safe for entry.

PREINCIDENT PLANNING

Confined space rescue involves extraordinary hazards. Specific decisions about a rescue operation are made based on the characteristics of the confined space. A preincident plan detailing potential hazards, mapping the area, and listing qualified response team resources can save time and lives. The final preincident plan should include the following considerations:

1. Gather as much information about the situation and the condition of the patient as possible. Locate responsible and knowledgeable resources for advice.
2. Ensure that an adequate number of trained rescuers and sufficient equipment have been requested, including special rescue teams, air supply and lighting trucks, and special drilling, forcible entry, or hazardous materials units.
3. Establish a clearly defined incident command network. Establish a safety zone. Clear the entrance and exit areas of everyone except essential personnel. Move all bystanders out of the safety zone.

4. Analyze the immediate environment of the confined space using gas detectors, if available, and information from knowledgeable people. If there is a flammable product in the area, find out the limits of its flammable range.
5. Begin a lockout procedure to reduce all hazardous conditions as much as possible. The term **lockout** means to shut off and secure all power sources. First, identify all sources of power, including electrical switches, hydraulic, steam, or pneumatic valves, and PTOs from external machines. Shut off, secure, and control these power sources to prevent their reactivation. No one should enter the area or have access to the controls of any power source unless the individual is part of the rescue team and in direct contact with the incident commander. When possible, use employees in large facilities to assist in identifying and securing all related power sources, and post a guard. Cap or close all product transport devices and valves. Disable all electric or hydraulically powered machinery within the confined space. Disconnect all steam or air-operated equipment.
6. Begin ventilation as soon as possible and eliminate any possible source of ignition if the atmosphere is determined to be **immediately dangerous to life and health (IDLH).**

    Do not enter an IDLH environment.

    Rescuers who enter this type of environment without the proper training and equipment place themselves in great danger of becoming victims.
7. Wear a self-contained breathing apparatus (SCBA) if the atmosphere is considered IDLH. All rescuers who enter a confined space must wear safety harnesses and safety lines. Use the "buddy" rescuer system in which line handlers control the safety lines of those who enter the environment. Also ensure that a system of signals via the safety line is agreed upon and understood before entering an IDLH environment. (**Note:** In underground pits and other confined spaces, conventional radio equipment may not work; therefore, a hard wire system such as field phones may need to be used, or a system of signals via the safety line.) Place rescuers with charged hoses at strategic positions. When there is no threat of fire or exposure to hazardous materials, minimum protective clothing, such as heavy coveralls, a helmet with a face shield, goggles, and gloves may be used.
8. Choose the best trained and most experienced rescuers for the operation. However, the most experienced rescuer at the incident should function as the safety backup. The safety backup is responsible for rescuing rescuers and should be fully equipped to enter the confined space, if necessary. Also, keep another rescue team in reserve, ready to enter at a moment's notice.

HAZARDS IN CONFINED SPACES

There are three types of hazards in confined spaces. Atmospheric hazards are determined by the shape and configuration of the area, the degree of ventilation, and the presence of hazardous gases. Physical hazards include the presence of or potential for fire, the accumulation of hazardous materials, mechanical entrapment, electrical exposure, or product engulfment. Psychological hazards are fears or anxieties that may profoundly affect rescuer performance and the outcome of the rescue.

Atmospheric Hazards

Atmospheric conditions hazardous to rescuers are those that present an unbreathable atmosphere. Air contains approximately 21% oxygen, 78% nitrogen, and 1% other gases. Humans cannot function normally in an atmosphere much outside of these levels. Of primary concern is the oxygen content. Any confined space that falls under 19.5% oxygen content must be considered IDLH. In areas of the country where alfalfa is ground and stored for making commercial feed, the storage structure will be flooded with nitrogen to preserve the original green color of the alfalfa. This reduces the oxygen content to approximately 1%, resulting in an IDLH environment.

Anyone who enters an oxygen-poor atmosphere may not immediately notice the effects on the body, particularly when concentrating on a rescue. The effects of hypoxia (low oxygen) vary (Table 9.1). But typically, the person becomes excited, agitated, or develops symptoms of intoxication. The person may rush to escape the area, which only increases the demand for oxygen. There are reported instances of people just sitting down and laughing. Disorientation, weakness, and lethargy prevent self-rescue from this type of situation.

TABLE 9.1   Effects of Reduced Oxygen on Humans

Percent of Oxygen in Air	Signs and Symptoms of Hypoxia
21%	None; normal concentration
17%	Increased respiratory rate/effort Some impaired muscular coordination (mild ataxia)
12%	Headache; dizziness (severe ataxia); fatigue
9%	Unconsciousness
6%	Respiratory/cardiac failure Death within minutes

CHAPTER 9   Grain and Silage Storage Facility Rescues

It is the lack of both adequate ventilation and inflow of sufficient fresh air that makes confined spaces so dangerous. In addition, a number of gases produced in agriculture can have a deadly effect on those working in these environments. While these gases are part of our daily environment and cause no harm at naturally occurring concentrations, they become hazardous when they are allowed to accumulate in confined areas.

In addition, oxygen can be consumed by many sources. In some settings, natural rotting vegetation consumes oxygen. Rodents or other animals may consume additional oxygen. In most incidents, however, methane, hydrogen sulfide, or other gases produced by decaying matter displace the oxygen and can cause death by suffocation.

Oxygen can also be removed by certain chemical reactions, such as the ensiling process, wet grain fermentation, or production of hydrogen sulfide from manure pits. Toxic gases are also a threat in confined spaces. Hydrogen sulfide, for example, is an extremely toxic gas that is heavier than air. It can displace oxygen as it rests in the low spaces of certain confined spaces. Hydrogen sulfide is more of a problem when there is agitation of effluents, such as in a liquid manure storage pit. This gas must be avoided as it can be fatal if even small amounts are inhaled.

Agricultural Gases Grain bins, silos, and elevators where the atmosphere is highly saturated with grain dust or flammable gases must be treated in the same way as vessels with flammable vapors. The dust to air mixture can easily be in the explosive range. A single spark can have catastrophic results. Table 9.2 shows some of the most dangerous gases present in confined spaces.

Carbon dioxide. The most common gas produced in confined spaces on farms is carbon dioxide, a waste product of human and animal respiration. It is colorless, odorless, and slightly heavier than air. Any confined space containing organic material may develop high concentrations of carbon dioxide, especially spaces below ground level. The pump for most household water systems on farms is in a well pit, 6' to 8' deep, lined with brick or cement, and equipped with a concrete cap and access opening. Since the lining is not gas tight and adequate ventilation is not present, carbon dioxide from oxidation from organic materials in the soil around the pit will displace the air over a period of time. If a rescuer enters the pit without proper ventilation, he or she may lose consciousness before realizing there is a problem.

Carbon dioxide is also produced by crops in storage. Corn, milo, and other grains give off carbon dioxide in amounts directly proportional to their moisture content. Wet grain respires greater amounts of carbon dioxide than dry grain. Once all of the oxygen is used, this process

TABLE 9.2 Gases Present in Agricultural Confined Spaces

Gas	Health Effects		Maximum Exposure Levels*		Physical Properties			Flammable Properties
	Acute	Long Term	Immediate Threat	Short Term Exposure	Density	Color	Odor	
Carbon Monoxide	Asphyxiant		1,500	400	Lighter than air	None	None	Flammable between 12.5% and 7.4% by volume of air mixture
Carbon Dioxide	Asphyxiant		50,000	15,000	Heavier than air	None	None	Nonflammable
Nitrogen Dioxide	Respiratory irritant	Permanent lung damage	50	No standards	Heavier than air	Reddish-brown	Strong, pungent	Nonflammable, but will support combustion
Nitric Oxide	Asphyxiant		100	35	Heavier than air	None	Strong, pungent	Nonflammable, but will support combustion
Nitrogen Tetroxide	Respiratory irritant	Permanent lung damage	50	No standards	Heavier than air	Yellow	Strong, pungent	Nonflammable, but will support combustion
Ammonia	Alkali burns	Permanent lung damage	500	35	Lighter than air	None	Strong pungent	Combustible, but difficult to burn
Methane	Asphyxiant		No standards	No standards	Lighter than air	None	None	Highly flammable 2% to 15% by volume
Hydrogen Sulfide	Asphyxiant Pulmonary irritant Coma Convulsions	Eye irritant Lung irritant	300	10	Heavier than air	None	Rotten eggs	Flammable between 4% and 44% by volume of air mixture

*Numbers represent parts of gas permissible per million parts of air; short term exposure is defined as 15 minutes, with a maximum of four exposures per 8-hour day, with 60-minute intervals between exposures.

stops. Additionally, fruits and tuber crops such as apples and potatoes also respire. To prevent spoilage of these crops, carbon dioxide is pumped into the storage facilities where these crops are kept.

Molasses tanks commonly found on feedlots and farms can also contain lethal quantities of carbon dioxide. Molasses is added to feed to make the feed more palatable to livestock. Warm days can heat the tank and cause increased bacterial action on the sugars, resulting in production of large quantities of carbon dioxide.

Carbon monoxide. Carbon monoxide, a toxic, colorless, odorless gas that is lighter than air, forms when carbon is only partially oxidized. It is commonly found in livestock housing facilities heated by propane or natural gas. The high dust levels and caustic gases present in the housing affect the heating units and cause uneven combustion of fuel. As a result, carbon monoxide is produced.

Carbon monoxide is a reducing agent, which means that it removes oxygen from many compounds. If you breathe air containing as little as 0.1% carbon monoxide by volume, the carbon monoxide will replace oxygen on the hemoglobin, which may lead to fatal oxygen starvation throughout the body.

Nitrogen dioxide. Nitrogen dioxide is produced by green crops when they are stored as silage. Shortly after crops are placed in a silo, a natural chemical fermentation process occurs. Corn, sorghum, and hay all contain nitrogen, which combines with oxygen to form nitrogen dioxide. This gas is so common in rural areas that it is called **silo gas**. It is produced for 2 or 3 weeks after the crops have been stored. The greatest production, especially with corn, occurs 1 to 3 days after storage.

Nitrogen dioxide is heavier than air and tends to collect at the surface of the silage and to flow down the silo chute into adjoining feed rooms or other low areas around the base of the silo. It may take the form of a yellow or pale orange vapor with a slight ammonia odor. It does not dissipate easily, and remains a potential hazard when the silo is opened for unloading.

Nitrogen dioxide presents an unusual hazard because it may not have an immediate effect on an individual. When combined with oxygen and moisture, nitrogen dioxide readily forms nitric acid, which often appears as a reddish-brown stain on concrete silos. Nitric acid causes severe irritation of the upper respiratory tract and may lead to pulmonary edema. There may be little immediate pain or discomfort, and other symptoms may not appear for days or weeks. Frequently a relapse, with symptoms similar to pneumonia, occurs 1 to 2 weeks after initial recovery. Therefore, it is very important that individuals who have been exposed to silo gas seek immediate medical attention.

Nitric oxide. Nitric oxide is a nonflammable gas that accelerates burning of combustible materials. It reacts with water to form nitric acid, which attacks respiratory tract tissues. If ammonia is also present, nitric oxide will react rapidly, and will also attack metals. The route of poisoning is by inhalation and/or skin or eye contact.

Nitrogen tetroxide. Nitrogen tetroxide is very similar to nitrogen dioxide in properties, reactivity (more reactive than nitrogen dioxide), and effects on humans. It is heavier than both carbon dioxide and nitrogen dioxide, so it will be found at the lowest points in any confined space. The route of poisoning is by inhalation, skin or eye contact, or ingestion.

Methane. Methane is a highly flammable, nontoxic gas that is another by-product of the silage fermentation process. It is also formed by bacterial action in manure storage areas. A single spark near a pocket of methane gas can cause an explosion. Methane is difficult to detect because it is odorless, but in concentrations above 5%, it can cause asphyxiation and explosions. Rescuers should assume that methane is present in all manure storage areas.

Hydrogen sulfide. Hydrogen sulfide is a very poisonous gas, and is considered the most dangerous by-product of manure decomposition. It is extremely corrosive and can paralyze the respiratory system at even small concentrations (500 parts per million). At concentrations of 1,000 parts per million, hydrogen sulfide can kill with a single breath. Hydrogen sulfide has a distinctive "rotten egg" odor, but because this gas deadens the sense of smell, the odor will seem to disappear after the first whiff. Hydrogen sulfide is heavier than air, and usually settles in low areas of the storage facility. High concentrations may remain even after ventilation. It is most prevalent in liquid manure storage pits after the pit has been pumped out. Hydrogen sulfide is released from the liquid when the contents of the pit are stirred or agitated.

Ammonia. Ammonia is a strong alkali that smells like common household bleach. It can be found in areas where there is a high concentration of manure, such as feedlots and poultry facilities. In small concentrations, ammonia can severely irritate the respiratory system; in high concentrations, it can be fatal.

Combating Atmospheric Hazards The best way to reduce hazardous atmospheric conditions in confined spaces is with thorough ventilation of the structure. This can often be done by using the ventilation system built into the structure. Ensure that the patient will not be injured when the ventilation system is started. One reliable and easy-to-use ventilation system is the smoke ejector found on most fire trucks. It will usually discharge between 5,000 and 10,000 cubic feet of air per minute (Figure 9.1). Always blow fresh air into the confined space. When blowing with forced air ventilation, always ensure that the air source is not polluted by the exhaust of a truck or other source.

Another type of ventilation is positive pressure ventilation in which fans are set up several feet from the entrance of the confined space. This technique increases ventilation because of the **venturi effect**, the increased volume of air created by a pressurized air stream. Also attempt to cross-ventilate the structure through doors or makeshift portals. Or use fans to blow fresh air in with the same number of fans on the opposite side to pull air out.

When making ventilation decisions, consider the content of flammable gases and liquids in a confined space. Flammable gases must have a specific mixture of gas and air to burn (flammable range). **The lower**

CHAPTER 9   Grain and Silage Storage Facility Rescues   185

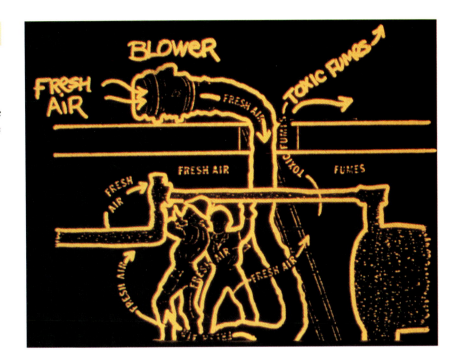

FIGURE 9.1

A smoke ejector can be used to ventilate a confined space. The air should always be blown into the confined space and never be drawn out of the space.

explosive limit (LEL) is the point at which a gas mixes with just the proper amount of oxygen to burn (Table 9.3). This is similar to the concept of a carburetor mixing the proper amounts of gasoline and air. If the confined space has too much gas compared to the air (too rich), an explosion or fire cannot take place. But once ventilation is begun, and the air-gas mixture falls and approaches the upper explosive limit, an explosion is possible.

This could also happen in a confined space incident when air is inducted into a flammable liquid storage tank via a hose stream used to reduce sparks from a circular saw used in the extrication. The venturi effect created might allow the air-gas mixture to approach the flammable range and be ignited by the sparks from the saw. The safest way to ventilate under these circumstances would be to breach the integrity of the tank wall by some other means, for example, a hydraulic spreader, cutter, or heavy air chisel.

The only alternative to ventilating a too-rich, flammable atmosphere is to enter the confined space with the proper breathing apparatus and protective clothing. Rescuers entering this type of a space add oxygen to the atmosphere, which may alter the mixture enough to make it explosive. Therefore, in this situation, extreme caution must be used when entering the confined space.

It may be possible to test the atmosphere with an acceptable testing device. The most important readings indicate a potential IDLH atmosphere: abnormal oxygen content and the presence of toxic and/or flam-

TABLE 9.3   Lower Explosive Limit

	Percent by Volume in Air Lower Limit-Upper Limit
Liquids	
Kerosene	0.7—5.0
Petroleum ether	0.1—5.9
Benzene	1.3—7.1
Gasoline	1.4—7.6
Liquified Gases	
Butylene (Butene)	1.65—9.95
Butane	1.86—8.41
Propylene	2.0—11.1
Butadiene	2.0—11.5
Propane	2.12—9.35
Gases	
Cyclopropane	2.4—10.4
Acetylene	2.5—81.0
Ethane	3.0—12.5
Methane (natural gas)	5.0—15.0
Hydrogen	4.0—74.2

The lower explosive limit (LEL) is the point at which a gas mixes with the proper amount of oxygen to burn. Adapted from *Combustion Flame and Explosion of Gases*, B. Lewis and G. von Elbe, Academic Press (1951).

mable gases and vapors. There are many different units available, and unfortunately, no two detectors operate in the same manner (Figure 9.2). More importantly, a gas detector that is being used by someone only marginally competent in its use can be a greater hazard than a help. A rescue team may develop a false sense of security if the person using the detector takes an improper reading.

The single best source of information regarding the proper use of a particular gas detector is the manufacturer. Insist on training time with the manufacturer before purchasing a new gas detector.

As stated earlier, entry into a confined space containing toxic gases or insufficient oxygen is one of the most hazardous situations rescuers encounter. Therefore, rescuers must be properly equipped and trained and must have practiced rescue procedures before considering entry into a confined space.

Each rescuer entering a confined space must wear a self-contained breathing apparatus (SCBA) unless he or she is absolutely certain that the atmosphere inside is breathable. Rescuers must also wear basic protective clothing such as gloves, eye protection, and appropriate head protection if possible. All rescuers entering the space must also wear a full safety harness and safety line. If the atmosphere is toxic, level A protection (maximum skin and respiratory protection) should also be worn.

Physical Hazards

Among the numerous physical hazards of confined spaces are the potential for entrapment, electrocution, drowning, fall-related injuries, crush injuries, or impalement on sharp objects. Locate and secure any mechanical, electrical, or product transfer device that could endanger the patient or the rescuers.

Combating Physical Hazards Locate the person or persons responsible for the structure. At a feedlot, this may be a manager or maintenance supervisor. The incident commander must establish direct communication with these individuals, and keep them close at hand throughout the rescue operation.

Locate and secure all electrical and mechanical devices in the confined space. This will require locking electrical boxes and posting a guard to ensure that someone does not inadvertently turn on a switch. Remove or block off any product lines, including chemical, steam, and water lines. Secure other apparatus affecting the confined space.

Under extreme circumstances, such as a very hazardous environment with the potential for explosion or when hazardous material exposure is possible, the time the rescuer spends in the confined space should be short. The rescuer should take all the previously mentioned precautions and make a very rapid access to the patient. Once access is gained, a hasty connection can be made to the patient by the wristlet method (Figure 9.3), if the exit is no more than 200' away, if there are no obstructions, and if the patient is not trapped in grain. This method involves carrying a 10' to 15' loop of nylon webbing and attaching it to the patient's wrists using a girth hitch. This will enable a quick retreat by the rescuer, while the patient is dragged out by rope.

FIGURE 9.2

a. A properly used gas detector will indicate if the atmosphere of the confined space is hazardous.

b. Lower the gas detector into the confined space to obtain the reading.

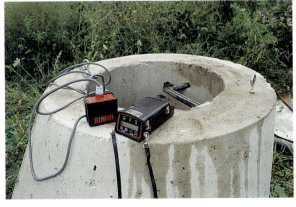

a.

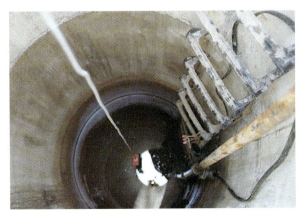

b.

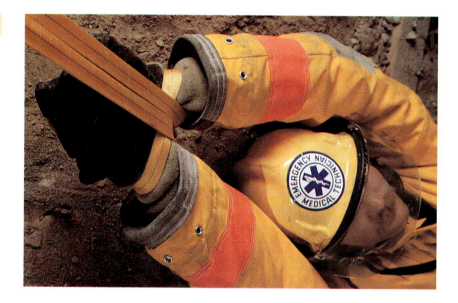

FIGURE 9.3

The wristlet method is one technique for quickly removing a patient from a confined space.

Of all the considerations required when making personnel decisions for confined space entry, the single most important factor is the level of training and experience. Qualified rescuers should have spent many hours training in confined locations so they are familiar with and able to handle the physical and psychological hazards present, and have the medical expertise necessary to assess and stabilize the patient.

While any rescuer entering a confined space must be well trained and experienced, the most experienced rescuer at the incident should function as the safety backup. The safety backup is responsible for rescuing rescuers. He or she should be fully equipped to a minimum of level B (some skin protection and excellent respiratory protection) plus safety harness and safety line and be ready to enter at any sign that a rescuer is having difficulty. Safety line handlers do not enter the confined space as do safety backups, but they must be physically capable of supporting the rescuer inside and removing him or her if necessary. One handler per safety line is usually inadequate for removing a rescuer in trouble.

Psychological Hazards

Perhaps the most challenging aspect of confined space rescue involves the psychological stress generated by the many potential hazards. Rescuers may experience a high level of anxiety when entering a tight enclosure under emergency conditions with limited escape options, especially in the presence of electrical hazards, hazardous materials, and a toxic atmosphere. Training and experience can prepare rescuers to assist those that have been injured or disabled in confined spaces.

One of the most significant psychological hazards for rescuers entering a confined space is anxiety produced by wearing an SCBA. All SCBAs have breathing resistance unless they are set to full flow. As the rescuer inhales, he or she must produce enough negative pressure in the mask and hose to activate the regulator diaphragm. The partial vacuum is readily sensed by the rescuer, which may produce anxiety and increased respirations. Hyperventilation may even develop. Setting the unit to bypass of full flow may also increase anxiety since the noise of the rushing air is very loud. Concern about "using up" the air supply adds to the problem. Some rescuers become claustrophobic from just wearing the SCBA in addition to their protective clothing and gear. Frequent training, including physical activity while wearing the SCBA, is absolutely necessary to combat anxiety.

Combating Psychological Hazards Every person has some anxiety when entering a confined space. This anxiety is a normal and natural part of the self-preservation instinct. The way to control anxiety in a confined space is to train under realistic conditions with a qualified instructor. As rescuers train, they will become more comfortable in unusual surroundings and can then concentrate on the goals of access, patient care, and extrication.

The safety of the rescuer must always come first. Rescuers must answer *yes* to three questions before contemplating entry into a confined space.

1. Am I absolutely sure that this area is safe?
2. Do I have access to and familiarity with the specialized equipment required to enter and work in a confined space?
3. Am I trained in and do I feel comfortable with confined space entry and rescue?

If the answer to any of these questions is *no*, rescuers should not attempt the rescue until the situation improves and they can answer *yes* to all three questions.

FLOWING GRAIN ENTRAPMENT

Moving or flowing grain presents potential entrapment and suffocation hazards. Problems may occur in flat storage areas, bins, trucks, or wagons, as well as in trench or upright silos. Grain transport equipment, commercial elevators, and grain processing facilities are also common incident sites. Incidents in flowing grain fall into four primary categories:

- Engulfment in a column of flowing grain
- Entrapment or suffocation in a grain transport vehicle
- Collapse of a horizontal crusted grain surface
- Collapse of a vertical crusted grain surface

FIGURE 9.4

The grain in a bin flows inward from the top center. An unloading auger at the bottom of the grain bin transports the grain outside.

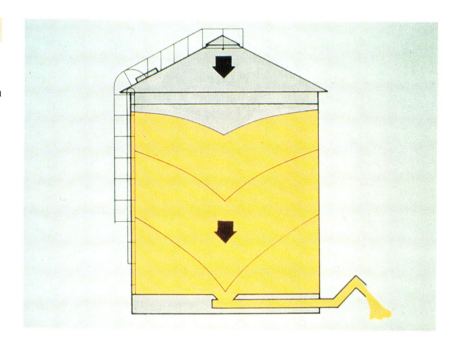

Grain is loaded into storage bins from the top and removed from the bottom. Grain bins are usually circular and constructed of heavy-gauge, galvanized, corrugated steel. There are usually three openings: the top cap, in the center of the cone-shaped roof; the scuttle door, also on the roof and reached by an access ladder permanently mounted to the bin's outside wall; and a ground-level door that is usable only when the bin is totally or nearly empty. In addition, the bin may be equipped with a sweep auger to level the grain as it is loaded, and an opening in the center of the floor to allow the grain to be removed by an unloading auger.

The most common mishap is entrapment or suffocation caused when an individual is drawn into a flowing column of grain. When a grain bin is being emptied by an auger or by gravity, the grain flows in a funnel-shaped path from the top center vertically down to the floor opening. The outlet for most on-farm storage bins is located in the center of the bin floor, so the grain flows down the center (Figure 9.4). As the column moves downward, the upper layers of grain roll inward toward the center. The flow velocity increases as grain flows from the bin wall at the top of the grain mass down to the small vertical column, until it approaches nearly the rate of the unloading auger.

Entrapment is similar to being drawn into a water whirlpool. The rate of inflow at the center top is so great that escape is nearly impossible. For example, an auger with an 8" diameter will move 52 cubic feet of grain per minute—enough to totally submerge a 185-lb person in just 8 seconds. Once engulfed in the flow of grain, the victim is rapidly drawn to the floor of the bin, perhaps even into the unloading auger (Figure 9.5).

FIGURE 9.5

Engulfment can happen quickly. A person weighing 185 lb occupies about 7 cubic feet of volume. Grain flows about 52 cubic feet per minute. Thus, this person would be totally engulfed in just 8 seconds.

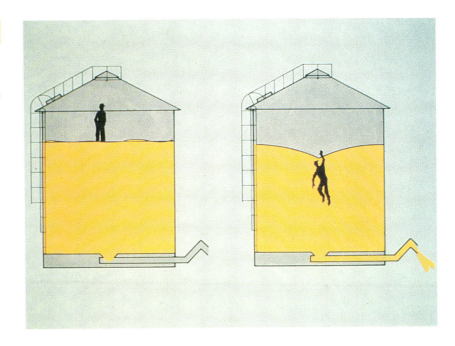

The condition of the grain may play a major role in the survival of an entrapped individual. It may be that entrapment in spoiled grain is less likely to be fatal because the caked masses of grain form open air pockets and reduce the grain pressure on the body.

Incidents with grain transport vehicles, such as trucks equipped with grain beds and gravity-flow wagons, often involve small children. The child may be buried as grain is loaded into the vehicle from a combine or storage bin, or the child may fall into the grain as it is being unloaded. A child can become completely submerged in grain in just 2 to 3 seconds.

Spoiled, dirty, or wet grain expands to form a hard upper crust or surface that looks solid and capable of supporting the weight of an individual. As grain is unloaded, this crust hides or "bridges" voids under the surface (Figure 9.6). If an individual enters the bin and attempts to walk on the crusted surface, the additional weight will cause the crust to collapse, and the individual may be partially or completely submerged. Oftentimes, the victim will not be located directly below the point where he or she was last seen. Shifting grain may cause the victim to move 4' to 5' horizontally from the point of entry.

Grain will have more space between individual kernels (fluffing) any time it has been recently handled. With time, the kernels settle, and the same amount of grain will occupy a slightly smaller volume. Fluffed grain provides less support than settled grain. Individuals will sink to their knees attempting to walk on grain that has just been put in the bin or has moved while being removed from the bin. After the grain settles,

FIGURE 9.6

Grain can form a hard top crust that appears to be firm enough to walk on. However, this crust can crack unexpectedly and engulf the person in grain if a cavity had formed under the crust.

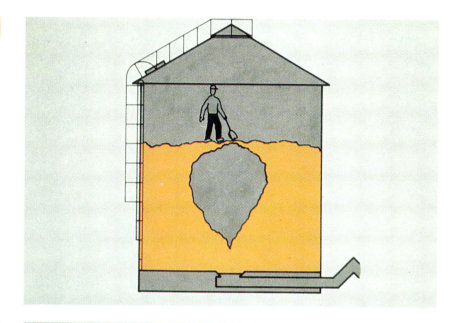

FIGURE 9.7

Grain can cake in large vertical columns against the bin wall. A person who tries to loosen the grain by tapping it with a shovel can be completely buried when the mass collapses.

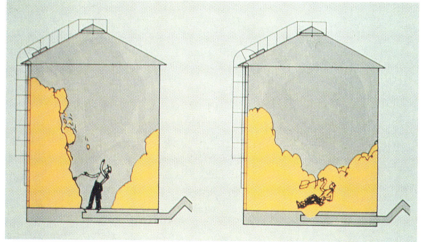

the same individual may only sink to ankle or midcalf depth. Heavier people, such as rescuers wearing protective clothing and an SCBA, will sink more. Grain provides more support for walking the longer it has been sitting without being handled, moved, or agitated.

Horizontal grain crusts are not the only danger in a grain bin. A partially empty bin may have a pile of grain against a wall. Grain in good condition will pile at an angle of 30 degrees with the floor, but spoiled or caked grain can stand almost vertical, and may be as much as 20' to 30' above the bin floor. An individual who attempts to dislodge the grain by poking it with a stick or shovel may cause an avalanche and become engulfed by the falling grain (Figure 9.7). This type of incident is common at large grain handling facilities.

Rescuers who are called to a grain entrapment incident should always assume that a victim entrapped in grain is alive, even if he or she is completely submerged. Successful rescues have taken place in which the victim was completely engulfed in 10' of grain for over 2 hours. Do not start the unloading auger or open the gravity flow gate of a grain bin or wagon for any reason. The victim may be drawn into the unloading auger or become wedged in the opening and sustain further injury.

Grain bins do not usually contain the number of toxic gases present in silos or other confined space structures. While carbon dioxide is found in grain bins, it will quickly dissipate once the bin is open and the ventilation fan started. However, grain dust and mold spores from spoiled grain can cause severe allergic reactions and respiratory problems for both patients and rescuers. If the victim is visible, conscious, and not having any difficulty breathing, rescuers should use filter masks rated for toxic dusts as respiratory protection to filter out dust and mold spores, along with the safety harness and safety line. If the victim is not visible or is unresponsive, rescuers should assume the atmosphere is toxic and wear an SCBA, safety harness, and safety line.

Extrication Technique

Securing the Scene.

1. **Establish a safety zone.** The first step in any rescue operation is to establish a safety zone. As you approach the scene, look for any potential hazards. Do not permit any open flames, including smoking, in or around the site. The safety zone should encompass an area of at least 50' from the bin in all directions. The safety zone should be expanded if there is a possibility of fire or explosion. Plastic barrier tape and light stakes should be used to outline the safety zone.
2. **Escort bystanders out of the safety zone.** Escort neighbors, co-workers, family members, and other bystanders out of the safety zone as soon as it is marked. One member of the rescue team should be assigned to communicate with the patient's family and friends throughout the rescue operation. Remember that communication with the family is a crucial part of the operation.
3. **Visually inspect the grain surface without entering the bin.** This inspection is done to determine if the victim is visible. If not, turn on the ventilation fan, if the bin has one and someone at the scene knows how to operate it. The fan will increase the flow of fresh air through the grain and may contribute to the air supply of a completely submerged victim. It will also help reduce dust levels during the extrication efforts. If the fan is equipped with a heating system or drier, ensure that it is not activated when the fan is started. The fan will be very loud, which makes coordinating rescue efforts difficult. The preincident plan should include a way to communicate in this situation.

Accessing the Patient—Partial Submersion.

1. **If the victim is not completely submerged, lower a rescuer into the bin, using a safety harness and safety line.** Reassure the victim

and calm him or her to prevent uncoordinated self-extrication efforts. Secure a safety line to the patient, around the chest beneath the armpits. *Do not try to pull the victim free using the rope or harness.* The pressure of the grain on the victim is so great that simply pulling with a rope will not move the victim; the victim must be dug out of the grain.
2. **Check the patient's airway.** The airway should be checked for lodged grain, and oxygen should be administered with the appropriate device and flow rate for the patient's condition.
3. **Construct a shield around the victim.** The shield should be made of plywood forced vertically into the grain. Three sheets may be used to form an overlapping triangle, or four sheets in a square or rectangle with overlapping edges (Figure 9.8). A section of snow fence covered with canvas also makes a lightweight, portable shield.
4. **Begin scooping the grain from inside the shield once the shield is in place.** Overlapping the edges of the shield provides self-bracing as the grain is removed. Additional lateral bracing may be necessary to prevent the walls of the shield from collapsing inward. This is a slow process, since space

FIGURE 9.8

Construct a shield around the patient with plywood or a section of snow fence in order to scoop out the grain from around the patient.

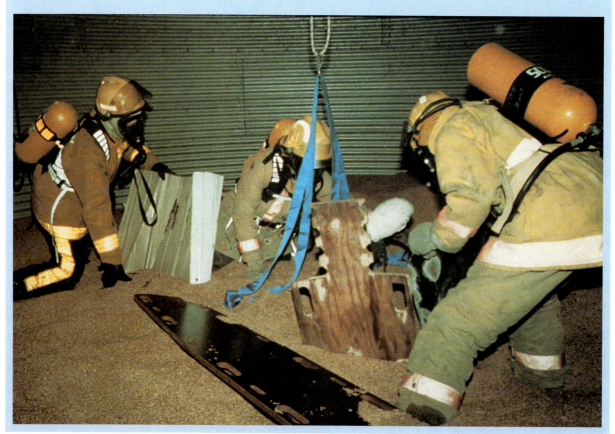

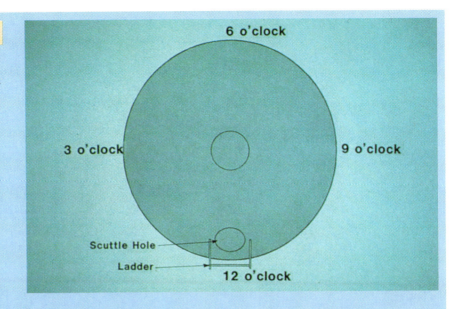

FIGURE 9.9

Establish reference points in a grain bin so all rescuers can communicate more effectively when extricating the patient.

around the victim is limited, and the digging must be done by hand or with small shovels or buckets.

5. **Conduct a primary assessment.** As soon as you reach the patient, begin the primary assessment. Check the patient's airway, breathing, circulation, and disability (ABCD).

   Assess breathing effort and lung sounds. If the patient is breathing, administer high-flow oxygen via a nonrebreathing mask. If the patient's respirations are under 10 or over 30 breaths per minute, assist ventilations with a bag-valve-mask device. If the patient is not breathing, use a pocket mask to initiate ventilation.

Accessing the Patient—Complete Submersion.

1. **If the victim is completely submerged, cut the bin walls and allow the grain to flow outward symmetrically.** This will move the grain down and away from the victim without changing the victim's position. *Do not turn on the unloading auger to remove grain.* Extrication in this situation requires removal of the grain from the bin in a rapid, orderly fashion. The large amount of grain and its natural flow make efforts to dig out a buried victim useless.

2. **Assign one team member to stay at the scuttle door and watch for the victim.** To provide a reference point for the extrication team, call the scuttle door "12 o'clock." Directly opposite would be 6 o'clock, with 3 o'clock to the left of the scuttle door and 9 o'clock to the right (Figure 9.9).

3. **Use heavy-duty air chisels to make V- or M-shaped cuts on opposite sides at the same level in the wall panels.** These cuts should be 30" to 40" across, and located at the highest ring below the grain surface, as long as the chisel operator can stand on the ground. Do not cut through fasteners or stiffeners (Figure 9.10). If two cuts are insufficient, make two more cuts equally distant from the first two cuts. Lower openings can be made as the grain level drops.

4. **Bend the metal with a large hammer or sledge to allow the grain to flow out freely.** Be sure to wear heavy leather gloves. To slow or stop the grain flow after the victim becomes visible, bend the metal back into place. Remove the grain accumulating out-

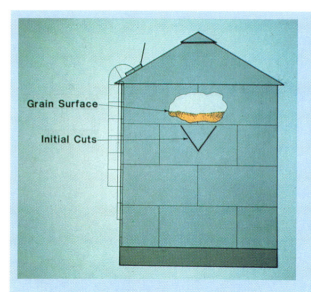 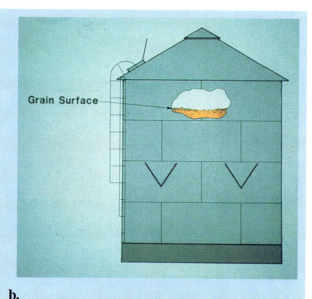

FIGURE 9.10 a. To extricate a partially or fully engulfed patient, make V-shaped cuts in the grain bin wall to remove grain from around the patient.
b. Avoid cutting the stiffeners on the grain bin wall.

side the bin, if necessary, during the extrication. A tractor with a front-end loader may be used, although this will add to the noise and confusion.

5. **Lower a rescuer into the bin once the victim is visible.** Remember the rescuer must be equipped with a safety harness and safety line.
6. **Conduct a primary assessment.** As soon as you reach the patient, begin the primary assessment. Check the patient's airway, breathing, circulation, and disability (ABCD). Assess breathing effort and lung sounds. If the patient is breathing, administer high-flow oxygen via a nonrebreathing mask. If the patient's respirations are under 10 or over 30 breaths per minute, assist ventilations with a bag-valve-mask device. If the patient is not breathing, use a pocket mask to initiate ventilation.

Victims trapped in grain transport vehicles may be wedged at the discharge opening, blocking the flow of grain. Following the same procedure above, cut openings in the bottom or sides of the vehicle to allow the grain to empty. If the vehicle is small, scoop shovels may be used to empty the grain.

Table 9.4 illustrates some of the most common injuries that result from confined space incidents.

SILOS

Silos are familiar structures on many farms and are used to preserve and store feed (Figure 9.11). Conventional silos vary in construction, and may be made of poured concrete, concrete blocks, or wood. Some may

TABLE 9.4 Common Injuries Involving Confined Spaces

Mechanism of Injury	Result	Typical Injuries
Fall or entrapment in confined space	Suffocation and/or trauma from fall	**Anoxia or hypoxia** due to low oxygen levels and/or high concentrations of toxic gases; **Fall injuries** depend on distance fallen; **Chest injuries** (broken ribs, possible flail chest); **Spinal injuries** (usually to cervical spine, injuries to lumbar and thoracic spine also possible); **Open or closed fractures**
Entrapment in flowing grain 1. "Quicksand" when grain is being unloaded from bin or gravity wagon 2. Collapse of grain "bridge" 3. Grain stuck to walls falls on victim 4. Overturned truck/wagon 5. Containing structure collapses	Suffocation; possible trauma; possible hypothermia	**Mechanical suffocation** due to inability to expand chest/diaphragm; **Airway obstruction** by grain; **Toxic atmosphere**; **Hypothermia**

FIGURE 9.11

Silage can be stored in oxygen-limiting silos, concrete silos, or in a trench or bunker.

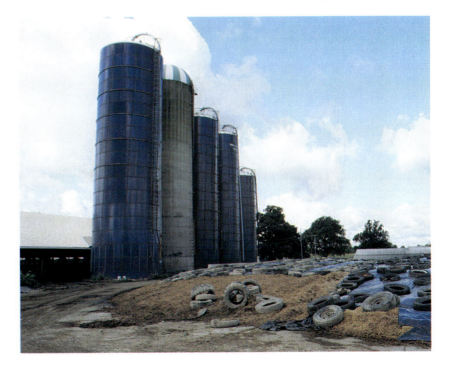

have a roof or cap while others have an open top. These open silos may have an electrically operated unloading device that rests on the top of the silage and blows a layer of silage down a chute to feed the livestock. This chute covers a series of unloading doors that go up the side of the silo.

Oxygen-limiting silos are sealed structures, constructed of steel coating with glass on the inside and blue epoxy on the outside. They have an unloading mechanism at the bottom and a small vent or access door at the top that also permits entry. However, an SCBA is required for anyone to enter these silos safely.

A third way to store feed is in a bunker or trench covered with plastic to prevent spoilage. These bunkers may be as deep as 30'. Hazards associated with these storage trenches and bunkers include entrapment in tons of silage and/or rollover of a packing vehicle such as a tractor.

Silos are dangerous because of the toxic gases they contain. As silage ferments, a variety of gases, including carbon dioxide, methane, and nitrogen dioxide, are released. The most dangerous of these is nitrogen dioxide, often called silo gas. A description of silo gas is presented earlier in this chapter. Because this gas is heavier than air, it may linger at the bottom of the silo long after the silage has ceased to ferment. Yet it remains dangerous even in small concentrations.

Rescuers should use extreme caution when working in and around silos, especially if the silos have been filled within the previous month. Wear an SCBA for respiratory protection against silo gas when working in and around open silos, and at all times when working in a sealed silo. Gas masks or simple respirators do not provide protection from silo gas.

Rescuers entering a silo should also always wear a safety harness and safety line controlled by an outside line handler. A life belt and hook should also be worn if rescuers must climb silo ladders. The rungs of the enclosed chute ladder double as door handles and do not provide a secure footing. Silage clinging to the walls could fall and injure the rescuer or the victim. One line handler on the outside should be assigned to each rescuer inside. A backup rescuer wearing an SCBA, safety harness, and safety line should stand by outside to assist if necessary.

Preincident planning for silo rescues should include determining the height of the tallest silo in the area and ensuring that there is enough rescue rope to lift a victim out, regardless of the level of silage in the structure. An incident involving a silo is considered a high-angle rescue. Rescuers should practice high-angle rescue and keep in mind the hazards associated with this type of operation.

Another part of the preincident plan should include a standard set of signals so the inside rescuer will be able to communicate with the line handler. These signals should be standardized for the team and practiced frequently. Radio communication may be impossible because of

SCBAs, so a series of tugs on the line may be most useful. A sample system is presented below.

> One tug by handler means "Are you OK?"
> One tug by rescuer means "Yes, I'm OK."
> Two tugs by rescuer means "Give me more line."
> Two tugs by handler means "I understand."
> Three tugs by rescuer means "Take up the slack."
> Four tugs by rescuer or handler means "Emergency—get out!"

Extrication Technique

Two rescue teams should be used for all silo rescues—an inside team and an outside team. A system of communication, either by radio or standard set of signals, should be established.

Securing the Scene.

1. **Establish a safety zone.**
2. **Escort bystanders out of the safety zone.**
3. **Turn off and secure the power source.** Before entering the silo, locate the main power control for the unloader, turn it off, and secure it so that it cannot be turned on again. If the switch cannot be locked, assign a rescuer to guard it, or place tape over it so that the mechanism cannot be restarted during the rescue operation.

Accessing the Patient.

1. **If the victim is caught in the unloading mechanism, study the equipment to plan the best method of extrication.** All tools will need to be lifted up the enclosed chute or lowered down from the top of the silo. Any rescuer exposed to silo gas should be immediately relieved from duty and receive medical attention.
2. **Carry a portable oxygen system equipped with a nonrebreathing mask into the silo.** If the patient is breathing, apply the mask and set the flow as high as the regulator will go. If the victim is not breathing, use a bag-valve-mask device.

   If the mask is not available, the Sylvester method of artificial respiration, a method used before the development of current CPR techniques, may be the only way to get oxygen into the lungs. While not as effective as mouth-to-mask rescue breathing, the Sylvester method may provide adequate oxygen when used with a well-fitted nonrebreathing mask and high-flow oxygen to keep the patient alive until definitive treatment can be administered.

   Place the victim on his or her back, open the airway as with CPR, and apply a nonrebreathing mask with oxygen. The rescuer should kneel at the head of the patient and face the patient. Firmly grasp the patient's wrists, one in each hand, and place them on the sternum. Press down on the sternum, firmly but gently, forcing exhalation (Figure 9.12a). Now lift the patient's arms above the head to draw oxygen into the lungs (Figure 9.12b). Repeat this procedure once every 5 seconds (12 times per minute).
3. **Secure the patient to a litter, back board, or harness, depending on the injury and situation.** Patients with an altered level of consciousness, possible spinal injury, or mul-

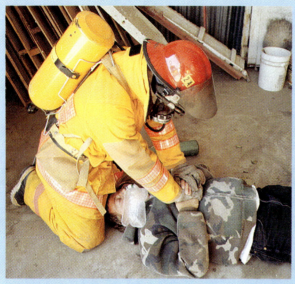 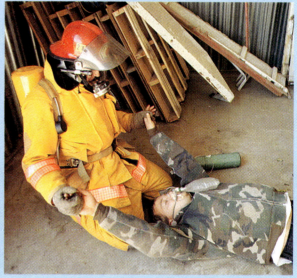

FIGURE 9.12
a. The Sylvester method of artifical respiration may provide sufficient ventilation to a patient during a confined space rescue. The rescuer applies gentle, firm pressure on the patient's sternum with the patient's wrists.
b. The rescuer then lifts the patient's arms over the head to move oxygen into the lungs.

tiple, long bone fractures should be fully immobilized on a long spine board. A foot board should be used when lifting or lowering the patient in a horizontal position. A harness should only be used on conscious patients with no airway problems or spinal injuries.

Removing the Patient.

1. **Lift the patient up from the inside and down on the outside of the silo.** In most cases, it will not be possible to lower a patient down the enclosed silo chute. Ensure that the rope is long enough to reach from the ground to at least 6' above the silo rim and back down to the ground, with adequate excess for securing the patient and for pulling.
2. **Rig a pulley or snatch block to the top of the ladder and run the rescue line through it.** Securely lash the ladder to the outside ladder or silo structure so that it extends at least 6' above the silo rim. Drop enough line inside the silo for the rescue team to secure the patient. Drop the rest of the line to the team outside the silo. Station another rescuer at this point to move the patient from inside to outside the silo, and to coordinate both rescue teams. This rescuer will have both visual and verbal access to both teams. While the inside rescue team packages the patient for extrication, the outside team should rig another pulley or snatch block to the base of the silo directly under the ladder lashed on top.
3. **Inspect the access door or opening in the top cap or roof of the silo, near the ladder.** If this opening is not large enough for the patient to pass through easily, enlarge it or cut a new one. Metal caps can be cut with a power saw or air chisel. Wooden roofs can be torn apart with power saws or wrecking bars. Both rescue teams and the patient must wear protective head gear to prevent injury from

falling debris, and both teams should be watchful for rotted or weakened wood. Do not use heat- or spark-producing tools if the potential for explosion is high.
4. **Pull the patient up from inside the silo.** The patient's ascent from inside and descent to the ground should be assisted and secured by two tag lines fastened to the back board, litter, or harness. The inside rescuer will either climb out (if the silo is equipped with an inside ladder), or be pulled out after the patient is removed. Be sure to monitor the air pressure in the inside rescuer's SCBA during the operation.
5. **Transfer the patient from the inside of the silo to the outside.** This transfer can be made through the door on the top of the silo, or through a removable door at the level of the silage. If the silo has a chute, and if space allows, lower the patient down the chute.
6. **Lower the patient to the ground.** The patient may be lowered down the chute or on the outside of the silo. Remember to use all precautions that any high-angle rescue operation may require. The outside rescue team will direct the lowering effort.

Silo Fires

Silo fires are caused by a chemical reaction called the **Maillard reaction.** Stored plant material continues to "breathe" for a short time after it is cut, and this respiration produces heat. As the plant material continues to ferment, more heat is produced along with the preservative acids until the plant material becomes stable or ensiled.

If the crop being stored has enough moisture content, the water in the forage will conduct the heat away from the silage mass and prevent overheating. If, however, the material is too wet (more than 40% moisture) or too dry (less than 25% moisture), the heat will not dissipate quickly enough and the internal temperature will rise. When the internal temperature rises above 130°F, the Maillard reaction occurs and may sustain itself. The heat begins to kill microorganisms and begins to break down the forage by a trapped oxidation process known as pyrolysis. This process produces flammable gases that can ignite when they come into contact with oxygen. The fire will slowly spread until it reaches the surface.

Silo fires do not usually create a significant amount of flame or pose immediate threat to other buildings. In addition, silo fires in conventional silos can usually be extinguished with only a few fire fighters. However, fires in oxygen-limiting silos are potentially hazardous and could lead to explosions. Several fire fighters have been killed while attempting to extinguish fires in oxygen-limiting silos.

The rescue team may be called upon to assist fire fighters in extinguishing silo fires. The rescuer who assesses scene safety should wear an SCBA because several potentially hazardous gases are formed during the ensilage process or as a result of a fire. If there is considerable smoke or if red hot embers are falling down the chute, rescuers will require full turnout gear and an SCBA.

Most fires in conventional silos occur in the top 10' of silage material, and are often found near unloading doors. The first indication of a fire is often a burning or burned unloading door. The silage will probably have a red glow with an occasional flame. Rescuers should clear the area of all livestock and people, and wet down the area around the silo to prevent the fire from spreading. One fire fighter, in full turnout gear with a safety harness and safety line, can usually extinguish all surface burning by dousing the fire from the silo blower platform.

Once surface burning is extinguished, several temperature readings of the silage should be taken to locate any hot spots and internal burning. The rescuer taking the readings should wear full turnout gear and SCBA, and should not step directly onto the silage. Wooden planks, large pieces of plywood, or ladders should be used to distribute the rescuer's weight over a larger area and minimize the risk of falling into a burned-out cavity.

A probe and thermometer can be easily constructed. The probe is made of 3/8" threaded pipe of various lengths capped by a 3" long machined pointed probe tip with four 3/16" holes drilled around it. The probe is inserted into the silage material, and a thermometer on a lightweight wire is lowered into the probe to take the readings. Temperatures of 180°F indicate smoldering or burning material; areas with temperatures between 140°F and 170°F should be rechecked every 2 or 3 hours; readings below 140°F are safe.

Once the hot areas have been identified, the probe can be used to funnel water to exact hot spots. Use the smallest hose available, perhaps even a garden hose may fit the probe. Injecting water may cause considerable smoke and steam, so the assigned rescuer should wear full turnout gear, an SCBA, a safety harness, and a safety line. The line handler should also be in full turnout gear to help handle the hose and stand by for safety. Remember that the water will add weight that may cause excess pressure on the silo walls.

After a silo fire is extinguished, the affected material must be unloaded. Damaged silage loses its nutritional value and may spoil. In addition, if any hot spots were missed, reignition is a possibility. A fire watch should be stationed at the unloading chute to extinguish any burning materials and wet down any charred or extremely dry materials.

Fires in oxygen-limiting silos are potentially very dangerous and could result in a devastating explosion. Any increase in the amount of oxygen in the silo could ignite the explosive gases formed by a silage fire, especially carbon monoxide. These fires cannot be hosed down since the oxygen carried in water droplets could trigger an explosion (Figure 9.13). Instead, the silo should be completely sealed and the fire allowed to die out. If sealing the silo does not extinguish the fire, liquid or gaseous nitrogen or carbon dioxide can be injected into the silo to displace the oxygen and cool the fire. Afterwards, the silo may need to be emptied.

LIQUID MANURE STORAGE

Farms generally use one of three types of liquid manure storage systems: a large tank located directly under the livestock housing area; an open lagoon or pond near the livestock housing area; or an aboveground, silo-type storage. Individuals may fall into the open storage and drown, or be overcome by the toxic gases released by bacterial action.

Manure storage tanks or pits should be considered as confined space situations. Therefore, rescue attempts should be undertaken with extreme caution. Rescuers should always wear an SCBA, a safety harness, and a safety line. Never enter any type of manure storage facility without a supply of air and assistance from a backup team using a safety line. Ventilate a manure storage facility as quickly as possible. Open windows or doors, activate the ventilation system, or use smoke evacuation equipment. Also ensure that the electrical supply to any storage facility is turned off. Rescuers and/or victims can be electrocuted due to a short in the pump inside the facility.

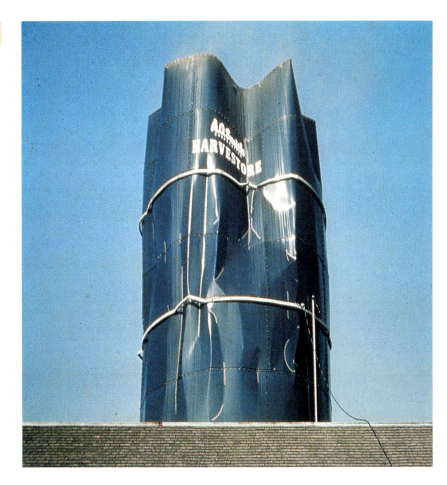

FIGURE 9.13

This silo exploded after rescuers attempted to extinguish a fire inside the silo with water. The oxygen from the water increased the amount of oxygen in the silo's atmosphere. The explosion killed one fire fighter.

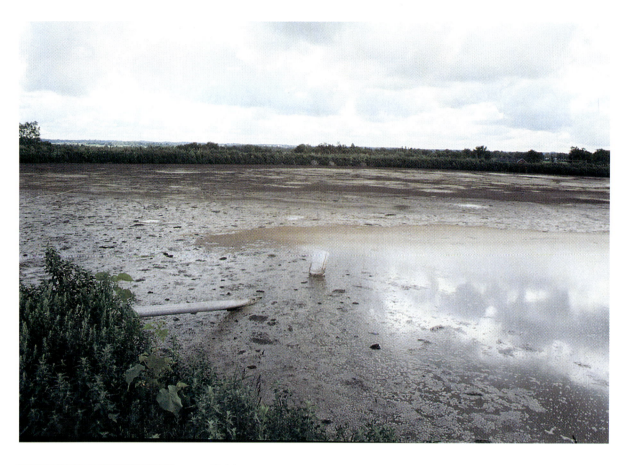

FIGURE 9.14

Drowning in an open manure pond can occur when a person attempts to walk on the crust that forms over the pond.

With open ponds, there is little danger of toxic gases. However, these areas may have a surface crust that looks solid but that will not support a person's weight. An individual who steps out on this area may fall through and drown (Figure 9.14). When drowning occurs, the area will have to be dragged, as the body will not float to the top. Rescuers will have to use a small boat or drag line to remove an individual from open manure storage.

SUMMARY

Grain and silage storage facility rescues must be considered confined space situations with a number of atmospheric, physical, and psychological hazards. A preincident plan is vital for a successful rescue, and each rescuer should be equipped with an SCBA, safety harness, and safety line.

Atmospheric hazards include a lack of oxygen, the presence of toxic gases, and the likelihood of an explosion because of the presence of grain dust or flammable gases. Carbon dioxide, carbon monoxide, nitrogen dioxide, methane, hydrogen sulfide, and ammonia are among the toxic gases encountered in these rescue situations.

Physical hazards include the potential for entrapment, electrocution, drowning, fall-related injuries, or impalement on sharp objects.

Psychological hazards include stress and anxiety when confronted with a confined space and with wearing an SCBA.

The safety of the rescuer must always come first in any confined space rescue situation. You must be sure that the area is safe, that you have the specialized equipment necessary, and that you are properly trained and comfortable with the techniques of confined space rescue before any rescue attempt is made.

CHAPTER 10

Animal Incidents

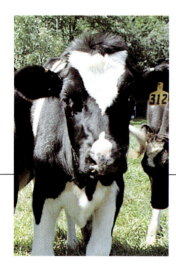

CHAPTER OUTLINE

Overview
Objectives
Animals
   Horses
   Cattle
   Pigs
Traps
Summary

KEY TERMS

Omnivorous: characteristic of some animals that will eat anything, plant or animal flesh, including human flesh.

Squeezing: incident in which an animal pushes a person against a wall or fence that may result in serious injury.

CHAPTER 10 Animal Incidents

OVERVIEW

Even though animals such as horses, cattle, and sheep are often considered domesticated, they can cause severe injury. A frightened animal remains a threat to rescuers as well. Planning is important to enable a swift, safe rescue.

Incidents involving animals may not be frequent, but they can be severe. Kicks may result in severe fractures, blunt trauma, concussions, and other injuries. Bites may produce deep lacerations, amputations, or serious infections; goring may result in penetrating injuries to the abdomen and chest. Extricating a patient from an animal incident requires special precautions to avoid further injury to the patient and to the rescuer.

Trapping incidents may require a search and other techniques of a remote rescue operation. This chapter describes incidents involving animals and traps. It also discusses safety precautions for rescuers.

OBJECTIVES

After reading this chapter, the rescuer should be able to:

- list the safety precautions that must be taken in dealing with animals.
- identify appropriate rescue techniques.
- recognize various types of traps and their mechanisms.

ANIMALS

While every animal presents a potential for injury, most farm animal rescue operations involve horses, cattle, and pigs. Animals are easily frightened by new people, shapes, and loud noises. As you approach the scene, turn off sirens and lights, and ensure that vehicles are either parked out of sight or at a distance. Approach all animals, especially dogs at the scene, with care to avoid frightening them and causing additional injury to the patient and/or the rescuers. A family dog can become very protective and try to prevent the rescue team from approaching the victim. Animals that are injured also pose a hazard to the patient and the rescue team. Injured animals must be restrained to prevent additional injury to the patient and the rescue team. Rescuers should exercise extreme caution if there is blood at the scene because animals often become frightened at the smell of human or animal blood.

All facilities that house animals are heavily contaminated with bacteria, viruses, parasites, and molds. Rescuers should maintain current immunization protection, especially for tetanus. Rescuers should also watch for tetanus and secondary infection of open wounds on the patient and advise the emergency department staff about environmental conditions.

Horses

Horses are responsible for about 80% of all injuries caused by animals. The horse may kick or bite the person, a rider may fall and be dragged behind the animal, or the horse may fall on the person, or **squeeze** the person against a wall or fence.

Kicks are the most common mechanism of injury. Kicks to the head may cause skull fractures or severe concussions (Figure 10.1); kicks to

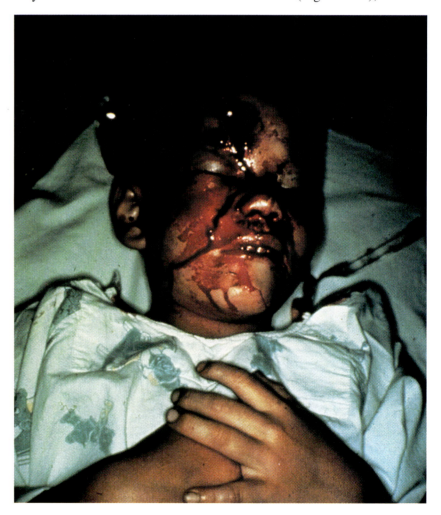

FIGURE 10.1

Kicks to the head may result in skull fractures or severe concussions.

the stomach or chest may result in blunt trauma to internal organs with severe internal bleeding, or possible respiratory compromise. Bites may also produce deep lacerations with underlying bone damage. Bites can also be complicated by tetanus, encephalitis, or rabies.

A rider who falls from a horse and is dragged behind it may sustain severe abrasions and contusions. If the rider is thrown from the horse, concussion and severe blunt trauma may result. A horse that falls on the rider can cause severe blunt trauma, extremity fractures, and spinal injuries. Additionally, the pommel on western saddles can produce extensive abdominal and pelvic injuries, including fractures, ruptured organs, and arterial damage.

Normally, a horse will react by running, bucking, or rearing when it perceives a threat and will stop when it thinks the threat is over. Consequently, rescuers may find a horse grazing near its fallen rider. Approach the horse quietly, and if you can reach the reins or lead rope, lead it safely away from the area. If the horse has a bridle, hold the bridle from the horse's left side.

A common injury occurs when the rider is preparing to mount a horse. As the rider swings his or her leg over the saddle, the horse tosses its head and strikes the rider on the left side of the face. The force of the blow may cause fractures to the cheek bones, eye sockets, forehead, and nose. Concussion is a strong possibility, and subdural and epidural hematomas are also common.

To prevent further injury to the patient, it is best to remove the horse from the situation, rather than try to remove the patient. Always approach an animal from the front, so it can see you. Speak in a calm, gentle voice to avoid startling the horse. Horses are afraid of being cornered or trapped, so if the incident occurred in a corral, stall, or some other enclosed space, and the patient is not lying near the gate, simply opening the gate to release the horse(s) may provide the space required to begin assessment and treatment. The animals will probably not go far, and can be rounded up later. If a family member is present and is familiar with the horse, rescuers should allow this person to approach and remove the animal.

However, if the patient is lying between the gate and the horse, the patient may have to be moved. Distract the horse by having someone approach the far end of the corral or stall with a bucket filled with a few handfuls of grain. That person should speak softly and calmly to the animal, and shake the bucket so the horse can hear the grain. While the horse is eating, another rescuer can quietly and slowly open the gate or crawl under the fence and pull the patient out.

In this situation, you may not have time to immobilize the patient. Using both hands, grasp the patient's clothing below the collar. Support the patient's head by cradling it in your forearms. Drag the patient back-

FIGURE 10.2

Use both hands and grasp the patient's clothing below the collar. Support the head by cradling it in your arms.

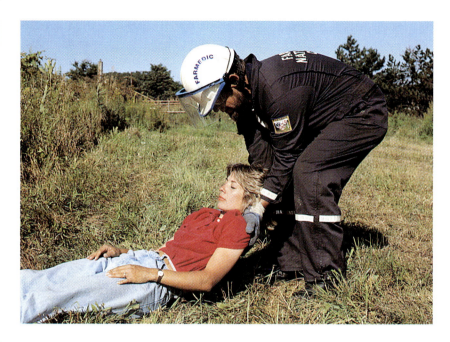

ward, keeping the head, neck, and spine as much in line as possible (Figure 10.2). Move the patient only the minimum distance necessary to reach safety.

Animals will often provide rescuers with clues to their disposition. For example, the position of a horse's ears can indicate anger, fear, interest, or relaxation. When a horse is angry, its ears are turned back and laid down on the top of the head. If the ears are pointed ahead, the body tense, the head high and the eyes concentrating, the horse is afraid of what he sees and will be ready for flight. If the ears are forward but the body is relaxed, the horse is interested but not afraid. When totally relaxed, a horse will have its ears turned to the side or slightly back, the head will sag slightly, and one hind leg may be raised.

Cattle

Dairy cattle can also cause major injuries. Almost one third of the incidents on dairy farms occur during routine chores. Dairy cows, normally docile, can become very aggressive, especially around newborn calves. They may butt, kick, trample, or crush a handler. Bulls may gore an individual causing penetrating injuries to the abdomen, chest, and pelvic area. One butt can produce a massive flail chest injury.

Beef cattle are traditionally less aggressive than dairy cattle, but the newer exotic crossbreeds may be larger, more nervous, and more prone to attack. Horned animals may gore an individual causing penetrating injuries; dehorned animals may butt resulting in severe blunt trauma to the chest, abdomen, and extremities.

Additionally, of all farm animals, cattle are most frequently affected by rabies. The disease may pass to humans without a bite if infected

CHAPTER 10 Animal Incidents

saliva from the animal gets on hands and arms and ente. stream through small cuts or abrasions. Because of this, rescuer. keep all immunizations current, especially tetanus immunizations, a. wear leather gloves when dealing with animals.

Incidents with cattle usually occur when the animals are being moved or loaded. Animals do not like small, enclosed spaces and may become extremely nervous. The animals may inadvertently step on, kick, or squeeze the handler against a wall. Squeezing against the wall of a stall or a fence may even occur if the animal does not seem nervous. Sharp hooves can cause multiple fractures of the foot; kicks may result in lower leg or pelvic fractures; and internal injuries, abdominal injuries, and rib fractures may occur if the handler is pinned against the pen or loading chute wall.

As with horses, it may be better and easier to remove cattle from the incident scene before attempting to remove the patient. It is important to let the animal know where you are at all times. A calm approach and soft voice will help relax the animal.

Once the patient is lying on the ground, a bull may become protective of its "prize" and try to prevent other people from reaching the patient. The team's response will depend on the situation. A conscious patient should be told to lie still and quiet. Any movement may cause another attack.

It may be best to open the gate and release the animal, or cause a distraction at the other end of the corral to give other members of the team time to pull a patient to safety. If the incident occurs in a wide field or open space, a car or rescue vehicle may be used as a protective barrier between the animal and the patient.

If the incident occurs in a chute or pen, make sure no other animals are permitted to enter the chute. The bottom rail of a chute side should be high enough to allow a person to crawl or be dragged out. Well-constructed chutes may even have upright openings large enough for a person to slip through, but too small for a bull to escape.

If rescuers are not comfortable handling large animals, request assistance from individuals experienced in handling animals. Consider contacting a veterinarian and/or animal control officer. As a last resort, consider destroying the animal. If possible, a family member, co-worker, or law enforcement officer should do the job, to protect the rescue team from a possible liability suit.

Pigs

Sows are extremely protective of their suckling young and will attack and bite anyone who enters the pen. Small children are usually most susceptible to this kind of injury. Complete amputation of the fingers or hands and extensive tissue loss is possible.

Additionally, pigs are **omnivorous** and will eat anything, including humans. An individual who enters a pen to feed or tend the pigs and has

TABLE 10.1 Common Injuries Involving Animals

Mechanism of Injury	Result	Typical Injuries
Animal incidents (kicked or stepped on by animal; fall from animal; animal falls on person; gores and bites)	Extremity fractures; concussion; crush injuries; blunt trauma; penetrating trauma; abrasions and contusions	**Head injuries** (basal skull fracture, depressed skull fracture, severe concussion, possible maxillofacial injuries); **Abdominal injuries; Fractures; Soft tissue injuries; Blunt trauma**

a heart attack or stroke may be unable to escape the pigs' voracious appetite and may suffer severe soft tissue loss.

Hog pens are built with wire or paneling flush to the ground. Because of this, it will be impossible to drag a patient out under the fencing, as is possible with cattle or horse pens. The animals will have to be removed before the patient can be rescued. Open the gate, use food as bait, or have a decoy attract the animals away from the patient. Once the animals are safely penned elsewhere, the rescue team can enter and proceed with primary assessment and stabilization. Use a long spine board to lift the patient out of the pen or to carry the patient to the transport vehicle.

Table 10.1 illustrates some common injuries that may result from incidents involving animals.

TRAPS

Although trapping is no longer the profitable occupation it was in pioneer days, many people continue to trap for sport and profit. There are three main types of traps: arresting traps, such as snares and spring steel traps, which grip animals but do not kill them; enclosing traps, such as box traps and nets, which imprison an animal without harming it; and exterminating traps, such as mousetraps and mole traps, which grip and kill the animal.

Trapping is governed by state laws, and regulations vary from state to state. Some states outlaw the steel traps with teeth. Because of the regulations limiting where and when people can trap, there are few incidents involving traps. However, these incidents still occur. A person may fall in a pit trap, break a leg and be unable to crawl out. Such a situation would call for high-angle rescue techniques. Extrications involving steel traps may require the assistance of a game warden or other trained individual who knows how the trap operates and can release it. If such a person is not available, it may be easiest to transport the individual with the trap.

SUMMARY

Incidents involving animals can be especially dangerous for rescuers; therefore, planning is necessary to ensure the safety of the rescuers and to avoid further injury to the patient. Rescuers should approach any incident involving animals with the utmost caution. Rescue vehicles should be parked out of sight, or at some distance, to avoid frightening the animal further. Rescuers should approach in sight of the animal, speaking quietly to reassure it. If food is available, it may be a good way to lure the animal away from the patient.

About 80% of all animal incidents involve horses that have kicked, bitten, thrown, or fallen on a person. Cattle kick and bite as well, but they may also butt, gore, or squeeze a person against a pen or chute wall. Pigs, especially sows, will inflict severe bites. An unconscious patient should always be quickly removed from a pigpen, since pigs are omnivorous and will eat human flesh.

If possible, remove the animal from the scene before attempting to extricate and stabilize the patient. All animal facilities are heavily contaminated with bacteria, viruses, and molds. Therefore, rescuers should be sure their immunizations are up-to-date, and should watch for signs of tetanus and secondary infection of open wounds. Notify the emergency department staff of the environmental conditions at the incident while en route to the hospital.

Although many of the most dangerous types of traps have been outlawed, trapping accidents still occur. Study the situation carefully before deciding on an extrication technique. If you are unable or inexperienced in working with traps, call for backup or transport the patient with the trap.

CHAPTER 11
Hazardous Materials

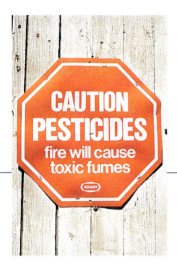

CHAPTER OUTLINE

Overview
Objectives
Definition of Hazardous Materials
Identification of Hazardous Materials
Anhydrous Ammonia
   Physical Properties
   Storage Requirements
   Mechanisms of Injury
   Personal Safety
   Management of Exposure
Pesticides
   Toxicity
   Exposure
   Personal Safety
   Major Incidents
Signs and Symptoms of Pesticide Poisoning
   Organophosphates and Carbamates

Fumigants
Organochlorines
Bipyridyls
Rodenticides
Hydraulic Fluids
   Mechanisms of Injury
   Personal Safety
Protection
   Time
   Distance
   Shielding
Decontamination
Management of Exposure
   Personal Safety
   Managing Ill or Injured Patients
   Contamination Control During Transport
Summary

CHAPTER 11 Hazardous Materials

KEY TERMS

Ammonium hydroxide: a highly caustic solution that corrodes metals and causes progressive chemical burns to soft tissue.

Anhydrous ammonia: fertilizer used to supply nitrogen to grain crops; it contains no moisture, but when combined with water forms the highly corrosive alkali ammonium hydroxide.

Bipyridyls: a common class of herbicide.

Boiling liquid expanding vapor explosion (BLEVE): an explosion of liquified compressed gas in which the compression heats the liquid in the tank, increasing vapor pressure until the tank ruptures.

Decontamination: the process of removing toxic and other harmful materials and properly disposing of them.

Fumigants: insecticides used to treat and protect stored grain, greenhouse crops, and stored fruits and vegetables.

Hazardous material: product or material that can cause damage or injury when released from its normal container or environment, or when exposed to another agent or environment.

Rodenticides: agents that kill, repel, or control rodents.

Shielding: all protective equipment used by the rescuer during a hazardous materials incident.

Toxicity: the level of poison in a pesticide.

OVERVIEW

Potentially hazardous materials can be found anywhere. In agricultural-rural settings, the most common hazardous materials include anhydrous ammonia, pesticides, and hydraulic fluids. Anhydrous ammonia, a commonly used fertilizer, will cause chemical burns and physical trauma if it contacts skin; absorption of pesticides may result in poisoning; hydraulic fluids, used to power many agricultural implements, may cause severe burns and blood poisoning, if injected into body tissue. Rescuers must be prepared to recognize and manage hazardous materials at all rescue sites. Part of this preparation is development of a preincident plan for a hazardous materials incident. Interagency drills are a particularly important way to prepare for an actual hazardous materials incident.

Agricultural-rural incidents involving anhydrous ammonia spills or pesticides may also cover large geographic areas. For example, a crop duster may crash and spill pesticides or a tractor or pickup truck pulling an ammonia tank may overturn, damaging the tank and releasing the ammonia. In these large-scale incidents, the rescue team is likely to call in a special hazardous materials team or even CHEMTREC. Most individual incidents of pesticide poisoning are mild, but sometimes trained help from an outside source is needed. Preincident planning, training, and information about the chemical involved are the keys to successful intervention in a hazardous materials incident.

This chapter outlines what can be expected during an incident involving hazardous materials. It also explains how to identify and contain hazardous materials. It is impossible to cover every chemical found on a farm within the boundaries of this text. Therefore, only the most common hazardous materials will be discussed. Remember that hazardous materials can range from the chemicals discussed in this chapter to dynamite. Ways in which rescuers can protect and decontaminate themselves and their patients are also described, as are ways to manage exposure to these materials.

OBJECTIVES

After reading this chapter, the rescuer should be able to:

- describe the initial assessment of an incident involving hazardous materials.
- identify hazardous materials warning signs, placards, and codes.
- describe physical properties of anhydrous ammonia and appropriate steps to take in the event of rupture or exposure.
- list commonly used pesticides and signs and symptoms of pesticide poisoning.
- identify indications of injury or poisoning from high-pressure fluid injection.
- list ways to protect members of the rescue team and patients from the dangers of exposure to hazardous materials.
- describe the steps for decontamination.
- discuss management techniques for exposure to hazardous materials.

DEFINITION OF HAZARDOUS MATERIALS

A **hazardous material** is a product or material that can cause damage or injury when released from its normal container or environment or when exposed to another agent or environment. Pesticides, fertilizers such as anhydrous ammonia, and hydraulic fluids are common hazardous materials found in agricultural-rural settings. Exposure to pesticides may result in chemical burns or poisoning. Anhydrous ammonia tanks may rupture, releasing vapors in the air that form ammonium hydroxide, a caustic alkaline solution. If this solution comes into contact with skin, the result may be tissue freezing, dehydration, and severe chemical burns. If a hose filled with hydraulic fluid breaks, the hot oil released will cause chemical and thermal burns. Even more dangerous is a leak that could force fluid through the skin without causing a wound. This could cause tissue necrosis and blood poisoning.

Farm machinery often uses hydraulic systems for power. Consequently, hydraulic fluid is present in every rescue operation that involves hydraulically powered equipment, such as a front-end loader. Even though this hazardous material is present at the site of an incident, there may be no immediate danger if it remains contained or controlled. However, the potential for a release, rupture, or spill remains. Ruptured hydraulic hoses can cause "grease gun" injuries. Rescuers must continually monitor the equipment and have a set plan for minimizing damage or injuries in the event of a release or spill.

Table 11.1 illustrates some of the injuries associated with hazardous materials exposure.

IDENTIFICATION OF HAZARDOUS MATERIALS

Though hazardous materials may fit into several classifications, they are identified by their primary hazard. The most common classes are shown in Table 11.2.

TABLE 11.1 Common Injuries Associated with Hazardous Materials Exposure

Mechanism of Injury	Result	Typical Injuries
Exposure to anhydrous ammonia	Freezes exposed tissue; chemical burns	Severe chemical burns to all exposed parts of the body; clothing frozen to skin; severe injury to lung tissue
Exposure to high-pressure liquids/fuels	Burns, if liquid is hot; subcutaneous or intravenous injection due to force of pressure	Thermal or chemical burns—both internal and external; embolic phenomena

TABLE 11.2 Common Classes of Hazardous Materials

◇ LABEL 1 — Domestic label / Domestic class number

Class Number	Nature of Materials
1	Explosives
2	Gases
3	Flammable liquids
4	Flammable solids
5	Oxidizers and organic peroxides
6	Poisons and etiological agents
7	Radioactive materials
8	Corrosives
9	Other regulated materials

Materials that fall into the "other regulated materials" classification may have a color-coded placard or warning label:

Red—flammables
Yellow—reactives (oxidizers)
Green—nonflammable gases
Orange—explosives
White—poisons
Blue—water-reactive materials
White on red—flammable solids
Yellow on white—radioactive materials
White on black—corrosives

While rescuers must be able to recognize the existence of potentially hazardous materials, they are not expected to stop spills or releases. Rescuers must have a basic knowledge of the effects of hazardous materials in order to make rescue decisions. However, a rescue team may need to delay entry to the scene until a team of hazardous materials specialists is available to assess the danger and assist in the management of the situation.

Knowing that a hazardous situation exists begins with the initial notification of the incident. Initial information should include the type of vehicle or facility involved; the presence of smoke or fire; the location of the incident; the topography of the location; a description of the scene; and the presence of warning or identification signs, placards, or numbers. Because placarding is required only for material that is transported on public roads, most chemicals and pesticides at the scene may not be easily identified (Figure 11.1). If the presence of hazardous materials is suspected, approach the situation with caution. Do not enter a scene containing potentially hazardous materials until the extent of the problem is known.

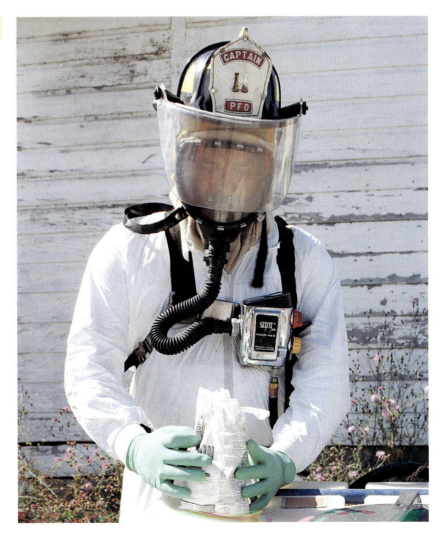

FIGURE 11.1

Approach incidents involving hazardous materials with extreme caution. Wear protective clothing and an SCBA when attempting to identify a chemical or pesticide.

Upon arrival, a visual survey of the area should be done from a safe distance upwind, preferably using binoculars. Maintain a safe distance until you are properly equipped to enter the scene. Look for evidence of a spill or release, such as the presence of damaged ground cover, unresponsive people or animals, chemical clouds or plumes, fire, or smoke. Anything out of the ordinary should be regarded with extreme caution and considered a potential hazardous materials incident.

ANHYDROUS AMMONIA

Physical Properties

Anhydrous ammonia is a fertilizer used to supply nitrogen to grain crops and to improve the food value of hay for livestock. Anhydrous means "without water," and anhydrous ammonia contains no moisture. However, it has a high affinity to water. Anhydrous ammonia is composed of 82.25% nitrogen and 17.75% hydrogen, and is not considered highly flammable.

At standard temperature and pressure, anhydrous ammonia is a gas, but it is stored under pressure in liquid form. As a liquid, anhydrous ammonia weighs slightly more than 5 lb per gallon, or 60% the weight of water. When released from its tank, 1 cubic foot of liquid will expand to 855 cubic feet of vapor. As a gas, anhydrous ammonia is lighter than air, with a density of 0.5963 grams per liter.

As anhydrous ammonia escapes from its tank, a white cloud will appear as the ammonia mixes with moisture in the air. On a hot, dry day the vapor will rise quickly; however, when the humidity is high, the anhydrous ammonia will attach itself to the water in the air, remain close to the ground, and not disperse readily. Visibility inside the cloud is zero, and patients and/or rescuers can become disoriented very easily.

When anhydrous ammonia gas comes into contact with water, 1,300 gallons of gas can be absorbed by 1 gallon of water. The combination of anhydrous ammonia and water forms **ammonium hydroxide**, a caustic alkaline solution that corrodes metals and causes progressive chemical burns of soft tissue.

Storage Requirements

Ammonia tanks and the tank control valves should be made of iron because anhydrous ammonia will attack copper, zinc, brass, or bronze alloys, resulting in heavy corrosion to the control valves. All anhydrous ammonia storage tanks are required to carry a 5-gallon container filled with water to irrigate burns (Figure 11.2). Individuals working around anhydrous ammonia should also carry a small squeeze bottle of water in a shirt pocket to irrigate any burns, especially of the eyes. The water in the squeeze bottle can be used to irrigate burns until the individual reaches a larger water supply, such as the container on the tank.

Anhydrous ammonia explosions or ruptures can occur either as a result of a **boiling liquid expanding vapor explosion (BLEVE)**, or be-

CHAPTER 11 Hazardous Materials

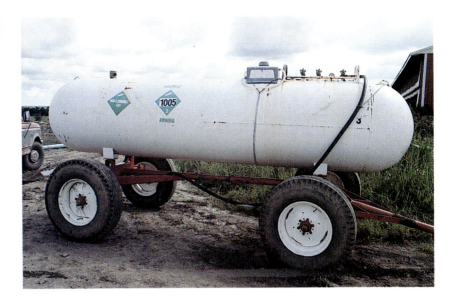

FIGURE 11.2

Anhydrous ammonia storage tanks carry a 5-gallon container of water to irrigate the eyes or skin in the event of a spill.

cause excessive pressure causes a hose to burst or a tank end to separate. The compression will heat the liquid in the tank, increasing its vapor pressure until the tank ruptures violently with a large release of energy. Because liquid ammonia expands as temperature rises, ammonia tanks should not be filled to more than 85% capacity. Each tank should be equipped with a level gauge that shows the percent of liquid in the tank, and a pressure gauge that indicates internal pressure.

A dangerous situation can occur if the same storage tanks, transport containers, and associated equipment are used for both anhydrous ammonia and liquid propane because of their similar vapor pressures. Anhydrous ammonia tanks use black iron fittings; propane tanks use nonporous bronze fittings. If ammonia is stored in a tank designed for liquid propane, the ammonia can corrode the bronze fixtures, which can cause leaks to occur. A mixture of anhydrous ammonia and propane gas that is subjected to burning from drying grain may emit a number of toxic gases, including carbon dioxide, carbon monoxide, and cyanide, during the combustion process.

Mechanisms of Injury

Anhydrous ammonia causes injuries in three ways. First, clothes and skin will immediately freeze when they come into contact with the liquid because the liquid stored in the tank has a temperature of –28°F when released. Second, chemical burns may occur if the anhydrous ammonia comes into contact with moist body tissue to create ammonium hydroxide. The eyes, which are 80% water, are especially vulnerable, as is lung tissue. This chemical burning process will continue until the ammonium hydroxide is completely diluted. Consequently, irrigation with water is the best immediate treatment. Third, dehydration may occur because anhydrous ammonia will remove fluid from the body tissue.

Personal Safety

Rescuers called to an incident involving anhydrous ammonia should approach from upwind, wearing full bunker gear (rubber boots, bunker pants and coat, lined rubber gloves, hood, goggles, helmet with face shield) and equipped with a positive pressure self-contained breathing apparatus (SCBA). The best way to disperse the ammonia cloud is to use a fire hose with the nozzle set for wide stream or fog spray. The water from the spray will attract most of the vapor, which will enable rescuers to approach and remove the patient and control the leak. The source of the leak can be identified from the visible stream of white vapor. An easy and effective way to plug an ammonia vapor leak is with an air bag. Simply belt the air bag to the tank and inflate the air bag. It will act like a plug and be a serviceable patch. If a fire hose is not available, and a rescuer must enter the cloud alone, a safety harness, safety line, protective clothing, and an SCBA must be worn.

Management of Exposure

Tissue damage due to chemical burns begins immediately. Therefore, continuous irrigation should begin the minute the rescue team reaches the patient—the more water, the better. Irrigating with water will dilute the ammonium hydroxide and attract any free ammonia present. If the water supply is limited or unavailable, juice, cold coffee, tea, or soft drinks may be substituted. The importance of continuous irrigation cannot be emphasized enough; it is essential that irrigation be started the minute the rescue team reaches the patient and should continue until the patient is delivered to definitive medical care. Irrigation for 15 minutes is usually sufficient for other types of burns, but with burns caused by anhydrous ammonia, irrigation should be continuous—from the time the team reaches the patient—until the patient reaches definitive medical care.

Anhydrous ammonia will travel to moist areas of the body, such as the armpits, groin, under tight clothing and watchbands, or inside shoes and boots. If clothing is frozen to the patient's body, begin irrigation immediately, literally dousing the patient with water. This will "thaw" the clothing, and enable it to be cut away from the body with surgical shears. Remove all clothing, including shoes or boots, and flush the entire body with water. The rescue team should wear protective clothing while treating the patient, including rubber gloves with a thin cotton lining to provide thermal protection.

A patient who has been exposed to anhydrous ammonia will be in considerable pain and have moderate to extreme dyspnea caused by chemical burns to every part of the body touched by the ammonia. The eyes will be especially affected (Figure 11.3), and the patient may have considerable traumatic eye injuries, such as ruptured globes, if struck by a stream of liquid ammonia. The patient's eyes will likely be tightly shut due to the pain, but it is important to force them open to begin irrigation.

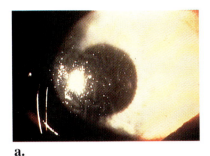 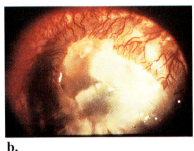 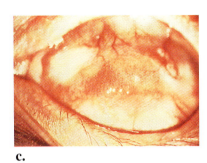

a. b. c.

FIGURE 11.3
a. A caustic burn of an eye caused by anhydrous ammonia. An ammonia burn is not easily diluted and continues to damage the eye.
b. Five days later the eye is seriously damaged.
c. Ten days later the eye is destroyed. Even after 24 hours of irrigation, the ammonia continues to damage the eye tissue.

An effective technique for irrigating the eyes can be improvised using a nasal cannula, infusion tubing, and normal saline solution or sterile water in IV bags or bottles. Apply the cannula over the bridge of the nose with the patient in a supine position. Insert the infusion line into the IV bag or bottle and connect it to the inlet of the cannula. Place an emesis basin under each ear to collect the solution. With this technique, about 100 mL/min of irrigation is provided, and the patient's eyelids can be held open with your fingers or by everting the lids with cotton swabs.

In addition to the eyes, the mouth and throat may also be burned from exposure to anhydrous ammonia. A conscious patient should constantly rinse these areas with water. An unconscious patient should be placed in a side-lying position to irrigate the mouth.

Do not apply salves, ointments, or dressings to a patient exposed to anhydrous ammonia. If oxygen is needed, use a nasal cannula set at high flow rather than an oxygen mask because the mask may trap ammonia against the skin. Elevate the head and shoulders so the irrigant may run off the patient's body, unless the eyes have been contaminated. In that case, the eyes will need to be irrigated as well so the patient will have to lie flat. Do not put anything on the skin until the body has been thoroughly irrigated. In situations involving anhydrous ammonia, 15 minutes of irrigation is not enough. Irrigation should continue until the patient is delivered to the nearest hospital burn unit. Again, the more water, the better. Rapid transport is necessary to help save the patient's sight; helicopter or air ambulance may be necessary.

Large-scale ammonia leaks pose a potential threat to those living or working downwind from the leak. If the leak cannot be controlled, these people should be evacuated.

PESTICIDES

Most farms use some type of pesticide, making the potential for an incident very real. By law, all pesticide containers must bear a label that provides the chemical makeup, the relative toxicity of the product, and emergency care instructions. These may be a primary source of information during a rescue operation.

Toxicity

Toxicity refers to the level of poison in a pesticide. Of more than 24,000 registered pesticides, only a few are highly toxic. Container labels are required to indicate the level of toxicity using three standard words. Low-toxicity pesticides are designated by the signal word "Caution"; moderately toxic pesticides are labeled "Warning"; highly toxic pesticides often show a skull and crossbones on the label along with the signal words "Danger–Poison" (Figure 11.4). Table 11.3 indicates the toxicity levels, product examples, and potentially lethal doses of some common pesticides. The lethal dose shown refers to an adult of average weight; it would be much less for a 50-lb child, and might be slightly more for a 200-lb adult.

Exposure

In order for pesticide poisoning to occur, the pesticide must be taken into the body. Toxic materials are absorbed by the body in three ways:
- The mouth and digestive system (oral exposure)
- The skin (dermal exposure)
- The nose, mouth, and respiratory system (inhalation exposure)

Oral exposure is usually due to carelessness. An individual may try to blow out a plugged applicator or nozzle, or smoke or eat without washing after using a pesticide, or eat fruits or vegetables that have recently

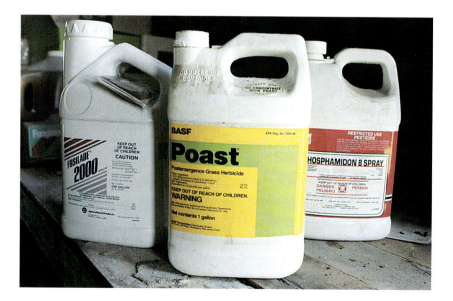

FIGURE 11.4

The label of a pesticide container will indicate the level of toxicity with the words "Caution," "Warning," and "Danger–Poison."

TABLE 11.3 Toxicity Levels of Common Pesticides

Key or Signal Word	Toxicity	Product Examples	Lethal Dose (oral dose to human of 150 lb)
Danger-Poison	Highly toxic / concentrated	Counter® Disyston® Parathion Furadan® Dyfonate®	Less than 1 teaspoon
Warning	Moderately toxic	Diazinon Sonalan® Lorsban® Dursban®	1 teaspoon to 1 tablespoon
Caution	Slightly toxic	2,4-D Sevin® Atrazine Malathion	1 oz to more than 1 pt

been sprayed. Children may also eat pesticides lying around in unmarked containers.

Dermal exposure can occur any time a pesticide is mixed, applied, or handled. A splash or spill can result in dermal exposure, particularly with liquid pesticides. The severity of dermal exposure depends on the toxicity of the pesticide, the rate of absorption through the skin, the amount of skin area contaminated, and the amount of time that the material is in contact with the skin.

Rates of absorption for dermal exposure differ for various parts of the body. For example, absorption is over 11 times faster in the scrotal area than on the forearm. Exposure of the scrotal area to pesticides approximates a direct injection into the bloodstream. Table 11.4 shows absorption rates for various body parts.

Inhalation exposure can occur when an individual is in a field or area while it is being dusted or sprayed, or as the pesticide is being mixed prior to application.

Personal Safety

Rescuers should avoid contact with any pesticide and should always wear protective clothing during a rescue operation involving a possible pesticide incident. Wear disposable water-repellent clothing, such as Tyvek coveralls, or a waterproof rubber coat to provide skin protection. Rubber gloves made of neoprene or nitrile, boots, a wide-brimmed hat, and goggles should also be worn. A self-contained breathing apparatus (SCBA) may be necessary if the pesticide is airborne over a large area (Figure 11.5).

Take time to carefully question family members or co-workers to try to determine the route of exposure. Locate the container and read the

TABLE 11.4 Absorption Rates

Body Part	Rate of Absorption
Forearm	1.0
Palm of hand	1.3
Ball of foot	1.6
Abdomen	2.1
Scalp	3.7
Forehead	4.2
Ear canal	5.4
Scrotal area	11.8

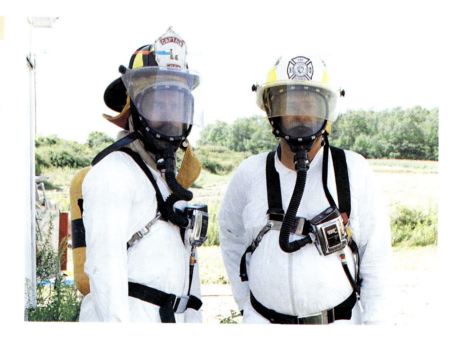

FIGURE 11.5

Rescuers entering a hazardous materials incident should wear appropriate protective clothing, including an SCBA.

label. Many containers will contain guidelines and/or requirements specifying the correct type of protective clothing and equipment to use. The container may also contain a statement of practical treatment or a "note to physician" describing the appropriate medical procedure for poisoning cases and may even indicate an antidote (Figure 11.6).

In all cases of pesticide poisoning, timely emergency medical treatment is vital to the survival of the patient. Some pesticides do not have a specific antidote; others can only be treated by a physician. Patient survival often depends on the speed with which emergency medical care can be initiated.

FIGURE 11.6

Some pesticide containers provide a "note to physician" that describes appropriate medical treatment for a poisoning and possibly an antidote.

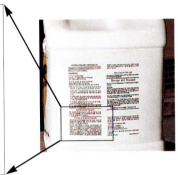

Major Incidents

Agricultural pesticides are applied in a number of ways. Some may be mixed in irrigation systems; others are sprayed by tractors, pickup trucks, or tank units; still others are applied from the air. If the incident involves an automobile accident, a tractor upset, or a plane crash, rescuers will have to deal with two situations—the extrication and rescue of the operator or pilot, and the release of pesticides in the air, onto land, and in water. In such cases, it is vital to know the type of pesticide involved, so that adequate protection for rescuers, bystanders, and the patient can be provided.

SIGNS AND SYMPTOMS OF PESTICIDE POISONING

Five common classes of pesticides pose the most significant health hazards to humans. They are organophosphates, carbamates, fumigants, organochlorines, and bipyridyls. All pesticides in a given chemical group will have similar effects on the body. It is important to know both the type of pesticide in use and the particular signs and symptoms associated with that pesticide.

Organophosphates and Carbamates

Organophosphates and carbamates are involved in most instances of pesticide poisoning. They are widely used in agricultural, horticultural, and household insecticides. Although the signs and symptoms of poisoning may vary slightly, both chemicals act in the same manner once in the body. Both will inhibit cholinesterase, an enzyme essential to the proper functioning of the nervous system.

Symptoms will begin shortly after exposure. In milder cases, symptoms can manifest anytime up to 12 hours after exposure, but usually within 4 hours. In acute cases, symptoms may appear during exposure.

Signs and symptoms associated with mild exposure to organophosphate and carbamate pesticides are similar to those for flu, heatstroke, heat exhaustion, or upset stomach. They include the following:

- Headache, fatigue, dizziness
- Loss of appetite with nausea, stomach cramps, and diarrhea
- Blurred vision and excessive tearing

- Constricted pupils
- Excessive sweating and salivation
- Slowed heartbeat, often fewer than 50 beats per minute
- Rippling of muscles just under the skin

The same signs and symptoms are associated with moderately severe cases of organophosphate and carbamate poisoning. However, because the chemical is affecting the nervous system, additional signs and symptoms will be present:

- Inability to walk due to weakness
- Chest discomfort and tightness or difficulty in breathing
- Marked constriction of the pupils (pinpoint pupils)
- Muscle twitching
- Incontinence
- Pulmonary edema with a productive cough
- Profuse secretion from the eyes, nose, mouth, and skin

Severe poisoning is indicated by incontinence, unconsciousness, and generalized seizure activity.

The order in which signs and symptoms appear may vary, depending on how the pesticide was absorbed into the body. If it was swallowed, stomach and other abdominal manifestations commonly appear first; if it was absorbed through the skin, gastrointestinal and respiratory signs and symptoms tend to appear simultaneously.

Fumigants

Fumigants are insecticides used to treat and protect stored grain, greenhouse crops, and stored fruits and vegetables. Methyl bromide and aluminum phosphide are two common commercial fumigants. Exposure to and absorption of these products is usually through inhalation. Soil fumigants are also used in greenhouses.

The signs and symptoms of fumigant poisoning will differ, depending on the product. However, headache, dizziness, nausea, and vomiting are common early signs and symptoms of severe exposure. The appearance of intoxication is also a sign.

Phosphine fumigants, such as aluminum phosphide, are most commonly involved in on-farm poisonings and during commercial or rail transportation. These products are sold in a solid form, such as tablets, pellets, or packed powder, and are usually used in confined spaces such as grain storage structures. Aluminum phosphide contained in commercial grain storage and grain in transit should be placarded. When this fumigant is exposed to the normal moisture content of air, phosphine gas is released. Phosphine gas depresses the central nervous system and irritates the bronchial and gastrointestinal membranes, making breathing difficult.

Early signs and symptoms of phosphine poisoning include fatigue, buzzing in the ears, nausea, an uncomfortable feeling or pressure in the chest, and general uneasiness. If a small amount of poison is ingested, these signs and symptoms may be the extent of the illness. Mild exposure is signaled by a sensation of cold, chest pain, diarrhea, vomiting, and fluid in the lungs. There may also be a cough, tightness in the chest, difficulty in breathing, weakness, thirst, and anxiety. Severe exposure is indicated by stomach pain, loss of coordination, cyanosis, pain in the limbs, dilated pupils, choking, and stupor. Severe poisoning leads to seizures, coma, and death.

Halocarbon fumigants, such as methyl bromide, affect the central nervous system in addition to the enzyme systems, heart, and liver. The manufacturer's label for methyl bromide cautions that gloves are not to be worn during application of this chemical, due to the strong reaction that would occur if the pesticide is trapped between the skin and gloves. Rescuers should keep this in mind during any incident involving methyl bromide. Respiratory protection is essential. Table 11.5 shows common signs and symptoms of fumigant poisoning and recommended treatment.

TABLE 11.5 Common Signs and Symptoms of Fumigant Poisoning

Type of Fumigant	Signs and Symptoms	Recommended Treatment
Phosphine Fumigants Aluminum phosphide Phosphine gas	**Mild exposure:** Cold sensation; chest pain; diarrhea; vomiting **Moderate exposure:** Coughing; tightness in chest; difficulty in breathing; weakness; thirst; anxiety **Severe exposure:** Stomach pain; loss of coordination; cyanosis; pain in limbs; dilated pupils; choking; stupor; seizures or coma	Move patient to fresh air. Keep patient quiet and in a semireclining position to facilitate breathing. If patient is still breathing, give 100% humidified oxygen by nonrebreathing mask. If breathing has stopped, give mouth-to-mouth or mouth-to-nose resuscitation. If there is no pulse, attempt CPR. Immediately transport to nearest emergency department.
Halocarbon Fumigants Methyl bromide	**Moderate exposure:** Nausea; dizziness; headache; unusual fatigue and weakness; blurred vision; slurred speech **Severe exposure:** Abdominal pain; mental confusion; tremors; convulsions; difficulty in breathing	If patient was exposed to these fumigants in a liquid form through skin contact, redness, blistering, and deep ulcers may also be present. In addition to moving patient to fresh air and giving oxygen, remove the patient's clothing and wash the skin surface immediately with soap and water.

Rescuers should be particularly cautious in dealing with fumigants. Because rescue operations involving these poisons usually occur in confined spaces, rescuers should always wear a self-contained breathing apparatus (SCBA), a safety harness, and a safety line (Figure 11.7). Extricating a patient from this type of environment always requires one inside rescuer wearing protective clothing, an SCBA, a safety harness, and a safety line, and one rescuer similarly equipped outside the confined space.

Organochlorines

Many organochlorines have been banned by the U.S. Environmental Protection Agency (EPA) because they are not readily biodegradable; therefore, they persist in the environment. Organochlorines include DDT, chlordane, and endrin. Although they are no longer commercially available, these chemicals may be stored on farms in old, leaking containers without labels.

Organochlorines affect the central nervous system as stimulants or convulsants. They are readily absorbed through the skin and stomach lining. If the patient ingested the poison, nausea and vomiting will be the first symptoms. If the poison was absorbed through the skin, the first signs and symptoms will be apprehension, twitching, tremors, confusion, and convulsions.

Other early signs and symptoms include excitability, dizziness, headache, disorientation, weakness, and a tingling or prickling sensation on the skin. As the poisoning proceeds, there may be loss of coordination, recurrent convulsions similar to epileptic seizures, and unconsciousness.

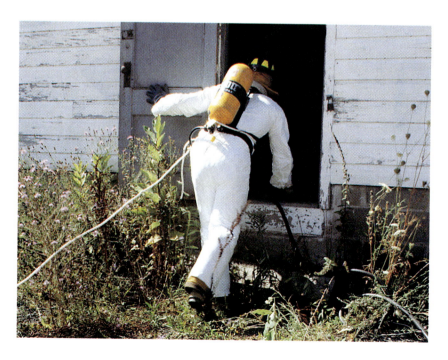

FIGURE 11.7

A rescuer entering a confined space in a hazardous materials incident should be attached to a safety line.

To avoid cross contamination, rescuers should wear neoprene or nitrile gloves and protective clothing, such as Tyvek coveralls, along with appropriate foot, eye, and head protection. Emergency care includes removing the patient's contaminated clothing immediately and bathing and shampooing the patient to remove the pesticide from the skin and hair. If the route of entry was oral, and the patient is still conscious, contact medical control for instructions.

Bipyridyls

Bipyridyls are herbicides used frequently on farms. The most common bipyridyls are gramoxone, paraquat, and diquat. Of the three, the least harmful is gramoxone. It has a strong odor and contains an emetic. This means it is also the least likely to be accidentally ingested, and if it is ingested, the emetic will make the person vomit so the poison will not cause much harm to the body.

Paraquat is the most toxic of the bipyridyls. It irritates the skin, causing it to become dry or cracked. Repeated exposure produces chronic abnormal cell growth in the skin and fingernails (which often turn black), as well as in the nasal mucosa, lungs, cornea, and lens of the eye. Ingesting paraquat causes severe irritation to the mucous membranes of the mouth, pharynx, esophagus, and stomach. The patient may feel an immediate burning sensation, followed by nausea, pain, and diarrhea. Repeated vomiting generally follows, with restlessness and hyperexcitability.

Ingestion of 6 to 8 oz of paraquat can cause fatal fluid accumulation in the lungs within 24 to 72 hours. Smaller doses will result in decreased urine production during the first 6 days and jaundice due to liver damage. These initial signs and symptoms may moderate over the next several days, and the patient will appear to improve. However, the poison will continue to spread throughout the body, concentrating in pulmonary cells, and causing irreversible and progressive lung damage. The result is respiratory failure due to the rapid growth and development of abnormal fibrous connective tissue over the alveolar surfaces of the lungs, preventing proper lung functioning.

There are no specific antidotes to counteract the effects of significant exposure and absorption of paraquat and other bipyridyl herbicides. If rescuers arrive within an hour of ingestion, administering fuller's earth or bentonite will help, as will inducing vomiting. If the absorption is through the skin, wash the skin immediately with soap and water and flush the eyes, if affected, with water. Do not administer oxygen unless the patient is obviously having difficulty breathing. High levels of oxygen will accelerate fibrous tissue growth in the lungs, so do not administer supplemental oxygen unless the patient is having difficulty breathing.

Rodenticides

Rodenticides are agents that kill, repel, or otherwise control rodents, and include strychnine, zinc phosphate, and several types of anticoagulants. Strychnine is a deadly poison and is lethal in very small doses. Anticoagulant rodenticides have a good safety record because they contain such low concentrations that massive ingestion is necessary for symptoms to develop.

The most likely causes of strychnine poisoning in humans are suicide attempts and accidental ingestion by children. Strychnine is not easily absorbed through the skin, nor does it accumulate in the human body. However, it has an almost immediate effect on the central nervous system. The patient becomes hypersensitive to external stimuli such as loud noises, light, and sudden movements. These stimuli may trigger violent seizures and severe convulsions within 10 to 30 minutes after ingestion. During the seizures, the patient may stop breathing. Death results from asphyxiation.

If the patient has not begun convulsing, try to empty the stomach. If seizures have begun, do not induce vomiting. Instead, eliminate or minimize outside stimuli. Place the patient in a warm, dark room and reduce noise levels. With strychnine poisoning, it is better to bring medical support to the patient, rather than transport the patient to a medical center because the movement will trigger additional convulsions. Advanced life support providers should administer an appropriate anticonvulsant and intubate, if possible, until medical support arrives.

While strychnine affects the central nervous system, anticoagulants affect the blood. They block the production of prothrombin, thin the blood, and prevent the blood from clotting. Poisoning from these types of rodenticides usually occurs because a child finds and eats the bait. If a small amount is ingested, there may not be any signs or symptoms. Acute poisoning is indicated by nosebleeds, bleeding gums, rectal bleeding, abdominal and back pain, anemia, or hematemesis. Hemorrhaging may occur if very large quantities are ingested.

Basic level care includes administering oxygen, treating for shock, and transporting to definitive medical care, particularly if the amount of poison ingested is unknown or if the patient has a history of liver problems or clotting dysfunction. A pneumatic antishock garment (PASG) should only be applied under the direction of medical control. Advanced life support providers should initiate an IV with blood volume expanders and draw blood for typing, crossmatching, and coagulation studies.

HYDRAULIC FLUIDS

Many types of farm equipment use hydraulic operating systems, which contain hydraulic fluid under extremely high pressure (2,000 to 2,700 psi or more). An engine-driven hydraulic pump generates energy that is transmitted through external hoses and transformed into linear or rotary motion by hydraulic cylinders and motors. The pump is equipped with a

CHAPTER 11 Hazardous Materials

relief valve to limit the maximum system pressure. Manual control valves start, stop, and direct the flow of fluids.

Mechanisms of Injury

Injuries can occur when an individual is running a hand along a hose or cylinder, looking for leaks by feel in the hydraulic system (Figure 11.8). The individual may also be checking fuel injectors or cleaning hands or clothing with an air gun. If the system is under pressure (3,600 psi), finely atomized hydraulic oil can be injected through the skin from a pinhole leak in a hose. Hydraulic oil or diesel fuel is injected through the skin without creating an open wound.

These injuries are extremely painful because hydraulic fluids are petroleum-based hydrocarbons that contain highly caustic antifoaming and anticorrosive additives. These additives irritate the skin and body tissue and may be toxic when introduced internally. In addition, the high temperature of the fluid will cause internal thermal burns.

Within minutes, the skin around the injection site will discolor to an unusually bright blue. Swelling of the affected area develops rapidly. Within 30 minutes, lack of oxygen to the blood and tissue necrosis will cause the skin to turn black. Occasionally, the fluid will travel along the soft tissue planes and bones of the hand and wrist several inches from the injection site, settling in the soft tissue of the palm or forearm. It may even penetrate completely through the hand, with an entry and exit point, usually an open wound.

Immediate treatment should focus on keeping the liquid localized so it does not spread into the bloodstream. The petroleum-based chemicals and additives could cause death if they reach the bloodstream. Keep the patient calm. Do not elevate the extremity above the level of the heart, or give the patient anything to eat or drink. Remove any rings or watches. Use insulated cold packs to cool the affected area, treat the patient for shock secondary to pain, and provide rapid transport to definitive medical care. Surgical removal of contaminated tissue (debridement) will be necessary once the patient reaches the hospital. Advanced life support providers at the scene should initiate an IV in an uninjured limb. *If within their scope of practice*, they may add pain medication.

A less serious injury can occur if a hose or fitting breaks completely, showering the individual with hot oil (200°F or more). Thermal injuries

FIGURE 11.8

a. This patient's hand was lanced, and the hydraulic fluid was allowed to drain from the hand.
b. The hand eventually healed.

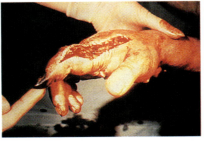
a.

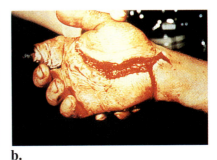
b.

may be exacerbated by chemical burns and contamination. Wash first-degree burns with soap and cool water; flushing alone will not remove the oil from the skin. If the eyes are injured, flush continuously during assessment, treatment, and transport. Use the same system to irrigate the eyes as that described for exposure to anhydrous ammonia.

Personal Safety

Rescuers at the scene should wear protective gear, including helmets with face shields, goggles, coats, boots, and heavy leather gloves. This gear will also protect rescuers from injury while using their own hydraulic extrication equipment. Naturally, the equipment must be examined carefully as part of planning and preparation, but hose or fitting failures may still occur, especially if the equipment is operated at or above its rated capacity. Always wear leather gloves when checking a hydraulic hose for leaks. Leaks may be located by moving a piece of cardboard or a small mirror along the hose to see if fluid is being sprayed. Never run a hand (even a gloved hand) along a hose to find a leak.

PROTECTION

In any situation involving hazardous materials, both rescuers and patients must be protected from further injury or contamination. Rescuers must consider all potential hazards and develop a strategy to minimize the danger. The three main factors to consider when attempting to minimize exposure are time, distance, and shielding.

Time

The longer an individual is exposed to a hazard, the higher the probability of injury. Prolonged exposure also contributes to the degree of injury. When managing a rescue operation, consider the time factor. Rescue teams should be rotated to reduce exposure to an acceptable level and keep the exposure time to a minimum.

Distance

The greater the distance between the rescuer and a hazardous material means less exposure. Rescuers and other individuals not directly involved in the rescue operation, particularly bystanders, must be kept at a safe distance. This distance may vary from product to product.

Shielding

Shielding refers to all protective equipment used by the rescuer during a hazardous materials incident. Rescuers must be familiar with protective equipment and clothing necessary for a hazardous materials incident. Never assume that minimum protective clothing alone will provide adequate protection from a hazardous material.

Required protective garments and equipment vary according to the type of hazard and the degree of exposure. Table 11.6 shows the EPA four-level classification for protective equipment to assist rescuers in determining the level of protection required. Classification is based on the degree of protection provided to the skin and respiratory tract.

Levels C, B, and A require the use of special chemical-resistant clothing, gloves, eyewear, and so on. Most rescuers do not have this type of equipment immediately available. Those who do must select gear based on the most likely route of entry of the hazardous material: absorption, inhalation, or ingestion. Most rescuers will use level D or possibly level B protection.

Level D clothing can be adapted to provide additional protection for very short periods of time. For example, if a rescuer is wearing fire service protective equipment, using a hood, turnout pants, and gloves with long gauntlets will help. Turnout gear, however, provides minimal protection against exposure because it is designed only for fire, heat, and water protection. The use of bands or duct tape around areas where openings occur, such as wrists, ankles, waists, and zippers, will help reduce exposure. Chemical-resistant gloves, disposable booties, and an SCBA enhance this level of protection. However, remember that this type of equipment provides only limited protection and should be used only in the event of lifesaving emergency. Street clothing does not provide any significant protection.

A major problem with using substitute protection is that the hazardous material may enter and pass through the materials, thereby reducing effective working time. In addition, substitute materials, especially natural fibers, may create absorption and contamination problems. Many materials are damaged by both corrosive and noncorrosive hazardous materials. For example, the Nomex material used in fire protective clothing can be damaged when the material comes in contact with petroleum products, which are considered noncorrosive hazardous materials. The petroleum product attaches to the Nomex and will con-

TABLE 11.6 EPA Classifications of Protective Equipment

EPA Level	Degree of Protection Provided	Protective Garments and Equipment
D	Minimal skin and respiratory protection	Minimum protective clothing, including boots, helmet, gloves, and eye protection
C	Some skin and respiratory protection	Chemical-resistant coveralls, gloves, eye protection, respiratory protection
B	Some skin and excellent respiratory protection	SCBA, chemical-resistant coveralls, gloves, eye protection
A	Maximum skin and respiratory protection	Totally encapsulated system with SCBA

tinue to adhere to the Nomex, regardless of washing. When heated, the petroleum product will vaporize, creating a hazardous, flammable condition that can endanger the wearer.

The degree of protection required is determined by the data collected in the early stages of the incident. If the type(s) of hazard, the required task(s), and the type(s) of protective equipment available are known, the rescue team can make an informed decision about the advisability of entering the hazardous area to perform the required work.

The label on the container of an agricultural chemical or pesticide can provide vital information from which the team can make decisions about how to proceed. The label will provide protective clothing and equipment guidelines and/or requirements for the specific chemical. The toxicity of the product influences the selection of the clothing and equipment.

DECONTAMINATION

Exposure to hazardous materials can be reduced by proper contamination control. Disposable water-repellent clothing, such as Tyvek coveralls, will help limit contamination of usual work clothes. These items can then simply be disposed of properly without further treatment after the rescue. **Decontamination** is the process of removing toxic and other harmful materials and properly disposing of them. It is an important part of all incidents involving hazardous materials, regardless of the materials involved or the size of the incident. Containment and decontamination must be included in the initial planning of all hazardous materials incidents.

Three generally accepted methods of decontamination can be used when dealing with people: dilution, absorption, and chemical washes. When dealing with materials, a fourth option, disposal and isolation, can be used.

Dilution uses copious amounts of water to flush hazardous residues from personnel and equipment. The runoff water must be contained and disposed of properly. The addition of a mild detergent may speed the decontamination process.

Water is the most commonly used solution for dilutional decontamination. Other common solutions are listed below:

1. Sodium carbonate (washing soda)—5% to 10% aqueous solution; a good water-softening agent and effective for inorganic acids.
2. Sodium bicarbonate (baking soda)—5% to 10% aqueous solution; an amphoteric (behaving either as an acid or a base), it is effective with most acids and bases.
3. Trisodium phosphate (TSP, Oakite)—5% aqueous solution; a good water-softening agent, detergent, and general rinse solution.

4. Combination—an aqueous solution of 5% sodium carbonate and 5% trisodium phosphate.
5. Calcium hypochlorite (HTH)—10% aqueous solution; a disinfectant, bleaching and oxidizing agent that requires considerable care in storage, preparation, and application. When heated above 212°F, HTH will explode. It will also react with water or steam to produce toxic, corrosive fumes and can react vigorously with reducing materials. This product is used to purify water and treat swimming pools.

Absorption is used primarily for equipment, but has limited application for people. Materials such as anhydrous fillers, soil, and other commercially available products are used to pick up the contaminant from the surface of equipment and people. Absorbents should be used only by trained personnel.

Chemical washes alter the hazardous material to a nonhazardous by-product. These can be used to wash down equipment, and some may be used on people.

Disposal and isolation is the process of discarding contaminated materials by packing and shipping them to an approved dump or incinerator. In some cases, equipment cannot be decontaminated and must be disposed of, no matter how expensive or irreplaceable.

Before using a piece of equipment in a hazardous materials incident, ask the following questions:

1. Will the equipment withstand the required decontamination process?
2. After decontamination, can the equipment be sterilized, if required?
3. Can the equipment be tested for residual contamination?

If the answer to any of these questions is "no," the equipment may have to be disposed of after the incident. That can be an expensive proposition, particularly if the equipment was not really needed for the rescue operation.

Decontamination should be done initially at the incident site. In an incident involving pesticides, check the label on the pesticide container for information on decontamination. Each label is required to provide a statement of practical treatment, which may include decontamination instructions. Clothing contaminated with highly concentrated and/or highly toxic pesticides should be discarded using disposal directions found on the pesticide container label.

Decontamination of contaminated protective gear should be done in a step-by-step process, beginning with the removal of the outer layers of clothing without touching the contaminated portion(s). Gloves and respiratory protection should be worn throughout the process. Assistants should wear the same kind of protective clothing as the rescuers. Final decontamination may require a total body wash. Rescuers should shower immediately after returning to the station.

The following guidelines for laundering can generally be used with low-concentration or slightly toxic pesticides:

1. Wear waterproof gloves when removing or handling pesticide-contaminated clothing. Wash the gloves thoroughly before removing them, and then dispose of them carefully. Do not use them for any other task.
2. Collect the clothing separately from all other laundry. Wash the contaminated garments as soon as possible, separately from all other laundry.
3. Always pretreat contaminated clothing. Soak in water, hose down out of doors, or use a commercial prewash product.
4. Launder clothing (do not dry clean) using hot water and a phosphate (powdered) or heavy-duty liquid detergent. Wash water should be at least 120°F, and preferably 140°F. Increase the amount of detergent to 1.25 times the recommended amount, especially if the fabric was previously treated with a water-repellent finish. If water is moderately hard, increase the amount of detergent used to at least 1.75 times the recommended amount. Wash only a few garments at a time, using a full water level and a normal (12-minute) wash cycle. (Note: Some chemicals have a unique response to laundering. Paraquat is an example. The presence of salt ions in water will facilitate decontamination. Adding one-quarter cup of salt for each 5 gallons of water significantly improves the ability of laundering to lower residues. Check the container label or contact the manufacturer for more information.)
5. Use fabric starch and if possible, line dry. Pesticide residues cling to fabric starch and will be washed away in subsequent wash cycles. Starch also inhibits the penetration of pesticides into the clothing fibers. Line drying is recommended because many pesticides will break down in sunlight.
6. Wash clothing more than once to draw out excess residues. Clothing contaminated with only slightly toxic pesticides may be effectively decontaminated in one to three machine washings. More washings are needed for clothes contaminated with more toxic or more concentrated pesticides. If excessive contamination has occurred, burn or bury the clothing.
7. Clean the washer after use. Wash down the inside of the tub and run a cycle (with or without detergent) before using the machine to launder other items.
8. Hang protective clothing, such as turnout coats that might not be successfully laundered, in moving air to maximize evaporative dissipation.

No research has been done on decontaminating leather or rubber, so these guidelines do not pertain to items made of these materials.

MANAGEMENT OF EXPOSURE

Patients exposed to anhydrous ammonia, pesticides, hydraulic fluids, or other hazardous materials may also have traumatic injuries or other illnesses as a result of the incident. Avoid aggravating those injuries during management of the hazardous exposure.

The most common problem for rescuers is determining whether to give priority to the patient's medical condition or to manage the situational hazard. If both a rescue team and a medical team are on the scene, the rescue team can turn its attention to the situational hazard after moving the patient to safety, and the medical team can focus on stabilizing and treating the patient. However, even the medical team may have to decide whether measures to control hemorrhaging, shock, respiratory, or cardiovascular problems are of greater or equal urgency than those to treat the hazardous materials exposure.

All required assessment and treatment measures have to be performed in rapid sequence or by simultaneous team action. Patients sustaining an injury during such an incident require a modified approach if a hazardous exposure is known or suspected. If the patient is stable, he or she must be decontaminated prior to treatment. In many incidences of pesticide exposure by absorption, decontamination is the primary treatment, such as in a rescue operation in which anhydrous ammonia is involved.

Personal Safety

Rescuers should train while wearing protective equipment in order to become proficient at providing medical care during a hazardous materials rescue operation. This will also help the team understand its limitations. For example, in a situation involving anhydrous ammonia, a patient must be moved to an uncontaminated area as quickly as possible. But preparing the patient for movement may not be easy when rescuers are wearing protective equipment. Cardiopulmonary resuscitation (CPR) cannot be performed easily when rescuers are wearing protective equipment, and may not be possible in a toxic gas situation.

Rescuers can best protect themselves in hazardous materials situations by knowing the extent of the situation before attempting the rescue. Preincident planning is vital. Learn all you can by questioning bystanders, examining the situation carefully, and using circumstantial evidence to measure the risk. If the risk of working in the hazardous atmosphere seems acceptable, all equipment and personnel should be protected as much as possible within the limits of the operation. Anticipate treating all individuals involved in the operation as possibly exposed and contaminated.

Managing Ill or Injured Patients

If patients with traumatic injuries or other medical illnesses are exposed to certain hazardous materials, decontamination should be accomplished as soon as the situation permits. Lifesaving measures for a traumatic injury or some medical problems must be given priority over immediate decontamination despite the possible increase in chemical injury to the patient caused by the delay. The general principle is as follows: better blistered and living than decontaminated and dead.

The recommended sequence for emergency action when a contaminated patient has other injuries or illnesses is listed below:

1. Control respiratory failure with assisted ventilation.
2. Control massive hemorrhaging (bleeding) with pressure dressings.
3. Administer an antidote or treatment, if available.
4. Decontaminate the face.
5. Remove contaminated clothing as soon as possible, and always before the patient is moved indoors or into the transport vehicle.
6. Decontaminate the skin (with the most sensitive areas first) where required.
7. Provide additional emergency medical care for shock, wounds, and illnesses that are so severe that delay may endanger the patient's life.
8. Manage and stabilize injuries.
9. Transport to definitive medical care.

Always alert the receiving facility as to the type of exposure, the extent of potential contamination, and the degree of decontamination accomplished on site. Hospital personnel may then be adequately prepared and protected. Remember that rescuers must be protected during the decontamination process according to the principles outlined earlier in this chapter.

Hazardous materials exposure may cause rapid changes in a patient's condition; therefore, continuous monitoring is required. Medical personnel should be prepared for and able to recognize the potential changes caused by the patient's exposure.

Contamination Control During Transport

In incidents involving anhydrous ammonia, pesticides, and hydraulic fluids, rapid transport to the nearest medical facility equipped to handle the emergency is vital. During transport, the patient should be considered contaminated even though decontamination procedures were conducted at the site. Transport personnel should wear appropriate protective clothing and continue contamination control procedures during transport. This may involve wrapping the patient in an impermeable sheet, or continuous flushing of the skin.

Ambulances or other transport vehicles should be prepared before transporting a contaminated patient. The transport should be made in a vehicle with a partition between the driver and patient compartments to prevent exposing the driver to the hazardous materials. To reduce contamination in the vehicle, drape the inside of the vehicle with plastic, remove all unnecessary items, and seal cabinet drawers and doors with tape before loading the patient.

Remember to maintain contamination control at all times. Proper cleaning and/or disposal of protective clothing and equipment used during the rescue will also ensure that adequate contamination control is maintained.

Secondary exposure of people not actually involved in the incident could lead to serious illness and occasionally results in death. However, in many of these situations, rescuers did not properly use effective contamination control procedures. As a result, they carried the hazard into their homes.

SUMMARY

Incidents involving hazardous materials can be dangerous to rescuers, but they can be managed. Agricultural pesticides are powerful and dangerous chemicals. Rescuers must be prepared to make an initial assessment of the rescue site, and to plan the rescue operation carefully. Three factors must be considered:

- Protection for both rescuers and patients
- Contamination control
- Management of exposure and injuries

Anhydrous ammonia is a fertilizer that forms ammonium hydroxide when it contacts water. This caustic chemical will cause chemical burns, tissue dehydration, and tissue freezing. Water—and lots of it—is the only way to dissipate anhydrous ammonia.

Incidents involving pesticides may require special precautions, based on the toxicity of the product. An important source of information for rescuers is the pesticide label itself, which should contain an indication of toxicity and directions for treatment. Pesticides labeled "Caution" have low toxicity; those labeled "Warning" are moderately toxic; and those marked "Danger–Poison" are highly toxic. Rescuers must be able to recognize the signs and symptoms of pesticide poisoning and must take prompt action to prevent serious consequences.

Hydraulic fluids under high pressure are another hazardous material encountered by rescuers in agricultural-rural settings. Because rescue equipment often uses hydraulic fluids and is under considerable pressure, rescuers must be careful to check all valves, fittings, and hoses before a rescue.

CHAPTER 12

Medical Care in the Rescue Setting

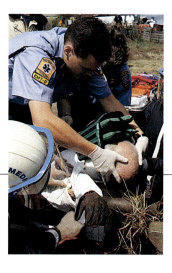

CHAPTER OUTLINE

Overview
Objectives
Rescue and Medical Care
Extended Transport
Information Gathering
Personal Safety

Communications
    Radio Communications
    Written Communications
Deceased Persons
Summary

KEY TERMS

Extended incident: situation in which the time from the initial injury to definitive medical care is longer than 2 hours.

Golden hour: the period after an injury in which the patient's body is able to compensate for the injury and remain relatively stable.

LAST: acronym that presents the four separate phases of rescue (Locate, Access, Stabilize, Transport).

SOAP: acronym that represents a method of relaying patient information commonly used by medical personnel (Subjective, Objective, Assessment, Plan).

CHAPTER 12 Medical Care in the Rescue Setting

OVERVIEW

There are important distinctions that set rescue emergency medical care apart from conventional, ambulance-based, rapid-transport emergency medical care. Rescue emergency medical care places greater demands on rescuers in terms of their medical training, individual responsibility, and ability to assess situations and make decisions. In agricultural-rural settings, a long period of time usually elapses from the time the incident occurs to delivery of the patient to definitive medical care. Response and patient transport times may also be extensive. Rescuers may even be required to improvise equipment and use medical procedures that differ from conventional, rapid-transport situations.

This chapter reviews common problems that rescuers may encounter and basic emergency procedures that rescuers may perform during rescue operations. It emphasizes the steps that need to be taken in every rescue situation. In addition, the extended transport often required in agricultural-rural areas will affect how emergency medical care is administered.

In some areas, a special medical team will work with a rescue team; the rescue team will have primary responsibility for scene safety, access, and extrication while the medical team will have primary responsibility for medical care, stabilization, and transport. In some areas, one team will perform both functions. In any situation, it is important that each team understands the other's functions. The greater the rescuer's understanding of anatomy, physiology, and basic emergency medical care, the more effective he or she will be as a rescuer. The greater a medical team's understanding of the principles of extrication, the more efficiently they will be able to work with rescuers and provide needed care. It is also critical that rescuers operate under medical control and perform only those procedures and use equipment that is within their scope of practice.

This text assumes that rescuers have a basic knowledge of conventional, rapid-transport emergency medical care and basic life support procedures such as cardiopulmonary resuscitation (CPR). For additional specific information and review, consult *Emergency Care and Transportation of the Sick and Injured*, published by the American Academy of Orthopaedic Surgeons, and *Standards and Guidelines for Cardiopulmonary Resuscitation*, published by the American Heart Association.

> **OBJECTIVES**
>
> After reading this chapter, the rescuer should be able to:
>
> - identify common problems encountered during a rescue operation.
> - list the basic procedures performed during a rescue operation.
> - describe the effects of extended transport.
> - explain the information-gathering process during a rescue operation.
> - identify important principles of rescuer safety.
> - describe medical communications during a rescue operation.
> - describe requirements regarding handling deceased persons.

RESCUE AND MEDICAL CARE

In an agricultural-rural rescue operation, cooperation between the rescue team and medical team is critical. During a rescue operation, the rescue team must often simultaneously rescue the patient and provide medical care. If a separate medical team accompanies the rescue team to the incident, rescue and medical care efforts must be coordinated. Each rescue technique must be evaluated for its effect on the patient's condition, and, as a result, rescue and/or medical priorities may change during the rescue. For example, are the dangers so great that the patient must be moved to a safe area before any medical care is provided? Should an IV line be started before or after the patient is extricated? Is the patient protected from the hazards of the rescue operation?

While theoretically there are four separate phases of rescue signified by the acronym **LAST** (**L**ocate, **A**ccess, **S**tabilize, **T**ransport), in many rescue situations the phases will overlap. The stabilize phase typically includes providing medical care to the patient. However, medical care will often begin before the stabilize phase and must continue after it.

The stabilize or medical phase continues during transport of the patient. Basic life support and all other treatment procedures initiated during the stabilize phase must continue while the patient is being transported to definitive medical care. Therefore, rescuers must consider the effect of all transport techniques on the patient's medical condition.

The primary objective during transport is to maintain the patient in a stable condition. Therefore, the patient's physical and mental status must be monitored during transport. The importance of ongoing evaluation of the patient's condition cannot be overemphasized. To do this effectively, at least one rescuer or medical care provider must be assigned to monitor the patient during transport.

EXTENDED TRANSPORT

Conventional, ambulance-based, rapid-transport emergency care, based on the U.S. Department of Transportation National Standard Curriculum, assumes a quick response, speedy access to the patient, expeditious assessment and stabilization, and rapid transport to definitive medical care. During agricultural-rural incidents, however, the transport of a patient to definitive medical care may be delayed or may require an extended period of time. Depending on the specific incident, it may be hours or days before a patient is delivered to definitive medical care. This extended time frame may be caused by delay in discovery of the incident, patient entrapment, difficult patient access or extrication, travel time to and from the incident site, or adverse environmental conditions such as weather or flooding.

Extended incidents are situations in which the time from the initial injury to definitive care is longer than 2 hours. A number of potential extended incident situations in which rescuers may need to provide emergency medical care are listed below:

- Entanglement in farm machinery or overturns
- Entrapment in confined spaces
- Hazardous materials incidents
- Storms or hazardous weather conditions
- Long transport time
- Natural disasters such as earthquakes or flooding
- Structural disasters such as a building collapse or cave-in
- Difficult terrain

An extended incident may affect rescuers in a variety of ways, including:

1. Assuming additional patient care responsibilities. Instead of a brief period of responsibility for patient stabilization, rescuers may have to provide some of the medical assessment and care that might ordinarily be done at the hospital. During a rescue operation, there may be prolonged periods without direct communication with medical control or others having higher level skills. Rescuers must rely entirely on their training and experience.

2. Exercising definitive assessment skills and perspectives. Rescuers must develop assessment techniques and skills so they can detect subtle, hidden, or late-appearing signs and symptoms that indicate serious medical management problems not commonly seen during rapid transport.

3. Anticipating problems. During extended incidents, a patient's condition may deteriorate. Rescuers must be able to detect immediate medical problems and anticipate those that may develop. Anticipating and recognizing signs of deterioration may help in preventing or delaying them.

4. Improvising equipment. In most extended incidents, equipment will be limited. In rural areas with difficult access, it may not be possible to carry enough equipment or have enough personnel to meet every possible medical need. Therefore, rescuers must be able to improvise equipment and solutions. The rescue team must be able to use equipment that can serve many different purposes.

5. Basing patient assessment on clinical signs and symptoms rather than on readings from diagnostic equipment. During a rescue operation, there may be limited equipment to aid in patient assessment. The environment may prevent the use of routine diagnostic tools. Rescuers must use their senses of sight, hearing, touch, and smell to detect the often subtle changes in the patient's condition.

6. Extending the "golden hour" for patients with traumatic injuries. The **golden hour** is the period after an injury in which the patient's body is able to compensate for the injury and remain relatively stable. After this period, morbidity and mortality increase tremendously as the critically injured patient becomes increasingly unstable. This period of danger does not end until definitive medical care, such as surgery, is provided. Rescuers must learn those techniques within their scope of practice that will help to extend the patient's "golden hour." These may include the use of a pneumatic antishock garment (PASG) or advanced life support (ALS) techniques such as IV fluids, intubation, or medications.

7. Coping with increased stress. Extended incidents put rescuers at greater risk for emotional stress from greater patient care responsibility and fatigue. Psychological stresses are often a factor if patients suffer or die despite the best efforts of the rescue team. It may also be difficult to face long-term exposure to dead bodies.

8. Attending to basic personal needs of the patient. During extended incidents, rescuers must provide the patient with food and water, ensure the patient's physical comfort, provide emotional support and reassurance, and attend to personal hygiene, including urination and defecation. Rescuers must also prevent the patient from becoming chilled, overheated, or dehydrated.

9. Modifying rapid-transport procedures and techniques. During extended incidents, the patient's condition may deteriorate beyond conditions normally found in conventional, rapid-transport situations.

CHAPTER 12 Medical Care in the Rescue Setting

The environment may change the patient's response to treatment, or severe environmental conditions may affect the manner in which rescuers can provide patient care. For example, rescuers may need to modify traditional approaches to the following: when to stop CPR; how to realign certain types of dislocations; how to manage open wounds; and when to remove impaled objects.

Remember, do not perform procedures or use equipment beyond your scope of practice. Operate under local medical protocols that are approved by medical control.

INFORMATION GATHERING

Rescue operations are often hampered by missing, incomplete, or unreliable information. This may occur because communications are difficult or impossible. The reporting party may be excited, confused, or frightened. Or a reliable observer may not be able to reach the scene to confirm the facts.

When the initial report of an incident comes in, gather as much information as possible, particularly the following:

- Description of the incident
- Potential hazards to the rescue team or the patient(s)
- Condition and number of patients
- Potential required equipment, both for the rescue and emergency care

The information-gathering process should continue even as the rescue team responds to the scene. As additional information becomes available on the nature of the incident, the team must be prepared to adapt to the changing conditions. The dispatcher should continue gathering information on the incident and advise the team of any significant changes.

PERSONAL SAFETY

The most important aspect of any rescue operation is the personal safety of the rescue team, as well as the safety of everyone else involved in the operation. It is essential that rescuers avoid becoming victims of the incident themselves. If any member of the team is injured, there is a greater burden and additional risk to all others involved in the rescue operation.

The first step in ensuring rescuer safety is to evaluate the scene. This begins when the first notice is received. The person taking the call must ask the caller about any local hazards. Before leaving for the scene, the team must gather appropriate gear and equipment for protection against any local hazard and against other general or long-term threats such as the weather.

Upon arriving at the scene, the rescue team must evaluate the site before entering it. An unstable or threatening scene must be stabilized before the team enters, regardless of the patient's condition. If two members of the rescue team enter a silo filled with silo gas without proper breathing apparatus to rescue a patient, the local media will most likely report three deaths rather than one.

After entering the scene, rescuers must protect the patient from further injury from threats, including overhead power lines, hazardous materials, falling objects, animals, or extremes in weather. This may mean moving the patient before beginning treatment. Rescuers must also protect the patient from any dangers inherent in the tactics used in the rescue operation, such as flying debris, heat, noise, or force.

Before transporting the patient, evaluate the evacuation route, pinpoint potential hazards, and take appropriate precautions or actions to neutralize the hazards.

Members of the rescue team must also constantly evaluate one another's mental and physical states. Overexcited or fatigued rescuers are a danger to themselves, other rescuers, and the patient.

COMMUNICATIONS

Accurate and definitive communications between rescuers and a medical facility are important for good patient care. In an extended incident, rescuers may need additional guidance or instruction from medical control on the care of the patient as the medical or rescue conditions change. When this communication is possible, a rescuer must be able to describe the patient's condition to medical control in an accurate, intelligent, and precise manner. During extended incidents it is also important to provide dependable, concise follow-up assessments, describing changes in the patient's status over time.

A second important reason to provide accurate and definitive communications is to obtain assistance in the field. This assistance might include higher-level medical expertise, a second or third rescue team, more physical help for transporting patients or equipment, specialized rescue equipment or transportation such as helicopters, and relief for fatigued rescuers. Good communications also help the receiving medical facility prepare for the arrival of the patient.

A comprehensive medical communications system helps rescuers discipline themselves to perform complete and accurate patient assessments, which are necessary during extended incidents. Reporting complete information provides an additional advantage in a rescue operation. An accurate assessment and precise communication of the patient's condition improves the chances for a successful rescue operation and the patient's survival.

Before communicating the patient's condition, write down the information to be delivered in a systematic way. This written information will help a rescuer transmit a complete message in the most effective, efficient manner possible. A written record of the patient assessment and planned treatment also provides necessary documentation of patient care.

Radio Communications

During a rescue operation, use the radio only to request assistance, to report the initial assessment of the patient, or changes in the patient's condition or the status of the rescue operation. Stay off the air unless there is new information to transmit. Following these guidelines, rescuers maintain a professional demeanor, decrease their work load and that at the receiving facility, keep the frequency clear for other radio traffic, and save battery power.

Written Communications

Diligent documentation of patient care is essential in all rescue operations. Litigation is increasing in rescue emergency care, even for those rescuers who are volunteers. Memory is not dependable. Write down everything found during the patient assessment and everything done for or to the patient. In a legal sense, if it is not written down, then it was not done. Although rescuers may wish to use their state's model ambulance run sheets for documentation in a rescue situation, it may be more convenient to use a smaller, modified form that prompts rescuers to collect all the essential information.

The **SOAP** format is a logical and efficient method of documenting patient information that will improve communications discipline. It is commonly used by all levels of medical personnel to provide a **S**ubjective description, an **O**bjective description, an **A**ssessment of the problems, and a **P**lan for medical treatment (Figure 12.1).

In extended incidents, careful documentation will improve continuity of patient care, especially if additional or advanced-level rescuers relieve the original team, and when the patient arrives at the receiving medical facility.

DECEASED PERSONS

Rescuers must follow their state's statutory requirements that relate to such actions as declarations of death and the removal of dead bodies. In some rescue environments, the officials normally responsible for declaring death or giving permission to remove a body may not be able to reach the scene. In some of these cases, they may give verbal permission to rescuers to do so. Rescuers must document this permission.

FIGURE 12.1

The SOAP format organizes information in a logical sequence to describe the patient's condition, assess the problems, and plan medical management.

> **S** Subjective
> **O** Objective
> **A** Assessment
> **P** Plan
>
> **S Subjective**
> A listing of the patient's symptoms and history (what the patient or bystanders have told you).
>
> **O Objective**
> Results of the patient exam and vital signs (what you have found from your observations and examination of the patient).
>
> **A Assessment**
> A list of problems and anticipated problems that you develop using your training and experience to assess the subjective and objective data you just collected.
>
> **P Plan**
> Treatment plan for each listed problem or anticipated problem.

However, the best approach is to establish written protocols on handling the deceased before such an incident occurs.

Before removing a body, completely document the scene and situation with photographs, sketches, and a written description.

SUMMARY

There are basic steps that must be taken in every rescue situation. An extended incident, however, presents unique problems, such as providing ongoing medical care until the patient is delivered to definitive medical care. Because of the prolonged period of time in an extended incident, the patient may develop more severe medical problems than would be seen during a conventional, ambulance-based, rapid-transport situation. Rescuers must use their assessment skills for long-term evaluation of a situation.

Anticipating problems, improvising equipment, and managing stress are essential skills for rescuers in an extended incident. In addition, gathering information, evaluating rescuer and patient safety, and establishing accurate communications are necessary components of any rescue operation. But they are especially crucial during an extended incident. Rescuers must also be prepared to handle deceased persons and therefore, must understand the legal requirements for doing so.

CHAPTER 13

Patient Assessment in Rescue Medical Care

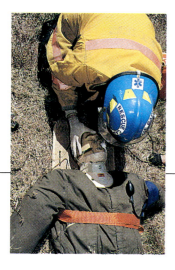

CHAPTER OUTLINE

Overview
Objectives
The Patient Assessment
    System
  Scene Survey
  Primary Survey

Secondary Survey
Vital Signs
History
Assessment
Plan
Summary

KEY TERMS

AMPLE: acronym used for recording a patient's history (Allergies, Medication, Pertinent medical history, Last meal, Events).

AVPU scale: method by which to measure level of consciousness based on four factors: Alert, Verbal, Pain, Unresponsive.

Patient Assessment System (PAS): seven-step assessment system based on the widely used SOAP format.

Primary survey: examination that covers immediate life-threatening conditions, commonly known as ABCD (airway, breathing, circulation, disability).

Secondary survey: complete head-to-toe examination of the patient, to be completed before beginning any treatment other than basic life support (BLS) or advanced life support (ALS).

CHAPTER 13 Patient Assessment in Rescue Medical Care

OVERVIEW

Patient assessment is the critical first step in any emergency medical situation. But in an extended incident, thorough patient assessment is even more important because rescuers are responsible for the patient for a longer period of time. In addition to managing the patient's current condition, rescuers must anticipate and be thoroughly prepared to manage any additional problems that may develop while the patient is in their care.

Patient assessment does not end with the initial examination. In an extended incident, patient assessment is an ongoing process that continues for as long as the patient is in the rescuer's care. Even if the patient is stable, reassessments should be done every 15 to 20 minutes. The more severe the injuries or potential injuries, the more frequently the patient must be reassessed.

This chapter explains the seven-step Patient Assessment System (PAS). Each step, which includes specific procedures for assessment and reassessment, is described in detail. In addition, a sample case history is presented to illustrate the development of a problem list with an accompanying management plan that addresses each real and potential problem.

OBJECTIVES

After reading this chapter, the rescuer should be able to:

- describe the importance of patient assessment in an extended incident.
- list the seven steps in the Patient Assessment System (PAS).
- identify common procedures that a rescuer should use to evaluate and re-evaluate the patient's condition.
- list methods for identifying problems, and then develop a plan to manage current or potential problems.

THE PATIENT ASSESSMENT SYSTEM

To ensure that no critical aspect of the patient's condition is missed, patient assessment must be done using a methodical, step-by-step system. One such assessment method is known as the **Patient Assessment System (PAS)**. The PAS is a seven-step system based on the widely used SOAP format. The first four steps of the PAS are as follows:

1. Scene survey
2. Primary survey

3. Secondary survey
4. Patient history, including vital signs

These first four steps provide the necessary information for the next three steps, the assessment and planning phases:

5. Assessment of problems
6. Plan for treatment
7. Continuing reassessment of patient

The PAS provides a framework for many of the activities involved in emergency medical care, including patient triage, assessment and management, patient monitoring and reassessment, communications discipline, and records/documentation.

Scene Survey

Hazards The first step in assessment is to survey the incident before entering the scene. The safety of all those involved in a rescue—both rescuers and patients—is the primary concern during any rescue operation. A survey of the scene may take a little extra time, but it may prevent additional injuries or death and avoid complicating the rescue operation. Surveying the scene includes identifying any threats or hazards to the safety of the patient or the rescue team. Such threats may include unstable objects or unsecured equipment, fires, downed power lines, frightened or wild animals, the presence of poisonous gases or other hazardous materials, or unsafe human situations such as a crowd of bystanders.

Do not enter a rescue scene until all the threats and hazards have been stabilized, neutralized, or secured. Do not approach or enter a rescue scene unless you have the appropriate protective clothing, equipment, and training. And when threats or hazards at a rescue scene have been identified, notify all other rescuers about their existence.

Mechanism of Injury or Illness As you enter the scene, briefly survey the area for indications of the mechanism of injury or illness. Rescuers with some knowledge of the factors involved in producing the injury or illness will have a better idea of the nature and extent of the patient's potential injuries. Knowledge of the mechanism of injury or illness will also assist hospital personnel in treating serious injuries. The typical mechanisms of injury that suggest major trauma in agricultural-rural incidents include falls of more than 15'; tractor or combine overturns; entanglements in augers, balers, or PTOs; falling objects; and crush injuries.

Some typical injuries that might be revealed by knowing the mechanism of injury include spinal and abdominal injuries caused by tractor overturns. The force of the overturn would cause spinal injuries, and the trauma of striking the steering wheel or penetration by a gear handle would cause abdominal injuries.

Primary Survey

The purpose of the **primary survey** is to uncover immediate life-threatening conditions that affect the three major body systems—the circulatory, respiratory, and nervous systems (both central and peripheral nervous systems). It includes assessing the ABCs—airway, breathing, and circulation. To these, add a "D"—disability—which includes conditions such as spinal injuries that could lead to disability.

The ABCD elements of the primary survey can be performed in sequence or simultaneously, but they all must be covered before beginning the head-to-toe physical exam. Stop and treat any problems found in the primary survey ("red flags") as you find them (Table 13.1). Only if there are no problems ("normal responses") can you continue with the physical exam.

Basic life support (BLS) and advanced life support (ALS) are performed only if there are problems or "red flags" in the primary survey. Local protocols, available resources, scope of practice, and level of training will determine the level of care that may be provided in a given circumstance as you strive to maintain the circulatory, respiratory, and nervous systems.

Rescuers involved in extended incidents need to be aware of the changing attitudes regarding the management of cardiac arrest sec-

TABLE 13.1 ABCD Elements of a Primary Survey

Normal Responses	Red Flags
A AIRWAY The patient's airway is clear so that he or she can breathe.	Air is not moving in or out (the airway is obstructed).
B BREATHING The patient is breathing, and/or ventilation is adequate.	The patient is not breathing, and ventilation is not adequate.
C CIRCULATION The patient has a carotid pulse, and there is no severe bleeding.	The patient has no carotid pulse, and/or there is severe bleeding.
D DISABILITY There is no mechanism for possible spinal injury, AND there is no obvious spinal injury, AND the patient has a normal pain response, AND the patient's level of consciousness is classified as alert.	There is a mechanism for spinal injury, AND/OR there is an obvious spinal injury, AND/OR the patient has an altered pain response, AND/OR the patient's level of consciousness is limited to responses to verbal or painful stimuli or the patient is unresponsive.

ondary to traumatic injuries and in settings where there will be a period of time greater than 30 minutes until advanced life support can be initiated. Refer to local protocols and current American Heart Association standards in these areas.

Secondary Survey

Physical Exam The head-to-toe exam of the patient should be completed before beginning any treatment other than BLS or ALS. Avoid focusing on a dramatic injury such as a fracture or skull laceration. If you do, you may miss other injuries that might be more serious but less obvious, such as spinal injury or blunt trauma and internal injury to the chest or abdomen. Visually inspect the site of any injury. To do this, pull or cut clothing away from the injury site. Long-term exposure in a severe environment, such as snow or a hot open field, could worsen the patient's condition. Therefore, move the patient out of a severe environment as quickly as is possible.

To ensure that nothing is missed or omitted, you must consistently conduct the exam in a logical order such as area by area. You may adopt a different order, but make certain you do so in a way that prevents the possibility of overlooking a potential injury, as shown in Table 13.2.

Once the entire exam is completed, you may need or want to return to a specific area for further inspection.

Vital Signs

Changes in a patient's vital signs over a period of time can provide important clues about the patient's progress or deterioration. Be cautious about relying on only one set of vital signs or a single exam to indicate that a patient is doing well. For example, low blood pressure may be a *late sign* of shock. When a patient's blood pressure begins to drop, he or she may already be in a great deal of trouble. An increasing pulse rate might have provided an early warning of impending shock. What is more important is the *change* and *pattern of change* in vital signs over time. If transport time is extended, continue to monitor the patient's condition en route to the hospital. Frequent reassessments will allow you to recognize clinical patterns, such as hypovolemic shock, as they develop.

Time Every time that you take a set of vital signs, document the time and values. A series of vital signs has no meaning unless the time is recorded.

Blood Pressure If possible, record both systolic and diastolic blood pressure because the relationship between the two is important in some medical conditions. However, environmental conditions or lack of equipment may prevent you from recording the diastolic pressure.

A significant change in blood pressure will usually result in changes in the pulse rate. If the patient is alert and oriented, and the pulse rate is steady and normal, then it may not be necessary to recheck the blood

TABLE 13.2 Area by Area Physical Exam

Head	Chest	Legs
Eyes	Abdomen	Arms
Ears	Pelvis	Neurologic
Nose	Genitalia	Back
Mouth/Throat		Buttocks
Neck		

pressure as often as with an unstable patient. This can be an important practical matter during an extended or difficult evacuation.

Pulse Record the pulse according to rate. Use terms such as "regular" or "irregular" that have meaning to other people, and avoid subjective terms such as "weak" and "thready."

Respiration Record the respiration rate and describe it in terms such as "regular" or "irregular," "easy," or "difficult." If the patient is able to speak without difficulty, he or she is probably not experiencing any serious respiratory difficulties.

Level of Consciousness Describe the patient's level of consciousness as precisely as possible. Avoid vague descriptions such as "semiconscious." One commonly used measurement of level of consciousness is the **AVPU scale**.

- **A** **Alert.** The eyes open spontaneously. The patient answers questions in a clear and appropriate manner. The patient can state the date, the location, and his or her own name. The patient is oriented.
- **V** Responds to **Verbal** stimulus. The eyes do not open spontaneously. The patient is not oriented to time, place, and person. There is some manner of response when spoken to.
- **P** Responds to **Painful** stimulus. The patient does not respond to verbal stimuli, but does move or cry out in response to pain.
- **U** **Unresponsive** (unconscious). The patient does not respond to any stimulus.

"Alert" patients are often described by their behavior such as hysterical, disoriented, frightened, relaxed, calm, or cooperative.

FIGURE 13.1

Use a methodical system to record assessment findings.

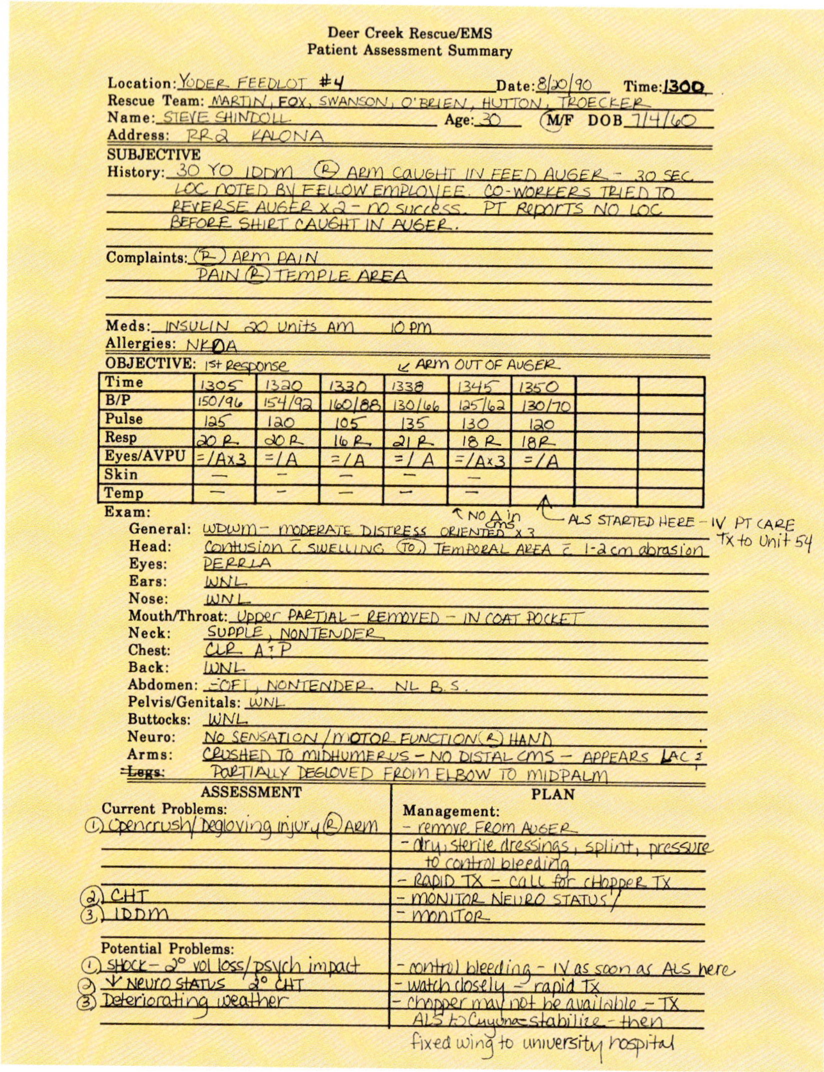

```
                    Deer Creek Rescue/EMS
                    Patient Assessment Summary

Location: YODER FEEDLOT #4            Date: 8/20/90    Time: 1300
Rescue Team: MARTIN, FOX, SWANSON, O'BRIEN, HUTTON, TROECKER
Name: STEVE SHINDOLL           Age: 30   (M)/F  DOB 7/4/60
Address: RR 2  KALONA
SUBJECTIVE
History: 30 YO IDDM  (R) ARM CAUGHT IN FEED AUGER - 30 SEC
         LOC NOTED BY FELLOW EMPLOYEE. CO-WORKERS TRIED TO
         REVERSE AUGER x 2 - NO SUCCESS. PT REPORTS NO LOC
         BEFORE SHIRT CAUGHT IN AUGER.

Complaints: (R) ARM PAIN
            PAIN (R) TEMPLE AREA

Meds: INSULIN  20 units AM   10 PM
Allergies: NKDA
OBJECTIVE: 1st Response          ← ARM OUT OF AUGER
```

Time	1305	1320	1330	1338	1345	1350		
B/P	150/96	154/92	160/88	130/66	125/62	130/70		
Pulse	125	120	105	135	130	120		
Resp	20 R	20 R	16 R	21 R	18 R	18 R		
Eyes/AVPU	=/Ax3	=/A	=/A	=/A	=/Ax3	=/A		
Skin	—	—	—	—	—	—		
Temp	—	—	—	—	—			

```
Exam:                      ↑ NO A in          ← ALS STARTED HERE - IV  PT CARE
                              EYES x 3                             TX to Unit 54
  General:  W/W/W - MODERATE DISTRESS  ORIENTED x 3
  Head:     CONTUSION c̄ SWELLING (TO) TEMPORAL AREA c̄ 1-2 cm abrasion
  Eyes:     PERRLA
  Ears:     WNL
  Nose:     WNL
  Mouth/Throat: UPPER PARTIAL - REMOVED - IN COAT POCKET
  Neck:     SUPPLE, NONTENDER
  Chest:    CLR  A&P
  Back:     WNL
  Abdomen:  -OFI, NONTENDER.  NL B.S.
  Pelvis/Genitals: WNL
  Buttocks: WNL
  Neuro:    NO SENSATION/MOTOR FUNCTION (R) HAND
  Arms:     CRUSHED TO MIDHUMERUS - NO DISTAL CMS - APPEARS LAC c̄
  Legs:     PARTIALLY DEGLOVED FROM ELBOW TO MIDPALM

            ASSESSMENT                    PLAN
Current Problems:                  Management:
① Open crush/degloving injury (R) ARM   - remove FROM AUGER
                                   - dry, sterile dressings, splint, pressure
                                     to control bleeding
                                   - RAPID TX - call for CHOPPER TX
② CHT                              - MONITOR NEURO STATUS
③ IDDM                             - monitor

Potential Problems:
① SHOCK - 2° vol loss/psych impact  - control bleeding - IV as soon as ALS here
② ↓ NEURO STATUS  2° CHT            - watch closely - rapid TX
③ Deteriorating weather             - chopper may not be available - TX
                                      ALS to Cuyuna - stabilize - then
                                      fixed wing to university hospital
```

Temperature It is important to know the core body temperature of a patient, particularly in environmentally caused conditions, such as hypothermia and heat exhaustion. Oral and skin temperatures are not always accurate measurements of the patient's temperature. The most accurate way to assess temperature is with a rectal thermometer, but conditions may not permit you to use one. If it is not possible to take a rectal temperature, estimate temperature by clinical signs and history.

Skin Color/Temperature/Moisture The condition of the skin and the appearance of the nail beds are indicators of blood perfusion to the skin and extremities, the body's shell. For example, decreased perfusion will change the color of the lips from deep to pale red. Skin color is not a reliable indicator of core temperature, nor is it a reliable indicator in parts exposed to the cold.

History

The patient's history is recorded using the acronym **AMPLE**.

- **A** Allergies
- **M** Medication
- **P** Pertinent past medical history
- **L** Last meal
- **E** Events (what happened to the patient?)

The patient's history should include any preexisting illness or significant previous injuries, particularly to the same body parts.

Assessment

The scene survey, primary and secondary assessments, and history provide a data base of information that can be used to assess the immediate problems and potential problems facing the patient. Develop a list of all the problems and anticipated problems that you determine from your evaluation of the information.

Plan

After developing a problem list, plan how to manage each current problem, and any anticipated problems that might arise.

The Patient Assessment Survey shown in Figure 13.1 was completed, using the SOAP format, for a 30-year-old, insulin-dependent diabetic man whose right arm became entangled in an auger. The entanglement resulted in crushing and degloving injuries from the midhumerus to the fingers in the right arm. He had a witnessed 30-second loss of consciousness that had resolved by the time the rescue team arrived.

SUMMARY

While patient assessment is an important first step in a rescue operation, it is also an ongoing process. Rescuers must be prepared to manage any medical problems that arise.

A methodical system, such as the Patient Assessment System (PAS), should be used to assess patients. The seven steps of the PAS are as follows:

1. Scene survey
2. Primary survey
3. Secondary survey
4. Patient history
5. Assessment
6. Planning
7. Reassessment

Each step has established procedures that enable rescuers to perform a thorough evaluation of the patient.

CHAPTER 14

Common Medical Conditions and Injuries

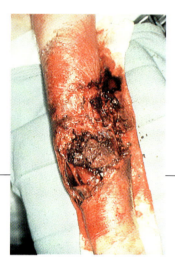

CHAPTER OUTLINE

Overview
Objectives
Injuries in Agricultural-Rural Settings
   Traumatic Injuries
   Polytrauma
   The Big Net Principle
Common Medical Conditions
   Respiratory and Cardiac Arrest
   Shock
   Autonomic Stress Reaction
Common Injuries
   Head Injuries

Closed Soft Tissue Injuries
Fractures of the Spine
Musculoskeletal Injuries
   Dislocations
Wounds
   Types of Wounds
   Impaled Objects
   High-Pressure Injection Injury
Burns
   Assessment
   Treatment
Patient Control
Summary

KEY TERMS

Autonomic stress reaction (ASR): temporary reduction in perfusion of the brain in response to extreme emotional situations, such as fear and bad news.

CHAPTER 14 Common Medical Conditions and Injuries

Big net principle: method of anticipating the worst case scenario to avoid overlooking injuries or complications.

Multiple trauma: incident in which there are two or more patients.

Perfusion: the circulation of blood within an organ or tissue.

Polytrauma: injuries that involve multiple body systems.

Rule of Nines: method used to determine the percentage of the total body surface area burned.

Shock: a condition of acute peripheral circulatory failure causing inadequate and progressively failing perfusion of tissues.

Trauma: the transfer of the energy of movement to the body tissues, resulting in injury.

OVERVIEW

The types of injuries and illnesses rescuers encounter in agricultural-rural settings are remarkably similar from incident to incident. Overturns of equipment cause crushing injuries. Entanglements in equipment may result in amputation or degloving injuries. Entrapment in grain or exposure to pesticides and other toxins may result in suffocation. Burns from fires or electrical injuries are also common.

This chapter discusses the types of injuries common in agricultural-rural settings. It also reviews some of the most common medical conditions that occur in association with these injuries. Assessment findings and appropriate management techniques for each are also discussed. While the chapter does not cover all situations, the most common injuries and illnesses are discussed in step-by-step fashion.

OBJECTIVES

After reading this chapter, the rescuer should be able to:

- describe the mechanisms of injury for common medical conditions and injuries encountered in an agricultural-rural setting.
- explain how to assess common medical conditions and injuries encountered in an agricultural-rural setting.
- describe appropriate treatment of common medical conditions and injuries encountered in an agricultural-rural setting.

INJURIES IN AGRICULTURAL-RURAL SETTINGS

Most patients in agricultural-rural incidents will have sustained some form of traumatic injury. To understand why particular injuries occur in certain instances, it is important to understand some basic laws of physics, as well as anatomy and physiology. Rescuers must be able to predict the type and severity of the injuries based on their knowledge of mechanisms of injury. By using this knowledge, they will also be able to anticipate the potential complications and conditions associated with these injuries.

Traumatic Injuries

Trauma is the transfer of the energy of movement to the body tissues, resulting in injury. To understand trauma, rescuers need to understand the laws of motion and kinetic energy, the energy of motion (Figure 14.1).

Understanding Traumatic Injuries To estimate the degree of trauma, you must understand the relationship between kinetic energy and the mass of the moving object and its velocity. The mathematical formula for this relationship is as follows: kinetic energy = (mass × velocity^2) ÷ 2.

In simple terms, if you double the mass involved in a collision, you will double the amount of energy that can cause tissue damage. That is why there is more damage to a tractor when it is hit by a semitractor trailer than when it is hit by a half-ton pickup truck. But if you double the velocity of the object, you quadruple the energy that can cause tissue damage. That is why there are many more broken parts when a tractor is hit by a car traveling 50 mph, than when hit by one traveling only 25 mph (Table 14.1).

Mechanism of injury. Trauma generally results from two types of forces—compression and deceleration. With compression injuries, tissue is crushed between two objects—for example, a hand caught in a baler. Deceleration injuries occur when the body stops suddenly but organs or tissues within the body continue until they strike another object.

FIGURE 14.1

An understanding of the laws of motion and kinetic energy will help in determining the type and severity of injuries encountered in the agricultural-rural setting.

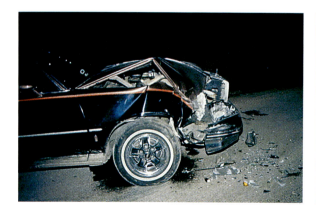

$$K.E. = \frac{MV^2}{2}$$

(M = mass)
(V = velocity)

TABLE 14.1 Kinetic Energy

Assume a 155-lb (70 kilo) object traveling at 30 mph, the kinetic energy (KE) would be:

$$\text{kinetic energy} = \frac{\text{mass} \times \text{velocity}^2}{2}$$

$$\text{kinetic energy} = \frac{(155) \times (30)^2}{2}$$

kinetic energy = 69,750

For comparison, look at what happens with changes in mass and velocity:

	155 lb (70k)	165 lb (75k)	200 lb (90k)
30 mph	69,750	74,250	90,000
40 mph	124,000	132,000	160,000
60 mph	279,000	297,000	360,000

An aortic tear caused by a fall from a height is an example of a deceleration injury. Most injuries will be a combination of these two forces, such as the ruptured spleen that occurs in an unrestrained driver whose automobile was traveling at a high rate of speed until it was stopped by a bridge abutment.

Compression injuries are frequently classified as blunt or penetrating trauma. In blunt trauma, the kinetic energy is spread over a greater area of the body. This compresses the soft tissues and ruptures or breaks underlying organs and bones. To understand how a direct impact on solid organs such as the spleen, liver, or kidney can cause lacerations and contusions leading to internal bleeding, remember that the solid organs are filled with fluid (blood). They behave much like a well-filled water balloon on impact. An example of a blunt injury is the ruptured spleen that results when the handlebars of a dirt bike hit the abdomen.

An impact will tend to move aside hollow organs such as the stomach and intestines so they are usually not seriously disrupted. They may also pop like a balloon if severely compressed when filled. The bladder will behave like a hollow organ when it is empty, but like a solid organ when full. Rib fractures can injure the lungs, which may also pop if compressed while the patient was inhaling.

Penetrating trauma is the result of a localized application of force that drives an object through the skin, injuring the underlying tissues. High-velocity penetrating injuries may have a zone of injury beyond the area of direct contact with the object such as the cavitation effect of a high-velocity gunshot wound. Do not rely on the size of the surface wound to assess the extent of injury in penetrating trauma.

A rotational injury is an indirect injury caused by twisting forces transmitted to a distant body part, such as when a shirt is caught in a PTO. A levering injury occurs when a lever effect disrupts structures at a distance from the point of impact. An example of a levering injury is a person who falls from a bicycle onto an outstretched arm which forces an anterior dislocation of the shoulder.

Anticipating Problems First survey the scene to determine the mechanism of injury, and then estimate the kinetic energy available to cause tissue damage. Next, think about the type and severity of injuries the patient might have sustained. Also anticipate complications that might develop before the patient arrives at definitive medical care.

For example, the lower abdomen, pelvis, and legs of a patient are trapped underneath an overturned tractor. Injuries could include a pelvic fracture, lumbar spine fracture and cord injury, femur fractures, and rupture of abdominal organs (liver, spleen, kidney, and bladder). Additional injuries might include crush injuries to the soft tissues of the buttocks and thighs. Complications of these injuries would include respiratory compromise from abdominal compression and possible hypovolemic shock when the tractor is lifted during the extrication process.

Additional problems result from the fact that the incident might have happened hours earlier, and remained undiscovered until the patient failed to return home for dinner. The "golden hour" is passed, and the setting itself presents problems in access and transport.

Because of the circumstances of the incident, the patient may be hysterical, uncooperative, withdrawn, disoriented, aggressive, rude, intoxicated, or otherwise difficult. Bystanders may have compounded the problem by attempting a rescue themselves before the team's arrival. Family members may also be in shock.

Environmental extremes, such as heat or cold, rain, blowing snow, high winds, or darkness will increase the difficulty of field management of trauma. Extremes in heat and cold can affect the nervous system, as well as sensitive higher functions such as judgment, problem solving, and even consciousness. These extremes can make assessment and treatment of traumatic injuries more difficult for both the rescuer and the patient.

The location and terrain of the incident may also complicate patient management. Confined spaces, leaking fuel, pesticides, live power lines, and sloping terrain make patient assessment, stabilization, and transportation difficult. They also pose hazards for the rescue team. In addition, the patient may require extrication from a confined building, an overturned tractor, a machine, or a confined space such as a manure pit before treatment of traumatic injuries can begin.

Time is a major enemy in the management of serious trauma. Urgent conditions require that the rescuer make important decisions with limited information. In many agricultural-rural situations, seconds count in saving lives or preventing serious long-term injury. Equipment may be limited or unavailable; therefore, equipment is frequently improvised.

Rescuers may experience extreme stress in situations involving trauma. Even experienced rescuers may be emotionally overwhelmed at the sight of severe bleeding, crushed body parts, angulated fractures, or other serious wounds. Under such circumstances, it is important for rescuers to rely on their training and basic knowledge rather than attempt to recall obscure or complex information. It is also critical to understand the basic mechanisms and principles of injuries and their management to perform effectively under stress.

Associated Conditions There are many situations in which trauma occurs simultaneously with other medical problems. Alcohol intoxication and drugs are major contributing factors to many traumatic injuries. In addition, alcohol and drugs complicate assessment and treatment of injuries. Intoxicated patients are often abusive, uncooperative, or hostile.

Trauma may occur in patients with chronic medical problems or even be caused or aggravated by chronic medical problems. For example, diabetics with open wounds have poorer wound healing and higher risks of infection. Patients with chronic heart disease have less cardiac reserve and are at greater risk of cardiac failure or collapse. Chronic heart disease may also result in heart attacks as a result of traumatic stress.

Very young or very old patients have lower tolerances for trauma. In children, a small blood volume creates a lower tolerance for acute fluid loss. At the same time, their proportionately greater surface area to body weight results in more rapid heat loss. The body tissues of the elderly are less elastic, making them more susceptible to a variety of injuries including broken bones and torn aortas. They also have an increased incidence of complicating chronic disease.

Assessment. Trauma has two components: external injury and internal injury. External injury may be difficult to manage but is relatively easy to assess. Internal injuries are generally more serious than external problems, more difficult to assess, and usually require surgical intervention for definitive management.

Management of internal injury requires an understanding of the following factors:

- Anatomy. Rescuers must have a three-dimensional perspective of the human body to know what organs and structures underlie the site of the injury and therefore might be affected by the injury.

- Kinematics. Rescuers need to know how kinetic energy is transformed into tissue damage and the reaction of body tissues to those damaging forces.
- Mechanisms of injury. Rescuers should be able to predict the type of injuries the patient might have, based on the mechanism of injury. Tables 14.2 through 14.11 illustrate several mechanisms of injury occurring in agricultural-rural settings and the resulting injuries. These tables also appear separately in their corresponding chapters. They are repeated here for easy comparison.
- Anticipated problems. After the initial assessment of the patient's injuries and conditions, rescuers should be able to anticipate potential problems that might develop during stabilization and transportation of the patient.
- Signs/symptoms pattern recognition. Rescuers should understand how these reflect the mechanism of injury, such as the pattern of hypovolemic shock and its progression.
- Patient Assessment System (PAS). A system to reevaluate a patient at intervals, such as PAS, will help identify problems even if the rescuer forgets to look for them. For example, the regular use of PAS may show the patient developing a hypovolemic shock pattern.

Polytrauma

Trauma often results in injury to more than one system or body part. Patients with multiple system involvement are referred to as **polytrauma** patients. This distinguishes them from incidents in which there are two or more patients, called **multiple trauma**.

On initial evaluation, all injuries may not be equally apparent. It is important to complete an initial assessment, even if the rescuer finds significant problems part way through the assessment. Stop only to treat immediately life-threatening problems found during the initial assessment and avoid focusing on the most obvious injuries. After completing the secondary assessment, begin management of the problems found in their order of importance. In situations involving trauma or serious injury, reassess the patient continually. Some injuries become apparent only after a span of time:

- Injuries may require time to develop. Examples include bleeding into a body cavity or soft tissues from blunt injury, or respiratory compromise from smoke inhalation.
- Autonomic stress reactions (ASR) can cause "pain masking" which diminishes with time. An example is pain and tenderness in the spine that becomes apparent during an extended incident but was not apparent during the initial exam of a confused, disoriented patient.
- Patients often focus on one injury at a time. An example would be a patient who complains loudly of pain in an open femur fracture but whose dislocated shoulder might go unnoticed for hours.

TABLE 14.2 Common Injuries Involving Tractors

Mechanism of Injury	Result	Typical Injuries
Tractor overturn—open tractor without ROPS Tractor overturn—closed cab without ROPS	Major crush injuries Laceration and shearing from torn metal in addition to crush injuries	**Chest injuries** (mechanical asphyxia, flail chest, pneumothorax, hemothorax, subcutaneous/mediastinal emphysema); **Abdominal injuries** (laceration of liver and spleen, rupture of hollow organs, penetrating wounds); **Spinal injuries** (fractures and dislocations); **Pelvic injuries** (fracture with associated internal bleeding, ruptured bladder, lacerated rectum); **Head injuries** (fractured skull, usually depressed, severe concussion, decreased level of consciousness)
Tractor overturn—ROPS-equipped cab	Major trauma if operator is ejected; deceleration injuries if operator not using seat belt	**Minor cuts and bruises** from broken glass and loose objects in cab

TABLE 14.3 Common Injuries Involving Combines

Mechanism of Injury	Result	Typical Injuries
Entanglement in snapping rolls	Fractures; amputations	**Traumatic amputation** of fingers, toes, hands, arms, legs **Fractures**
Header collapse	Crush injuries	**Chest injuries** (mechanical asphyxia, flail chest, pneumothorax, hemothorax, subcutaneous/mediastinal emphysema); **Abdominal trauma** (laceration of liver and spleen, rupture of hollow organs, penetrating wounds); **Spinal injuries** (fractures and dislocations); **Pelvic injuries** (fracture with associated internal bleeding, ruptured bladder, lacerated rectum); **Head injuries** (fractured skull, usually depressed, severe concussion, decreased level of consciousness)
Entanglement in straw walkers/choppers	Fractures; lacerations	**Fractures; lacerations**

TABLE 14.4 Common Injuries Involving PTOs

Mechanism of Injury	Result	Typical Injuries
Entanglement in power take-off	Clothing entanglement produces extensive soft tissue and severe deceleration injuries.	**Head injuries** (closed and open skull fractures); **Spinal injuries** (severe fractures and dislocations); **Chest injuries** (flail chest, sucking chest wounds, pneumothorax, hemothorax, tension pneumothorax, pulmonary contusion, myocardial contusion) **Abdominal injuries** (blunt trauma, internal bleeding, possible extensive evisceration); **Pelvic injuries** (fractures with internal bleeding, ruptured bladder, ruptured rectum, degloving or avulsion of external male genitalia); **Extremity injuries** (open fractures and dislocations; closed fractures with extensive comminution; soft tissue wrapped around PTO drive shaft; complete avulsion of hands, feet, lower arms, and legs; extensive degloving of large areas of skin)
Entanglement in secondary drive	Strangulation; hand fractures; avulsion of fingers and soft tissue; degloving of extremities; hair entanglement may result in scalping.	

TABLE 14.5 Common Injuries Involving Portable Augers

Mechanism of Injury	Result	Typical Injuries
Entanglement in portable augers	Amputation or deep lacerations from auger flighting; electrical burns if auger contacts overhead power lines; crush and shear injuries if auger collapses	**Head injuries** (concussion and/or fracture if auger collapses); **Spinal injuries;** **Chest injuries;** **Abdominal injuries** (evisceration if victim is small and auger is large); **Pelvic injuries** (if victim is small); **Extremity injuries** (amputation of fingers, toes, feet, arms, legs, hands; spaced, deep lacerations; spiral fractures; localized crush injuries); **Electrical injuries**

TABLE 14.6 Common Injuries Involving Conventional Balers

Mechanism of Injury	Result	Typical Injuries
Entanglement in rectangular baler	Crush injuries Hands and fingers caught in knotting mechanism	High incidence of fatality Severe lacerations; possible amputation
Entanglement in small round baler		

TABLE 14.7 Common Injuries Involving Large Round Balers

Mechanism of Injury	Result	Typical Injuries
Entanglement in compression rollers of large round baler	Crush injuries	High incidence of fatality
Entanglement in open throat round baler	Crush injuries	Incidence of fatality limited—very few since switch to open throat baler

TABLE 14.8 Common Injuries Involving Other Equipment

Mechanism of Injury	Result	Typical Injuries
Falls into tub grinder	Massive blunt trauma to body	High incidence of fatality
Entanglement in ensilage cutter	Amputation of extremities	Traumatic amputation Open fractures
Entanglement in potato digger	Shear injuries	Traumatic amputation Fractures
Entanglement in sugar beet harvester	Shear injuries	Traumatic amputation Fractures
Entanglement in cotton picker	Amputation; puncture wounds	Traumatic amputation Fractures
Entanglement in drive belts and chains of any equipment	Local compression injuries	Traumatic amputation Fractures Degloving injuries

TABLE 14.9 Common Injuries Involving Confined Spaces

Mechanism of Injury	Result	Typical Injuries
Fall or entrapment in confined space	Suffocation and/or trauma from fall	**Anoxia or hypoxia** due to low oxygen levels and/or high concentrations of toxic gases; **Fall injuries** depend on distance fallen; **Chest injuries** (broken ribs, possible flail chest); **Spinal injuries** (usually to cervical spine, injuries to lumbar and thoracic spine also possible); **Open or closed fractures**
Entrapment in flowing grain 1. "Quicksand" when grain is being unloaded from bin or gravity wagon 2. Collapse of grain "bridge" 3. Grain stuck to walls falls on victim 4. Overturned truck/wagon 5. Containing structure collapses	Suffocation; possible trauma; possible hypothermia	**Mechanical suffocation** due to inability to expand chest/diaphragm; **Airway obstruction** by grain; **Toxic atmosphere**; **Hypothermia**

TABLE 14.10 Common Injuries Involving Animals

Mechanism of Injury	Result	Typical Injuries
Animal incidents (kicked or stepped on by animal; fall from animal; animal falls on person; gores and bites)	Extremity fractures; concussion; crush injuries; blunt trauma; penetrating trauma; abrasions and contusions	**Head injuries** (basal skull fracture, depressed skull fracture, severe concussion, possible maxillofacial injuries); **Abdominal injuries**; **Fractures**; **Soft tissue injuries**; **Blunt trauma**

TABLE 14.11 Common Injuries Associated with Hazardous Materials Exposure

Mechanism of Injury	Result	Typical Injuries
Exposure to anhydrous ammonia	Freezes exposed tissue; chemical burns	Clothing frozen to skin; Severe chemical burns to all exposed parts of the body; Severe injury to lung tissue
Exposure to high-pressure liquids/fuels	Burns, if liquid is hot; subcutaneous or intravenous injection due to force of pressure	Thermal or chemical burns, both internal and external; embolic phenomena

The Big Net Principle

Assessing trauma in the field may present different clinical problems with varying degrees of seriousness in the same patient. It may be difficult or impossible to determine if the overall clinical picture of a patient is caused by a more serious problem or a possibly less serious problem. Some examples of this dilemma include the following:

- Is the patient's abnormal behavior due to a head injury or hypoxia, or is the patient intoxicated?
- A patient complains of pain and tenderness in the neck following a 15' fall. Are these signs and symptoms due to a muscle strain or could they be caused by a potentially unstable spinal injury?

In some cases, an event can have more than one possible result. It may be impossible to determine the final outcome during initial field management. Some examples include the following:

- The signs and symptoms of copperhead envenomation can be delayed for several hours. Has the patient been envenomated?
- A patient who fell 20' from a grain bin is confused and anxious, appears pale and sweaty, and has a pulse of 120/min. Is this condition due to ASR or hypovolemic shock? Will the patient get better or worse with time?

It would be easier to get answers to these questions in a hospital; the patient could be kept alive with advanced life support equipment and periodic observations. But in the field, equipment and manpower are not available. The patient may continue to deteriorate. It is best to assume that Murphy's Law is operating. That is, assume the worst possible case and plan patient management on that assumption. If the patient's condition improves with time, modify the treatment plan. An injury that is overtreated will rarely cause harm. If the worst case proves correct, the rescue team has anticipated the problems and is ready to manage them correctly. This method of anticipating the worst case scenario to avoid overlooking injuries or complications is known as the **big net principle.**

Treatment In trauma care, rapid management saves lives. Patients with major trauma are saved by definitive treatment within the first or second hour after the injury, also known as the golden hour. The golden hour refers to the initial period after a traumatic injury when a patient's body is able to compensate for his or her injuries. During this time, the patient's condition remains relatively stable. After this initial period, patient mortality and morbidity rapidly rise unless definitive trauma management has been successfully instituted.

The golden hour begins when the patient is injured. Less severely injured trauma patients may have 4 to 6 hours to be saved by definitive treatment. For effective treatment of serious trauma, rapid transport to a trauma center is imperative. That is why agricultural-rural incidents are often fatal. Hours may pass between the time of the incident and the discovery of the incident. The advantage of the golden hour is no longer there.

Ideal trauma management is rapid stabilization of the patient and immediate transport to definitive medical care. Unfortunately, in agricultural-rural rescue operations, definitive medical care is not always nearby or easily accessible. Even if access, stabilization, and/or transport are extended, the medical objectives and treatment principles are the same. And though the situation may go beyond the golden hour, there are holding actions that may extend the time available to maintain your patient. Such actions include application of a PASG and advanced life support techniques such as IVs and fluid therapy and advanced airway techniques, *if they are within your scope of practice.*

COMMON MEDICAL CONDITIONS

Respiratory and Cardiac Arrest

Rescuers must be familiar with current standards for the management of repiratory and cardiac arrests. Management of cardiac arrest due to traumatic injuries differs from that for primary respiratory and cardiac arrests. It is often difficult to estimate the probability that a patient will survive a cardiac arrest, except for those with severe physical injuries.

Possible causes of cardiopulmonary arrest associated with trauma include the following: severe neurologic injury with secondary cardiovascular collapse; hypoxia; direct injury to the heart or aorta; underlying or preexisting medical conditions such as cardiac arrhythmia, decreased cardiac output secondary to pericardial tamponade or a tension pneumothorax; major blood loss; and severe hypothermia.

Resuscitation should be attempted for patients in primary cardiac arrest with secondary traumatic injuries. For patients with primary traumatic injuries, management efforts should be directed at potentially reversible injuries and conditions that adversely affect ventilation, oxygenation, and cardiac output. Therefore, management would include endotracheal intubation and initiation of IV therapy, *if within your scope of practice*. Local protocols for management of hypothermia should also be initiated. If resuscitation is attempted, rapid extrication followed by rapid transport to definitive medical care is necessary.

Resuscitation should not be attempted for patients who have obvious, severe blunt trauma and no vital signs, pupillary response, or an organized or shockable cardiac rhythm.

There is a body of evidence developing that suggests that providing cardiac compression for patients in traumatic cardiac arrest has little effect on ultimate patient outcome. Another body of evidence suggests that unless ALS can be provided within 30 minutes of a nontraumatic, normothermic cardiac arrest, there is an extremely low probability that the patient will be resuscitated. Rescuers may encounter circumstances in remote environments or situations with long response or transport times before ALS can be started in which it is appropriate to withdraw BLS. State and local EMS authorities are encouraged to develop protocols for the initiation and withdrawal of BLS in situations where ALS is not readily available, with consideration given to local circumstances, resources, and risks to rescuers.

Shock

Shock is defined, in a strict medical context, as acute loss of capillary blood perfusion that results from a loss of pressure within the cardiovascular system. Shock is a condition of acute peripheral circulatory failure causing inadequate and progressively failing perfusion of tissue. As a result, the body cannot perform its normal functions. The term **perfusion** is defined as the circulation of blood within an organ or tissue. Therefore, a loss of perfusion means that organs and tissues are not receiving enough blood to work properly. Adequate perfusion in the body keeps the cells alive and healthy.

The severity of shock varies, depending on the type and degree of injury. Patients who have sustained a traumatic injury or heart attack will very often be in shock. Shock is also common in victims of auger entanglement. If not reversed, severe shock will often result in death. In rescue situations, shock always indicates a serious threat to life and as such requires aggressive treatment. However, field treatment is limited to measures that may briefly extend the time available to transport the patient to definitive medical care.

Mechanisms of Injury Shock is caused by three basic mechanisms: fluid loss, which results in hypovolemic shock; failure of the heart to pump effectively, which results in cardiogenic shock; and dilation of the blood vessels, which results in vascular shock. Whatever the mechanism, the common element is loss of perfusion pressure (Figure 14.2).

1. Hypovolemic shock. Loss of blood/fluid depletes the vascular system volume to the point that it is insufficient for perfusion. The volume loss may be the result of internal or external bleeding. The loss may also occur as a result of dehydration secondary to diarrhea or vomiting.
2. Cardiogenic shock. The heart muscle is damaged so that it is unable to pump the blood volume effectively. Perfusion pressure is lost even though blood volume is normal. Common mechanisms for cardiogenic shock include myocardial infarction, cardiac ischemia, tamponade, contusion, arrhythmia, and electrical shock.
3. Vascular shock. Normally, a large percentage of the blood vessels in the body are partially constricted. If all the blood vessels dilate, then the blood within them, even though it is of normal volume, is insufficient to fill the system and provide perfusion pressure. There are generally two basic causes of vascular shock: mechanical (spinal shock) and chemical (anaphylactic shock). In spinal shock, injury to the spinal cord causes loss of autonomic control over blood vessels. This results in vasodilation in all parts of the body. In anaphylactic shock, an allergic reaction results in a generalized vasodilation—dilation of all the vessels in the body—and subsequent loss of perfusion pressure to the body tissues.

Assessment The effect of all three mechanisms is identical. There is insufficient blood perfusing through the tissues to provide adequate nutrition and oxygen and to carry away waste. All local body processes are affected by shock.

FIGURE 14.2

There are three basic causes of shock and impaired tissue perfusion: (left) failure of the heart to pump effectively; (middle) fluid loss, usually a result of bleeding; and (right) dilation of blood vessels.

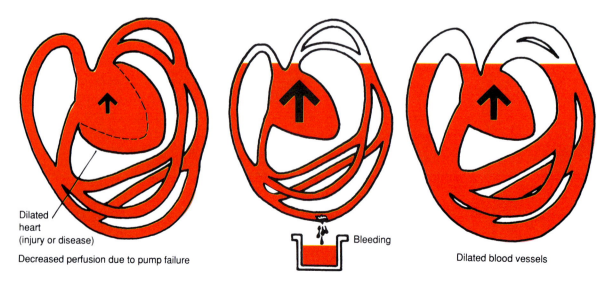

One of the most dangerous aspects of shock is that the patient's body may try to compensate for the loss of perfusion. As a result, the signs and symptoms of shock may not appear until the condition reaches a dangerous level. Rescuers must anticipate the possibility of shock developing based on the patient's history, mechanism of injury/illness, and physical findings. This means watching for the subtle warning signs of impending collapse of the cardiovascular system before the condition reaches a dangerous level. The signs and symptoms of hypovolemic or cardiogenic shock include the following:

- Agitation, anxiety, or a feeling of impending doom
- Increased pulse rate
- Diminished urinary output
- Gasping for air, "air hunger"

These signs and symptoms are the result of the body's compensation mechanisms that decrease blood perfusion in the extremities or body shell to provide additional perfusion to the brain and other vital organs of the body core. These clinical findings do not appear in vascular shock, since the peripheral vessels are dilated and unable to constrict and transfer the blood volume to the core.

One or more of these signs of shock may appear in the following situations: severe blows to the head or body; massive external or internal bleeding; fractures; an acute abdomen; stab or puncture wounds; gunshot wounds; spinal injuries; severe infection; or poisoning. Regardless of the cause, rescuers must always anticipate the development of shock, based on the patient's history, mechanism of injury, and physical exam. It is critical to promptly recognize the early signs of impending shock, take immediate measures to delay its onset, and provide rapid transport to definitive medical care.

General Treatment The following three steps are common in the treatment of all types of shock:

1. Give high-flow oxygen, if available. This increases the oxygen content of the limited blood perfusion to body tissues.
2. Position the patient flat with the legs slightly elevated to help perfuse the body core. This treatment is helpful but has limited effect.
3. Maintain normal body temperature. This is particularly important for any patient who is seriously injured, exposed to the environment, or unable to move and maintain body heat. This also applies in hot environments where increased temperatures can increase peripheral vasodilation and aggravate the shock.

Treating hypovolemic shock. The following three steps are to be included in the treatment of hypovolemic shock:

1. Stop the bleeding. Use direct pressure for external bleeding. A pneumatic antishock garment (PASG) may help stop bleeding in the pelvis and upper legs. Surgery is generally required to stop most internal bleeding.
2. Administer IV fluids, *if within your scope of practice.* Replace fluids with IV therapy using the 3:1 rule: 300 mL of electrolyte solution for every 100 mL of blood loss. Blood replacement is generally required after 2,000 mL of blood loss. Fluids taken orally are usually not absorbed fast enough to replace severe losses. Therefore, oral fluids must not be given to patients with suspected internal injuries or diminished level of consciousness.
3. Apply a PASG, if ordered by medical control.

The most important aspect in treating hypovolemic shock is stopping or slowing the flow of blood. To control bleeding, apply sufficient pressure to external bleeding points and splint major long bone and pelvic fractures properly to minimize internal bleeding. Monitor the patient's vital signs and urinary output. Remember that field management of hypovolemic shock is an attempt to provide a little extra time to get the patient to definitive medical care, which usually includes surgery.

If IV fluids are used in the management of shock during an extended incident, carefully monitor urinary output. This is done preferably with a Foley catheter, *if within your scope of practice and authorized by medical control.*

Treating cardiogenic shock. The following three steps are to be included in the treatment of cardiogenic shock:

1. Administer medications, *if within your scope of practice.* Certain medications can decrease the work load of the heart, restore normal heart rhythm, increase pumping strength of the heart muscle, and reduce ischemic pain.
2. Defibrillate to restore normal pumping rhythm, *as indicated by local medical protocol and if within your scope of practice.*
3. Administer IV fluids, *if within your scope of practice.* Start an IV and infuse fluids as slowly as possible to avoid adding additional work load to the heart. The IV line will be used primarily as an access route for medication administration according to local protocols or at the hospital. It is generally easier to start a line as early as possible before decreasing perfusion makes it even more difficult to locate an accessible vein.

Treat and transport patients with cardiogenic shock in the position in which they can breathe most easily. Monitor vital signs and urinary output. Use a portable cardiac monitor, *if within your scope of practice,* and the equipment is available and feasible to use.

CHAPTER 14 Common Medical Conditions and Injuries

Treating vascular shock. The following steps are to be included in treating vascular shock, depending on the type.

The following steps are appropriate for treating spinal shock:

1. Administer IV fluids, *if within your scope of practice*, using the same guidelines as for hypovolemic shock.
2. Apply a PASG, if ordered by medical control.

The following steps are appropriate for treating anaphylactic shock:

1. Administer medications, *if within your scope of practice*. Administer epinephrine by injection and oral or injectable antihistamines.
2. Administer IV fluids, *if within your scope of practice*, using the same guidelines as for hypovolemic shock.
3. Apply a PASG, if ordered by medical control.
4. Begin airway management. Administer high-flow oxygen, provide ventilatory assistance as needed, and prepare for possible intubation *if within your scope of practice.*

Autonomic Stress Reaction

The term psychogenic shock, when used to refer to an autonomic stress reaction, is misleading. This condition is different from true shock in that it is usually temporary and is not life threatening. It will also generally resolve with minimal intervention. The term **autonomic stress reaction (ASR)** is a better term for this parasympathetic reaction. ASR is commonly associated with emotional situations such as fear, bad news, good news, the sight of an injury or blood, the prospect of medical treatment, severe pain, and anxiety. In an agricultural-rural setting, ASR may affect family members who may have discovered the incident, or even inadvertently caused it. The severity of injuries in agricultural-rural incidents may also cause rescuers or other bystanders to experience ASR.

ASR results from a temporary reduction in perfusion of the brain as blood momentarily pools in dilated vessels in other parts of the body and the heart rate suddenly slows. ASR is usually self-correcting since the patient usually ends up in a horizontal position, thereby restoring the blood flow to the brain. A patient believed to be experiencing ASR should be placed in a supine position to improve blood flow to the brain. If ASR causes the patient to fall, the fall may cause other injuries, especially in an older patient. Therefore, it is important to check for injuries associated with a fall. When psychogenic shock involves an injury to the head, it is important to stabilize the patient, place the patient in a secure, supine position, and transport immediately.

Nausea, vomiting, confusion, fainting, and disorientation are common ASR responses to severe injury or stress. ASR can be a problem in rescue situations because it may cause confusing symptoms and mask real injuries. ASR can be confused with shock, and it may also coexist with shock. But ASR tends to improve spontaneously, while true shock does not.

ASR can have a positive effect on patient survival, and there have been numerous cases in which severely injured persons have performed heroic acts while under the influence of ASR. ASR tends to diminish with time and reassurance. A patient believed to be experiencing ASR should be reevaluated at regular intervals to ensure that ASR is not masking serious injuries.

COMMON INJURIES

Head Injuries

Increased Intracranial Pressure The terms closed head trauma or head injury are inexact but usually imply injury to the brain. It is important to distinguish closed head trauma from head wounds, which are scalp or facial soft tissue injuries without injury to the brain.

The rigid skull enclosing the brain prevents any expansion of brain tissue. Thus, any bleeding or swelling of the brain may result in increased intracranial pressure. Unless corrected quickly, increased intracranial pressure will result in permanent neurologic damage or death.

Mechanism of injury. Trauma is the most common mechanism of increased intracranial pressure seen in rescue situations. Lacerations, tears, or contusion of the brain or blood vessels in the skull may cause bleeding and/or swelling, resulting in increased pressure.

Much less frequently, increased intracranial pressure develops as a result of cardiovascular accidents (CVAs or strokes). These are localized infarctions that cause cell death within the brain and may result in bleeding or swelling. In addition, cardiac arrest or cardiogenic shock decreases brain perfusion resulting in increased intracranial pressure from edema, or extra fluid in and around the cells of the brain due to cell death.

Edema may also develop as a result of the vascular changes of hypoxia at high altitudes. This is called high altitude cerebral edema (HACE), a form of acute mountain sickness.

Assessment. Whatever the cause, increased intracranial pressure presents a relatively constant clinical pattern. Determine the patient's history. Has the patient sustained a blow to the head or suffered a cardiac arrest or CVA? Is the patient at high altitude?

With a positive mechanism of injury and an altered level of consciousness, assume that the patient has closed head trauma with increased intracranial pressure. Monitor and record the progression of the vital signs and other signs and symptoms. They may be helpful in predicting the outcome of the injury.

The following signs and symptoms will help confirm the assessment:

- Blood pressure will increase in a severe injury.
- Pulse will decrease with severe closed head trauma.
- Respirations may alter from normal breathing patterns after head injuries. Some patients may breathe more deeply or more rapidly than normal. Do not assume that head injury automatically means lower respirations. If the injury is severe, the breathing may be irregular or absent.
- Temperature will be variable.
- Skin temperature and moisture will be variable.

Level of consciousness and mental status are the most sensitive indicators of a change in the patient's condition. In the early stages after head injury, the patient may exhibit restlessness or signs of being intoxicated or combative. If the injury is severe, there will be a decreased level of consciousness as measured by the AVPU scale, described in chapter 13.

Assessing overall level of consciousness is a crucial step in evaluating a patient with a head injury. The patient's level of consciousness should be determined using the AVPU scale, immediately after the primary survey is completed.

Assess the patient's initial level of consciousness and note the time, and then recheck and document the level of consciousness every 10 minutes. Any change in level of consciousness, either positive or negative, is significant in a patient with a head injury. The level of consciousness may fluctuate—improving, deteriorating, then improving again over time. However, a progressive deterioration in the patient's response to stimuli usually indicates serious brain damage requiring prompt surgical treatment. Physicians need to know when loss of consciousness occurred and what the patient's responses have been, if any, during the rescue operation and during transport. The rescue team's neurologic evaluations of the patient will be compared with those obtained when the patient reaches definitive medical care. Therefore, it is critical to obtain a baseline evaluation as soon as possible during the rescue operation.

Headache is an early sign of increased intracranial pressure, but it may be confused as pain associated with trauma to the skull or neck. Vomiting is often also seen in early stages of increased intracranial pressure. Late signs include seizures, unequal pupils, and paralysis, which may be localized to one side of the patient's body. Decorticate or decerebrate posturing are always signs of very serious closed head trauma with high increased intracranial pressure.

A patient who has closed head trauma with increased intracranial pressure does not generally present a typical clinical picture for shock.

If the patient does exhibit a pattern of shock, look for additional injuries that might cause internal bleeding.

Treatment. High-flow oxygen must be given and the patient hyperventilated to reduce intracranial pressure. Since spinal injuries are often present in patients with closed head trauma, the cervical spine must also be protected. Arrange transport to definitive medical care (surgery) as soon as possible. Other field treatment options are limited and have little effect on patient survival. In these patients, respiratory failure often occurs before cardiac failure.

Concussions Injuries to the brain have a broad band of severity and do not always result in increased intracranial pressure. Concussions are generally minor injuries, ranging from temporary memory loss or confusion to a temporary alteration in level of consciousness. No treatment is indicated for a concussion. Patients should be monitored carefully for possible increased intracranial pressure and should not be allowed to return to activities where they would be at risk of additional closed head trauma until they have been examined by a physician.

All neurologic changes from a concussion will resolve within a few minutes. Therefore, any neurologic abnormalities that last for more than a few minutes should not be attributed to a concussion. Look for other causes for these changes. Confusion that does not clear completely is also a sign of a more severe injury that requires medical evaluation and intervention. Severe concussions may result in loss of consciousness for 15 to 20 minutes. Such injuries indicate a more severe brain injury that may require aggressive medical intervention.

Contusions Contusions are bruises to the cortex of the brain associated with severe concussions. They are characterized by longer periods of confusion, memory loss, or loss of consciousness. Contusions may result in focal neurologic defects if they are located in a sensory or motor area of the cortex. Coup contusions occur directly under the point of impact. Contrecoup injuries occur opposite the point of impact as a result of a bounce phenomenon. Bleeding into contused areas can result in a major neurologic injury from a mass effect. Contusions require evaluation by a physician.

Intracranial Hemorrhage There is no typical clinical picture for intracranial hemorrhage because of the great variation in location, size, and rapidity of bleeding that may occur. Patients who have intracranial bleeding may show focal neurologic defects and rapid deterioration. They require rapid transport to definitive medical care.

Scalp Lacerations Because the face and scalp both possess a rich blood supply, even small lacerations on the head, neck, and face can

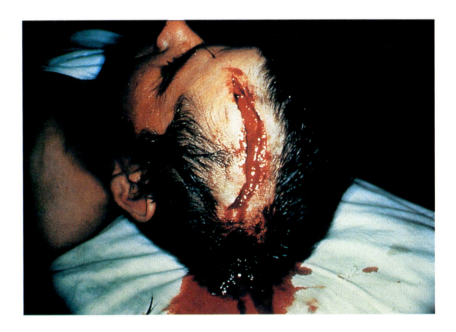

FIGURE 14.3

A scalp laceration will bleed profusely.

cause significant amounts of blood loss (Figure 14.3). In rare cases, blood loss from a scalp laceration may be severe enough to cause hypovolemic shock.

Bleeding from scalp lacerations can almost always be controlled by applying direct pressure to the wound with a dry, sterile dressing. Apply firm compression for several minutes in order to control the bleeding. Avoid applying pressure to underlying skull fractures, which may increase injury to the brain.

If a triangular or square flap of skin is protruding from the scalp, fold the flap back down onto its bed before applying a compression dressing. If the dressing becomes saturated with blood, apply a second dressing over the first to reinforce it. Continue to apply manual pressure until the bleeding is controlled (Figure 14.4).

Skull Fractures Skull fractures can result in serious injury to the brain and increased intracranial pressure. It is important to protect the skull from further injury during evacuation and transport.

All patients with skull fractures require total immobilization of the cervical spine because of the risk of associated spinal injury. One indication of skull fracture is a clear or pink watery fluid dripping from the nose, from the ear, or from an open scalp wound. This fluid is cerebrospinal fluid (CSF) and will leak to the outside only if both the covering of the brain (dura) and the skull have been penetrated. Leakage of CSF indicates serious injury. Do not attempt to pack the wound, the ear, or the nose because packing the drainage site could block the escape of fluid and cause additional pressure on an already damaged brain. The

FIGURE 14.4

If a laceration involves a flap of skin hanging from the scalp, fold the flap back down onto its bed and apply a compression dressing.

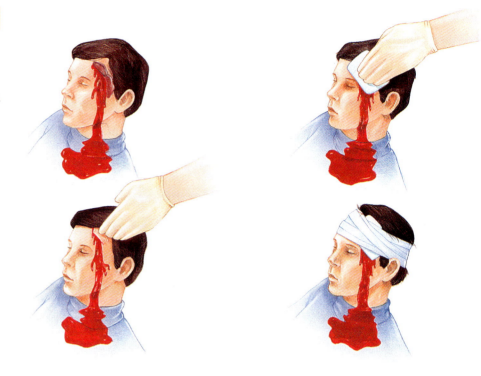

presence of the so-called gray matter of the brain in an open skull fracture is a poor prognostic sign.

Cover the wound with a sterile dressing to prevent further contamination and infection, but do not bandage tightly.

Closed Soft Tissue Injuries

Closed soft tissue injuries are considered either contusions or hematomas. However, contusions may also exist with open wounds such as lacerations and abrasions. Contusions may be minor, or they may be severe, such as in the brain with increased intracranial pressure or in the abdomen with a ruptured spleen, liver, or kidney.

A hematoma is a localized collection of blood beneath the skin that occurs from the rapid bleeding when larger blood vessels tear. The progression of swelling is the greatest during the first 6 hours following injury and continues for up to 24 hours. A hematoma can also occur following fractures or when the blood vessels to any organ in the body are damaged. In fractures of a large bone such as the femur or pelvis, large hematomas may form, containing more than a liter of blood.

The most important part of assessing any closed injury is examining for injury to underlying organs and structures. During extended transport, additional bleeding and swelling may cause problems, so frequent reexaminations are necessary.

Small bruises in most soft tissue injuries require no special emergency medical care and generally heal on their own. With more extensive closed injuries, swelling and bleeding beneath the skin can be extensive and may even result in hypovolemic shock.

Treatment during the first 24 hours is intended to minimize the swelling by following the principles outlined in the acronym RICE:

R Rest the injury by splinting the affected extremity and limiting its use.

I Ice applied as tolerated during the first 24 hours. Do not expose the skin directly to the ice or frostbite may result.

C Compress the injury and distal extremity. Isolated proximal compression can obstruct circulation to the extremity distally.

E Elevate the affected part above heart level to reduce bleeding and promote drainage.

If there is potential for underlying damage and further bleeding, monitor vital signs and urinary output.

Fractures of the Spine

The spinal column protects the delicate nerve tissue of the spinal cord. Unstable spinal injuries may damage the cord that the spine normally protects (Figure 14.5). Fractures and disruptions of the soft tissues, tendons, and ligaments that hold the vertebral bodies in alignment present similar patterns of injury and will be discussed in the next section. Such injuries are extremely serious because they can result in permanent paralysis. Major cervical injuries generally result in quadriplegia, which is complete or partial paralysis of all four extremities. Thoracic and lumbar injuries may result in paraplegia, which is a partial or complete paralysis of the lower extremities. *Up to 20% of all spinal cord injuries occur after the initial injury and are caused by movement of the unstable spine during extrication, treatment, or transport.*

While field treatment of spinal injuries is similar to that of other fractures, there are important differences. The long-term consequences of spinal injuries are much more serious than those of other fractures. Field management of spinal injuries requires great care.

Another concern in spinal injuries is spinal shock. This may result from an injury to the spinal cord causing the autonomic nervous system to lose control of dilation and constriction of blood vessels. This loss of autonomic control results in a generalized vasodilation below the level of the spinal cord injury. The resultant pooling of blood in the involved extremities results in a loss of perfusion pressure and decreased perfusion of the body core.

Common Mechanisms of Injury Spinal injuries may result from direct trauma to the spine, such as being entangled in a PTO. Or they may result from indirect trauma, such as fracture of the thoracolumbar junction in a patient who falls 20' and lands on his or her feet. Spinal cord

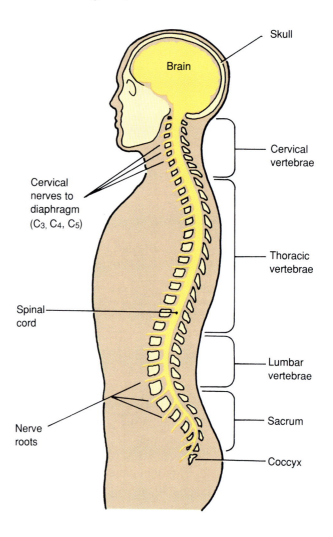

FIGURE 14.5

The spinal canal forms a protective covering around the spinal cord. Patients with suspected spinal injuries must be immobilized to prevent permanent damage to the spinal cord.

injuries result when the stability of the spine is disrupted to the point that it can no longer protect the cord.

A positive mechanism of injury is any mechanism of injury capable of causing a fracture to the spine. Examples include any head or facial injury, a direct blow or impact on the neck or back, or a fall of greater than 15'.

Assessment In rapid-transport situations, assume that the patient has a spinal injury if the mechanism of injury suggests a possible spinal injury. Ensure that the patient's spine is fully immobilized. A patient's pain response is usually abnormal immediately following a significant or major injury, so the signs and symptoms may be unreliable indicators of injury. In conventional, rapid-transport EMS, immobilizing a patient for a short trip to the hospital is not usually a problem. Sufficient resources are usually available to load and transport the immobilized patient without danger to the patient or the rescue team.

During extended incidents, providing full spinal immobilization can range from difficult to impossible. It can even be dangerous in certain severe environments or when using improvised equipment. During extended incidents, the rescue team will have the opportunity to repeat surveys and observe changes in the patient's condition. If approved by local medical control, there may be circumstances in which it is appropriate to manage the patient without full spinal immobilization.

Cervical spine injuries. The cervical spine is the most commonly injured area of the spine because it is the most mobile area of the spine and may be affected by blows to the head. Injuries to the cervical spine have a higher potential for more generalized damage to body function than other areas of the spine. The action of the diaphragm is controlled by the phrenic nerve arising from the third, fourth, and fifth cervical levels (C_3, C_4, and C_5). Injuries to the cervical spine may result in paraplegia, but they are more likely to result in quadriplegia.

Thoracic spine injuries. The area of the thoracic spine is the most stable area of the spine. Injury here is less common than in the cervical spine. Injury to the spinal cord at a thoracic level may result in paraplegia, but the upper extremities will be spared.

Thoracic spine injuries may be seen in patients who were wearing their shoulder harnesses incorrectly (under their arms) and were subsequently involved in an automobile accident. These patients also have a high incidence of abdominal injuries as a result of their improperly positioned restraints.

Lumbar spine injuries. The lumbar spine is more mobile than the thoracic spine, so injury here is more common, though less common than in the cervical area. Injuries at the thoracolumbar junction are frequently seen in deceleration injuries such as falls from a height. This is because of the relatively fixed thoracic spine and the stiffness of the large vertebral bodies in the lower lumbar region. Severe injuries may result in paraplegia.

Assessing for lumbar spine injuries should include checking for the following:

- Loss of motor and sensory function below the site of the injury
- Spinal shock
- Priapism in males, a sustained erection that often occurs with spinal cord injury
- Respiratory distress or failure from a cervical or high thoracic injury causing paralysis of the chest muscles

Remember that not all spinal cord injuries result in a complete injury to the spinal cord. Some patients will have an *incomplete cord injury* and show signs of partial paralysis and partial loss of sensation below the injury site. These patients must be reassessed often for possible progression or resolution of their symptoms. Report any changes to medical control and the receiving medical facility. Ensure that management of such a patient does not result in additional injury that converts a partial cord injury into a complete one.

Treatment The principles of treatment of suspected spinal fractures are essentially the same as those for any long bone/joint fracture: traction in position (TIP), hands-on stable, and splint stable.

1. **Traction in position.** The principles of spinal TIP are the same as TIP for long bones and joints. The injured spine is most stable in the normal anatomic "eyes forward" position. Transporting a patient with an injured spine that is out of normal anatomic position is often impractical and may increase the risk of additional injury. Discontinue TIP and stabilize in the position found if TIP causes a significant increase in *pain* or if movement of the distal part is met by *resistance*.

2. **Hands-on stable.** Hands-on stability applies to all unstable fractures, including fractures to the spine. When done correctly, log rolling and patient lifting are hands-on stable procedures to control an unstable spine during patient movement before immobilization. A spinal injury is more important to immobilize than an extremity injury. It is important to provide maximum stability to the spine when moving the patient. If a spinal injury is suspected, stabilizing the head and neck coordinates patient movement. Application of a cervical collar will help in obtaining hands-on stability.

3. **Splint stable.** Apply splints to all unstable fractures, including fractures of the spine. Spine boards are splints applied to the spine to hold it in a normal anatomic position. Short boards are splints applied to aid in patient extrication. They provide partial immobilization of the cervical and thoracic spines. Patients on short boards should be secured to a long spine board after extrication. Long spine boards provide immobilization for the lumbar spine, the pelvis, and the lower extremities.

Lifting, Extricating, and Moving Patients With Spinal Injuries The principles involved in accessing, stabilizing, and transporting a spinal injury patient are identical to those involved in managing unstable fractures of the extremities: traction in position (TIP), hands-on stable, and splint stable.

For example, to splint a thoracic spine injury, immobilize the thoracic spine, and include the cervical and lumbar spines, the pelvis, and both femurs. The legs should also be immobilized because the pelvis cannot be immobilized effectively if the legs are free.

In a patient with multiple injuries, a spinal injury is more important than an injury to any extremity. If a spinal injury is suspected, spinal immobilization takes precedence over control of the extremities.

Refer to local medical protocols for the specific clinical standards to follow in assessing and managing spinal injuries during extended incidents.

Musculoskeletal Injuries

Musculoskeletal injuries are among the most common problems seen in rescue work. Effective emergency care of musculoskeletal injuries decreases immediate pain, reduces the possibility of nerve or vessel injury, and improves the patient's chances for a rapid recovery with early return to normal activity.

In general, any incident in which the body has been thrown against a barrier, fallen on a hard surface, or been struck by a moving object has the potential to cause a fracture, dislocation, or sprain.

Extremity Fractures Fractures result in unstable bone fragments with sharp ends that can cause injury to adjacent structures such as nerves, blood vessels, and muscles (Figure 14.6). Fractures also result in internal bleeding because bones have a rich blood supply. Severe bleeding may be associated with fractures of the pelvis and femur. If a patient who has a fracture shows signs of impending shock, do not assume that the fractures are the only source of bleeding. Assess for internal injuries and bleeding.

FIGURE 14.6

Fractures can result in unstable bone fragments with sharp ends that can cause injury to adjacent structures such as nerves, blood vessels, and muscles.

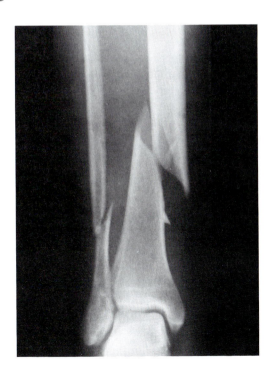

Open fractures may be caused by sharp fragments of bone protruding through the skin. They may also result from penetrating injuries through the overlying soft tissues to the bone, such as a gunshot wound. Open fractures are at high risk for serious infection. Larger wounds, contamination, and associated soft tissue and vascular injuries all increase the risk of infection.

Unstable bone fragments also cause pain in the periosteum, the membrane that covers the bones. This pain often produces an autonomic stress reaction, resulting in decreased blood pressure and pulse, clammy skin, and fainting.

The instability of long bone fractures is increased by movement of the joints at either end of the affected bone. Muscle imbalance and spasm may also cause significant movement. Fractured long bones are generally most stable in their normal "in-line" anatomic position where the muscle pulls are balanced. Stability is also improved when splints control the joint at both ends of the fractured bone.

Bleeding and swelling increase at the fracture site for the first 24 hours, with most swelling occurring during the first 6 hours.

One critically dangerous result of fractures is ischemia or reduced perfusion of the extremity distal to the fracture. Ischemia may occur for several reasons, including the following: swelling or angulation at the fracture site; injury to the vessels at the time of the fracture; movement during the reduction or splint application; movement allowed by improper splinting, or a too tightly secured splint. If the ischemia is prolonged (more than 2 hours), it may lead to tissue necrosis, or death of the ischemic tissue. Severe tissue necrosis may require amputation of the limb. Monitor the distal circulation of a fractured extremity frequently and loosen all dressings and splints on the injured extremity if circulation decreases.

Assessment. The objective of fracture assessment is to identify any potentially unstable injuries or injuries that have the potential to damage adjacent structures. Without x-ray films, the assessment of *fracture* is essentially the same as *possible fracture*. In the field, fractures and possible fractures are treated the same, as indicated in the following equations:

Positive mechanism of injury + Positive signs and symptoms = Fracture or possible fracture

Positive mechanism of injury + Negative signs and symptoms = No fracture

Nonspecific positive signs and symptoms include pain, tenderness and/or point tenderness, and swelling. Specific positive signs and symptoms include the inability of the extremity to move or bear weight immediately following the injury, a "snap" or "crack" sound at the time of the incident, an obvious deformity or angulation, or crepitus, a grating sound created when the moving ends of a fractured bone rub against each other. (Remember that even if a patient can move or use an extremity, it may still be fractured.)

Treatment. There are three phases of fracture management: traction in position (TIP), hands-on stable, and splint stable.

1. **Traction in position.** Fractures of long bones are most stable when in their normal anatomic alignment. The distal blood supply is also generally best maintained in this position. Stabilize the proximal part of the fractured bone. Apply gentle, steady traction to the distal part in the position found. While maintaining traction, slowly and smoothly move the distal part into its normal anatomic position.

    Fractures that involve joints are generally not improved by repositioning. The exceptions include fractures with loss of distal circulation or a severely rotated or deformed joint. In these cases, apply gentle traction and attempt to move the joint to its normal anatomic position. For most joints, this is the "midrange" position, midway between flexion and extension.

    Discontinue TIP and stabilize the injured extremity in the position found if TIP causes a significant increase in *pain* or if movement of the distal part is met by *resistance*.

    TIP can be used on open shaft fractures that have protruding bone ends. Before applying traction, gently cleanse the exposed bone ends by irrigating with a sterile solution. Then apply a dry, sterile dressing. The bone ends will often retract beneath the skin surface when traction is applied. Do not attempt to prevent this from happening. Be sure to report to the receiving medical facility that the bone ends were protruding before traction was applied.

2. **Hands-on stable.** Use hands-on stability of the fractured limb to control unstable injuries if the patient or injured limb must be moved before a splint is applied. Situations where hands-on stability might be helpful include lifting a leg to apply a splint or making a rapid emergency extrication from a hazardous location. Hands-on stability will also help stabilize an injured part during assessment or treatment of associated wounds.

    To understand hands-on stability, imagine moving a chain and keeping all the links in line with one another. Stabilize shaft fractures of long bones by maintaining position in the normal axis of the bone. Stabilize fractures involving joints in the position that is most comfortable for the patient. This is generally in the "midrange" position. The stability of joint fractures is usually not improved by traction along the axis of the limb. Release hands-on stability only when the injured part is immobilized with a splint.

    When moving a patient, the rescuer who is stabilizing the most unstable or serious injury coordinates the actions of other rescuers.

3. Splint stable. In the splint stable phase, a splint replaces hands-on stability to maintain the fracture in position and minimize additional injury and pain.

After splinting, monitor ischemia in the distal extremity by checking circulation, sensation, and movement (CSM). This is particularly important during extended incidents because of swelling that develops with time.

C Circulation
- Pulse
- Capillary refill (warm conditions only)

S Sensation
- Numbness
- Tingling
- Severe pain

M Movement
- Ability to move fingers or toes

General Principles of Splinting The steps for applying a splint are as follows:

- Always check the ABCDs and perform a thorough head-to-toe examination before beginning treatment of fractures.
- In most situations, remove clothing from the area of any suspected fracture or dislocation to allow inspection of the limb for open wounds, deformity, swelling, and ecchymosis.
- Note and record the circulatory (pulse and capillary refill) and neurologic (sensation and movement) status distal to the site of injury. Continue to monitor the neurovascular status until the patient reaches the hospital.
- Cover all wounds with a dry, sterile dressing before applying a splint. Notify the receiving hospital of all open wounds.
- Do not move the patient before splinting extremity injuries unless there is an immediate hazard to the patient or yourself.
- In a suspected fracture of the shaft of any bone, make sure the splint immobilizes the joint above and the joint below the fracture.
- With injuries in and around the joint, make sure the splint immobilizes the bone above and the bone below the injured joint.
- Pad all rigid splints to prevent local pressure.
- During application of the splint, use your hands to minimize movement of the limb and to support the injury site until the limb is completely splinted.

- Align a limb severely deformed from a fracture of the shaft of a long bone with constant gentle manual traction so that it can be incorporated into a splint.
- If you encounter resistance to limb alignment when you apply traction, splint the limb in the position of deformity.
- Immobilize all suspected spinal injuries in a neutral in-line position.
- When in doubt, splint.

Dislocations

A dislocation is a disruption of a joint that occurs when the supporting ligaments and capsule of the joint tear and allow the bone ends to separate completely (Figure 14.7). In some cases, a dislocation may be accompanied by a fracture. The term for this injury is a fracture-dislocation.

Because the surfaces of joints have sensory nerve fibers similar to those found in the periosteum, dislocations can be painful especially when muscle spasms cause movement across unstable joint surfaces. Muscle spasms and pain will increase with the length of time the joint is dislocated.

Dislocated joint surfaces can injure adjacent structures by direct impact, which causes a contusion. Dislocations can also obstruct vascular circulation by compression. Direct compression of nerves may result in permanent loss of nerve function. The effect on adjacent structures increases with the length of time the joint is dislocated.

FIGURE 14.7

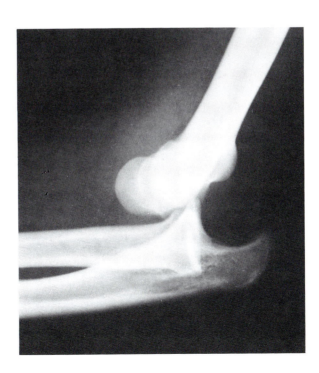

A dislocation occurs when the supporting ligaments and capsule of the joint tear and allow the bone ends to separate completely.

The joint cartilage has no direct blood supply but depends on the synovial fluid within the joint for nutrition. Without this nourishment, injury to the cartilage of the joint surface increases with the length of time the joint is dislocated.

Mechanisms of Injury There are two basic mechanisms for dislocations. In a *direct injury*, the force is applied directly to the joint area. This separates the bone ends within the joint. An example of a direct injury would be a patient falling directly on the shoulder, causing it to dislocate. A direct injury is often associated with the more serious fracture-dislocation.

An *indirect injury* occurs when the force is applied to the extremity distal to the joint. The dislocation results from a levering force at the joint. An example of an indirect injury would be the knee striking the dashboard. The force travels from the knee up the femur and levers the hip out posteriorly.

Assessment Field assessment of dislocations should be directed toward simple dislocations from indirect force. Base the assessments on the mechanism of injury or the patient's history of previous dislocations. The presence of *minor* associated fractures should not change the treatment plan.

Treatment In conventional, rapid-transport EMS, stabilize all dislocated joints in the position found, and then transport the patient to definitive medical care. Use traction in position (TIP) to attempt to reposition dislocations anatomically *only if distal circulation is impaired and if approved by medical control.*

During extended incidents, refer to local medical protocols for specific local clinical standards regarding the assessment and treatment of dislocations. Dislocations associated with direct force that could also cause severe fractures should be treated as joint fractures. Splint or stabilize in the position you find the joint.

If you have been properly trained in the procedure, consider an attempt at reducing a simple dislocation if an extended transport time is expected. Do not attempt reductions unless you have been trained and authorized to perform the procedure by a medical control physician and *the procedure is within your scope of practice*. Simple dislocations include indirect injury to the shoulder or to the patella and direct or indirect injury to the fingers.

Discontinue any attempts at reduction if pain increases significantly or if you encounter resistance to movement. In these cases, splint the joint in the injured position for transport. After reduction, recheck circulation and nerve function. Splint in anatomic position for transport.

WOUNDS

Wounds are injuries that disrupt the skin. Wounds may involve the underlying soft tissues such as fat, muscle, and connective tissue between the skin and underlying bones, joints, and organs, as well as the small vessels and nerves. Wounds are quite common in accidents and range from simple abrasions to serious lacerations, impaled foreign objects, gunshot wounds, and other more serious injuries. The three goals of wound management are as follows:

1. Control bleeding.
2. Prevent or control contamination and infection.
3. Protect the wound from further damage.

Types of Wounds

Abrasions An abrasion is a shallow wound that occurs when the skin is rubbed or scraped against a rough or hard surface. Blood may ooze from the injury, but the abrasion normally does not penetrate completely through the dermis.

Lacerations and Incisions In a laceration or an incision the skin is cut or torn, exposing underlying tissues and structures. A laceration may leave either a smooth or jagged wound through the skin. Bleeding and injury to the underlying structures will vary with the wound.

Some lacerations present a high risk of serious infection. These include the following:

- Animal or human bites
- Dirty or contaminated wounds or those likely to get dirty or contaminated
- Ragged, crushed, or contused tissue, such as a chain saw wound or PTO injury
- Injuries to a bone, joint, or tendon
- Wounds that are not immobilized

Puncture Wounds A puncture wound penetrates into underlying tissue with a minimum of skin disruption. Typical puncture wounds result from penetration with a knife, screwdriver, splinter, bullet, or any other pointed object. External bleeding from puncture wounds may not be severe, but internal bleeding may be significant. Puncture wounds carry a high risk of infection, especially if they cannot drain.

Gunshot wounds are a special form of puncture wound with unique characteristics that require special prehospital care. Gunshot wounds frequently are multiple, so the patient should be inspected carefully to identify the number and sites, including exit wounds.

Avulsions An avulsion is an injury in which a segment of tissue is torn completely loose from its attachments or is left hanging as a flap.

Amputations In an amputation, a segment of an extremity is completely detached. In some amputations, bleeding may be severe. If carefully preserved, an amputated part often can be reattached at the hospital.

Preserve an amputated part by placing it in a dry, sterile dressing. Place the part and moist dressing in a container, preferably sterile. Place the container in another cool container containing ice and water. Do not allow the amputated part to contact the ice and possibly freeze.

Amputations are common in agricultural-rural incidents. These amputations are usually severe, and a single limb may be in several pieces. Both the amputated pieces and the open end of the wound are likely to be very dirty, so the risk of infection is high (Figure 14.8). The rescue team must carefully search, often through grain or straw, to make sure all the missing parts have been retrieved. Before packaging the parts for transport, rinse them carefully in sterile saline solution. Then follow the procedures outlined above for preserving and transporting amputated parts.

Near amputation refers to a segment of an extremity that has been severed except for a small flap of skin. Try to maintain the attachment, and follow the procedures for amputations.

Assessment and Treatment Assess potential injures to underlying organs and structures and evaluate for continuing blood loss. Determine if the injury is at high risk of infection.

Well-positioned direct pressure will stop most bleeding within 15 minutes as normal clotting mechanisms are activated. The rescuer may need to cut the patient's hair or remove clothing in order to see the wound and apply direct pressure.

Persistent bleeding may result from inadequate pressure or pressure not applied directly to the source of bleeding. For rapid transport, it is generally better to widen the pressure dressing to attempt to cover the point of bleeding more accurately. In an extended incident or transport, remove the original, ineffective dressing to examine the wound, then reapply pressure directly to the bleeding site.

During short transport, a PASG can provide direct pressure to multiple bleeding sites in the patient's lower extremities. Air splints may be used for upper extremity injuries. When the patient is moved to a warmer or cooler environment or is evacuated by air medical transport, carefully monitor the pressure being applied to the extremity by any inflatable device.

Monitor the circulation, sensory, and motor status in the affected limb. If it is diminished, loosen the pressure dressing as long as bleeding does not restart. Do not remove the dressing in the event that the bleeding recurs.

CHAPTER 14 Common Medical Conditions and Injuries

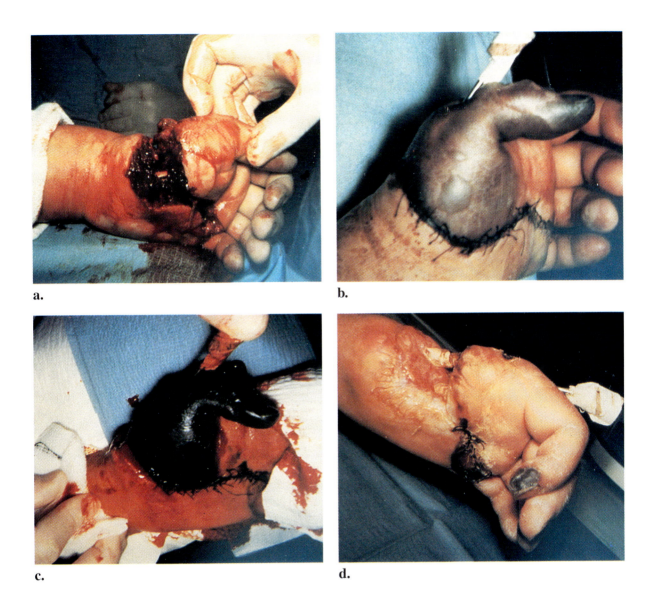

FIGURE 14.8

a. Body parts that are amputated in agricultural-rural incidents are heavily contaminated with foreign material. This hand was caught in an auger.
b. The thumb was reattached in an attempt to save it.
c. and d. The thumb was removed after it became infected.

Control bleeding by elevating the affected limb and splinting to prevent motion that might loosen clots or cause additional injury. Splinting also increases patient comfort and may make it easier to maintain elevation to decrease the swelling. Use ice in addition to direct pressure.

The use of arterial pressure points to control bleeding is rarely effective. However, in some agricultural-rural incidents such as an auger entanglement, it may be impossible to apply direct pressure until the extrication is complete. In these situations, the use of arterial pressure points may be necessary. Do not use hemostats to control bleeding unless in an operating room. Use tourniquets only as a last resort, and only if approved by medical control.

In avulsion injuries, gently irrigate the wound to remove debris, then carefully fold the soft tissue onto the wound if possible. If a flap of tissue has been completely avulsed, collect it and take it to the emergency department with the patient. It is often possible to reattach totally avulsed tissues. The most effective way of transporting the part is to wrap it in dry, sterile gauze and place it in a sterile container that, in turn, should be placed in a cool container. Do not allow the tissue to freeze.

In an agricultural-rural incident, open wounds are likely to be contaminated with foreign matter, such as grain and dirt. Both the wound and any amputated parts should be gently cleansed. Irrigate them with sterile saline solution if it can be done without restarting bleeding. Local medical protocols may instruct the team to use an antibiotic solution for the final rinse, or to use an antibacterial dressing.

Impaled Objects

The primary objective in treating a wound from an impaled object is to reduce the possibility of further injury from unwanted movement of the object. In a rapid-transport situation, the impaled object should be stabilized in place unless it is obstructing the airway. In an extended incident, it is sometimes best to remove the impaled object if it prevents safe and effective patient packaging or transport and if removal can be done simply, safely, and easily. Removal of an impaled object by the rescue team must be done only in special circumstances by trained rescuers under direct orders of the medical control physician.

High-Pressure Injection Injury

High-pressure injection injuries are extremely serious. They occur when finely atomized fluid is injected through the skin from a nozzle or a leak in a hose, valve, or fitting, without creating an open wound. These injuries may be extremely painful because of the severe soft tissue injury from the pressure or reaction to the material injected.

Within minutes, the skin around the injection site will become an unusually bright blue, due to lack of oxygen. Swelling develops rapidly. Within 30 minutes, tissue necrosis may cause the skin discoloration to turn black. Occasionally, the fluid may travel along the bones of the hands and wrist several inches from the injection site and settle in the soft tissue of the palm or forearm. It may even penetrate completely through the hand, with an entry and exit point.

Immediate treatment should focus on keeping the fluid localized, so it does not spread into the bloodstream, which could result in death. Keep the patient calm. Do not elevate the extremity above the level of the heart, or give the patient anything to eat or drink by mouth. Remove any rings or watches and apply insulated cold packs to cool the affected area. Treat the patient for shock secondary to pain and provide rapid transport to definitive medical care. Extensive debridement (surgical removal of contaminated tissue) will be necessary once the patient reaches the hospital. If advanced life support personnel are available, they should start an IV in an uninjured limb.

BURNS

Burns are among the most serious, painful, and dangerous of all injuries. They occur when the body receives more thermal energy than it can absorb without injury. The source of this energy is generally heat, but may also include toxic chemicals, electricity, and nuclear radiation.

The three major concerns with a burn patient are as follows:

1. Hypovolemic shock. The clinical pattern will begin within minutes or hours after the patient sustains the burn injury.
2. Respiratory burn or irritation. Swelling occurs during the first 24 hours after the patient sustains the burn injury.
3. Infection. Signs of infection in the burn patient usually begin to appear several days after the incident. But the degree of infection and the outcome are affected by early treatment and the way the patient is handled.

Assessment

Follow the steps described throughout this text for securing the scene and ensure that no member of the rescue team is at risk for burn injury from live power lines, toxic fumes, exposure to radioactivity, or outbreaks of fire and explosion. The first step in assessment is to stop the burning process. Move the patient from the burning area, and remove any smoldering clothing. If the skin and clothing are still hot, immerse them in cool water or cover them with a cool, wet dressing.

As in any other emergency medical response, check the ABCDs (airway, breathing, circulation, and disability). Indications of respiratory burn include singed facial hair or skin, or soot in the nostrils. If there is any possibility of respiratory burn, continue to monitor the airway. Respiratory burns generally cause problems 4 to 6 hours after the injury as swelling in the airway develops.

If the burn is the result of electrical contact, including lightning, monitor the patient for cardiac arrhythmias.

Examine the body. Do not let the severity of the burn injuries distract you from the possibility that the patient might have sustained other injuries at the time of the incident. For example, the patient may have sustained fractures as the result of falling or thrashing around, especially following an electric shock.

Estimate the severity of the burn. The actual depth of the burn and the surface involved are calculated together to determine the seriousness

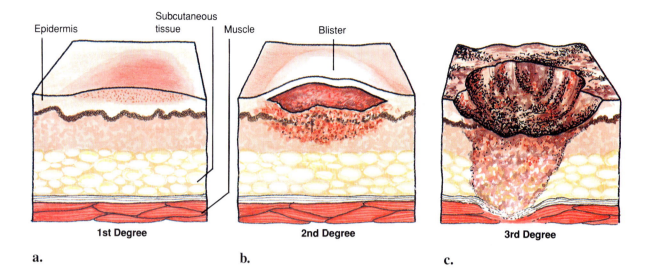

FIGURE 14.9

Three common degrees of burns.
a. A first-degree burn causes epidermal injury with redness of the skin.
b. A second-degree burn causes partial destruction of the dermis and is characterized by blisters.
c. A third-degree burn causes complete epidermal and dermal destruction, and may extend even deeper.

of the burn. There are three categories of burns (Figure 14.9). First-degree burns are those in which only the superficial part of the epidermis has been injured. The skin may turn red but does not blister or actually burn through. A sunburn is an example of a first-degree burn.

In second-degree burns, the epidermis and a portion of the dermis are burned without destroying the entire thickness of the dermis. A second-degree burn is commonly characterized by the formation of blisters.

Third-degree burns extend through the dermis into or beyond the subcutaneous fat. The area becomes dry, leathery, and discolored with a charred, brown, or white appearance (Figure 14.10). Clotted blood vessels may become visible under the burned skin, or the subcutaneous fat itself may be visible. In severe third-degree burns, superficial nerve endings and blood vessels are destroyed, leaving the burned area without feeling, although the surrounding areas will be extremely painful.

Estimate the area burned by the **Rule of Nines** (Figure 14.11). There are five factors that determine the seriousness of a thermal burn:

- The depth (first-, second-, or third-degree)
- The amount of Body Surface Area (BSA) involved (Rule of Nines)
- The involvement of critical areas (hands, feet, face, or genitalia)
- The patient's age
- The patient's general health, especially in the presence of other injuries or illnesses

Critical burns include any third-degree burns that involve the hands, feet, genitalia, or face, or any third-degree burns involving more than 10% of the body surface area. All burns complicated by fractures or any degree of respiratory injury are considered critical. Critical burns also include any second-degree burns involving more than 25% of the body

FIGURE 14.10

A severe electrical burn can split open the skin.

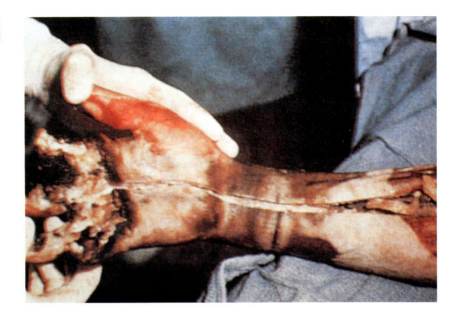

FIGURE 14.11

The percentage of body surface affected by a burn is estimated by the Rule of Nines. In the adult, most areas of the body are divided roughly into multiples of nine. In the child, relatively more area is taken up by the head and less by the lower extremities.

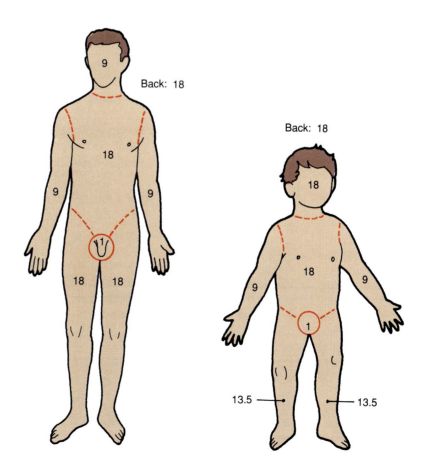

surface area or any otherwise moderate burn in an elderly or critically ill patient.

Moderate burns are less serious than critical burns, but they are dangerous and susceptible to infection and other complications. Moderate burns include third-degree burns involving 2% to 10% of the body surface area and second-degree burns involving 15% to 25% of the body surface area. First-degree burns, including sunburn, involving 50% to 75% of the body surface area can also be characterized as moderate burns.

Minor burns include third-degree burns involving less than 2% of the body surface or second-degree burns involving less than 15% of the BSA.

In children, any third-degree burn is considered critical. A second-degree burn of more than 20% of the BSA is considered a critical burn, and a second-degree burn of 10% to 20% of the BSA would be considered a moderate burn, as would any first-degree burn.

Treatment

Continue to monitor the patient's airway for signs of respiratory distress. A developing cough suggests impending airway problems. Administer oxygen according to local medical protocols.

Perform initial cooling with sterile dressings soaked in water to reduce injury to tissues and relieve pain. To avoid hypothermia in patients with greater than a 10% BSA burn, limit cooling to several minutes on each area.

Apply dry, sterile dressings to prevent contamination and relieve pain and treat any associated injuries. *If within your scope of practice,* begin IV fluid replacement if the burn area is extensive.

Treatment for Extended Transport In extended transport situations, continue soaks to areas of less than 10% of the BSA, as long as the patient is in pain. Cleanse the burn as you would an abrasion. After the wound has been cooled and cleansed, apply an antibacterial dressing according to instructions from medical control.

IV Volume Replacement During extended incidents in which the patient has second- and third-degree burns of greater than 20% of the BSA, begin IV fluid replacement *if within your scope of practice and if ordered by medical control.* For burn patients, the Brooke formula for fluid replacement, using lactated Ringer's solution or normal saline solution, is as follows:

$$2 - 4 \text{ mL} \times \text{kg body} \times \% \text{ burn} = \text{estimated fluid needs for 24 hours}$$

Give half the estimated fluid requirement in the first 8 hours, and the second half over the next 16 hours. Remember that this guideline is an estimate only. Adjust the actual volume and rate according to the patient's vital signs and urinary output. Use the same standards as for volume replacement in shock. Monitor urinary output using a Foley catheter, *if within your scope of practice and training, and if ordered by medical control.* Refer to local medical protocols for specific clinical standards regarding the treatment of burns during extended incidents.

PATIENT CONTROL

Patient care during extended incidents often requires sensitivity and kindness, attributes that are as important as medical skills and procedures. These attributes are less definable yet still important to a patient's well-being. Patient comfort and reassurance are important components of any medical treatment but are especially important in trauma care.

Because of the excitement, surprise, anger, stress, and pain that occur with injury, patients often become their own worst enemies. Fear or confusion may be translated into "uncooperative behavior" such as sudden, dangerous movements. Therefore, it is important to establish a trusting relationship and working rapport with patients.

A relaxed patient with a positive attitude will make treatment and evacuation easier for the rescue team. And it will also provide the patient with a better chance of survival and recovery.

SUMMARY

Rescuers will often encounter the same types of medical conditions and/or injuries from incident to incident. Therefore, it is important for rescuers to be able to recognize, assess, and treat the more common medical conditions and injuries. Some of these include shock, head injuries, wounds, burns, musculoskeletal injuries, fractures, dislocations, and traumatic injuries. Some of these conditions, such as shock, indicate a serious threat that requires immediate treatment. Others, such as concussions, may be minor and simply require monitoring for change during the rescue operation.

Rescuers must be able to assess patients, looking for signs and symptoms of medical problems. A careful assessment helps to differentiate among potential problems or injuries and indicates the seriousness of any possible medical condition.

For a rescue involving medical conditions and/or injuries to be successful, rescuers must be familiar with appropriate treatment measures for common medical conditions and injuries. This is especially true for those conditions that require immediate and aggressive treatment measures.

CHAPTER 15
Patient Packaging and Litter Evacuation

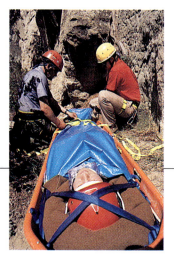

CHAPTER OUTLINE

Overview
Objectives
Packaging Considerations
Packaging for Litter
    Evacuation
    Packaging Spinal, Pelvic, or
        Lower Extremity Injuries
    Additional Packaging
    Airway Management
    Immobilization in Other
        Types of Litters
Special Treatment,
    Packaging, and Evacu-
    ation Considerations

IV Use in Rural Areas
IV Maintenance
Carrying Litters
    The Litter Team
    The Load Sling
Belaying the Litter
Moving a Litter Through a
    Confined Space
Basic Lowering Systems
    Lowering Devices
Hauling Systems
Summary

KEY TERMS

Belay: system of safety ropes attached to a litter that acts to support the litter in the event the litter starts to slip or fall during evacuation.

Bombproof anchor: one that is stronger than any forces that will be placed on the system during the rescue operation.

Brake bar rack: U-shaped frame in which one arm of the U is longer than the other. This rack helps control lowering large loads.

CHAPTER 15 Patient Packaging and Litter Evacuation

Brakeman: rescuer who controls the rate of lowering.

Counterbalance system: a simple 1:1 MA system commonly used in silo rescues.

Hauling system: system used to raise a patient to a higher elevation.

Lowering: controlled movement in which a patient is moved from higher elevation to lower elevation.

Rope handler: rescuer who assists brakeman by feeding rope and removing kinks in rope before they foul the brake.

OVERVIEW

Knowing how to package and transport patients in a safe and efficient manner is crucial to the successful outcome of a rescue operation. This chapter explains packaging and litter transport techniques.

The techniques of litter evacuation range from packaging the patient in the litter to moving the litter through and from the rescue site. This chapter also examines a variety of litter evacuation techniques. It offers detailed instructions on certain aspects of litter evacuation.

The chapter begins by describing packaging techniques, including securing a patient with lower extremity injuries and immobilizing the patient on a spine board. There is also a section outlining special packaging considerations. This section addresses patient protection and administration of IV fluids in rural areas, where it might be difficult for an ambulance to approach and where rescue teams might have to carry the patient to the ambulance. The chapter also analyzes the tasks of carrying and moving litters. The litter team, lowering systems, and hauling systems are also discussed.

OBJECTIVES

After reading this chapter, the rescuer should be able to:

- describe how to package a patient for transport.
- describe how to package a patient in a litter for transport.
- describe how to construct specific patient packages for evacuation by helicopter.

continued

- describe how to manage and maintain IVs during transport.
- describe how to carry a litter.
- explain basic techniques for belaying a litter.
- describe how to move a litter through a confined space.
- explain basic lowering and hauling systems.
- describe how to determine mechanical advantage in hauling systems.

PACKAGING CONSIDERATIONS

There are five major concerns in packaging the patient for transport. First, rescuers must package the patient to avoid additional injury. Second, rescuers must be concerned about patient comfort. The third concern is ensuring effective patient immobilization while allowing access for reassessment and continued treatment. Immobilization equipment must be adaptable and must fit within the size constraints of the specific transport system.

A fourth concern is the ability to move the patient. Once the patient is packaged comfortably in relation to his or her injuries, rescuers must be able to carry the patient and litter to the transport vehicle or other destination. For example, carrying the weight of a stretcher with only one hand will cause fatigue sooner than if the stretcher is carried with both hands.

The last concern, and equally important, is that the packaging must be compatible with the transport being used. For most helicopter transports, the litter and patient package must fit into the aircraft. Occasionally, the litter will be slung under the aircraft for a short distance transport when the rescue scene does not provide an appropriate landing zone. Rescuers involved in air medical operations need to discuss with the flight crew the types of stretchers that are acceptable for use in fixed-line flyaway operations. Certain types of litters, such as the solid plastic Stokes, have aerodynamic characteristics that make them unacceptable for such operations because of the high risk of injury or death to the patient.

PACKAGING FOR LITTER EVACUATION

The patient must be packaged so that he or she will not fall out even if the litter is angled or tilted. The patient also must not shift inside the "patient package" or the litter. If spinal injuries are suspected, the patient must be immobilized to prevent any movement of the spinal column. One method of securing a patient in a litter is to lace him or her in

CHAPTER 15   Patient Packaging and Litter Evacuation

with 1" webbing. Figure 15.1 illustrates the procedure for securing a patient in a plastic Stokes litter, using a 30' length of 1" tubular webbing. This procedure is also described below.

1. Find the center of the webbing. Attach the center to the railing at the foot of the litter, using a girth hitch.
2. With one rescuer on each side of the litter, pass the webbing back and forth across the patient. The webbing should be snug across the patient, but should not cause discomfort or impede circulation. On a metal basket, run the webbing around the major support members that attach the rail to the basket. On a plastic basket, attach the webbing by running it over the rope laced inside the basket by the manufacturer. Never run the webbing over the rail, as it may be damaged by abrasion as the litter is carried over rough terrain.
3. Do not allow the webbing to run across the neck of the patient. In a high-angle environment, extra tie-ins may be needed in addition to the straps designed for the litter.

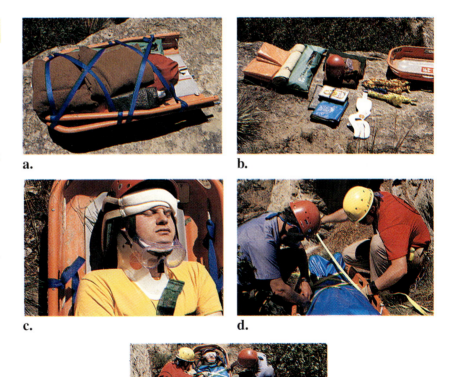

FIGURE 15.1

a. Store materials for packaging a patient in the litter.
b. Packaging materials include protective gear, padding, webbing, and immobilization equipment.
c. Immobilize the patient first to prevent any movement of spinal areas. Then, attach the center of the length of webbing with a girth hitch to the railing at the foot of the Stokes litter.
d. Two rescuers, one on each side of the litter, pass the webbing back and forth across the patient. The webbing should be snug across the patient, but should not cause discomfort or impede circulation.
e. Secure the webbing near the patient's head in a way that avoids running across the neck of the patient.

There should also be a separate tie-in that connects a safety harness on the patient to a belay system. This is a necessary safety system for the patient, in case the litter or other portions of the rope system fail.

If there is any chance that the litter will be tilted, foot tie-ins or a seat harness will be needed to prevent the patient from sliding down in the litter. Ankle hitch restraints can be used for patients who do not have lower extremity, pelvic, or lumbar spine injuries. Figure 15.2 shows how to secure the patient's feet with 12' to 15' of 1" tubular webbing, but *this technique must not be used if there are spinal, pelvic, or lower extremity fractures. The next section discusses the appropriate technique for such injuries.* The ankle hitch technique is also described below.

1. Lay the webbing behind the ankle. Then bring it around the foot and cross the webbing over the top of the foot.
2. Pull the webbing firmly toward the bottom of the litter and across on the bottom of the foot.
3. Bring the webbing up on the opposite side of the foot, through the previous crosses, and pull firmly toward the head of the litter.
4. Tie off the webbing on the litter rail supports or over the interior laced rope. It should be tight enough so that the patient will not shift if the litter is stood on end. The seat harness described below may be used to provide additional stabilization.

Packaging Spinal, Pelvic, or Lower Extremity Injuries

The ankle hitch method of securing a patient cannot be used if the patient has spinal, pelvic, or lower extremity injuries. For these patients, use 1" webbing leg loops or a climbing harness to prevent lengthwise movement. Both ends of the harness should be secured to the litter rail. The restraint system used should not compromise blood vessels or nerves.

FIGURE 15.2

Use foot tie-ins or a seat harness to prevent the patient from sliding down in the litter, if the litter is tilted.

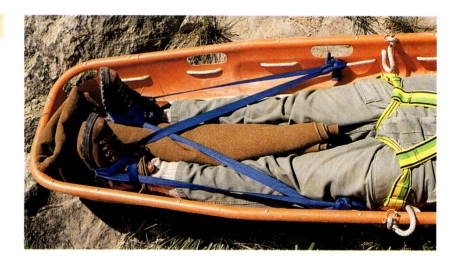

Patients with pelvic, chest, or spinal cord injuries pose a challenging situation. A combination of the two systems discussed above, with the addition of a nonconstricting chest restraint, can be adapted to meet the most difficult situation.

Additional Packaging

Even with webbing restraints, patients may shift in a litter. This is particularly true of patients who do not fill the litter, such as thin people and children. Side-to-side movement can be eliminated by adding enough padding to fill any spaces between the patient's body and the packaging device (litter, back board, stretcher).

Airway Management

As with other forms of emergency medical care, patient packaging for litter evacuation must include considerations for airway management. The patient must be packaged so that the total package can be rolled onto its side to allow for definitive care of the patient's airway, without any significant patient movement within the package, in the case of vomiting or airway threats. The patient must be secured so there is no shift along the spinal column. One possible solution in these situations is to immobilize the patient on a long spine board or the equivalent within the litter.

Immobilization in Other Types of Litters

Semirigid, conforming litters provide patient packaging by conforming around the individual. However, the patient must not shift inside these litters. Package the patient by packing soft materials such as clothing in any spaces between the litter and the patient's body.

Some litters have additional means for securing the patient, such as attached D rings or carrying straps.

SPECIAL TREATMENT, PACKAGING, AND EVACUATION CONSIDERATIONS

Many agricultural-rural incidents take place in the open, such as in the middle of a field or farmstead. Consequently, during rescue and packaging, a patient must be protected from environmental hazards such as cold, heat, and wetness. In addition, whenever patients are packaged for a high-angle rescue, such as from a silo, they become vulnerable to two other hazards: they may fall, or they may be hit by falling objects, such as clumps of material stuck to the sides of the silo. Keep all of these hazards in mind when packaging patients for transport.

A patient immobilized in a litter is more at risk from environmental hazards than is the rescuer. Patients are unable to generate heat from muscle activity; their only shelter is that provided by rescuers. Also, a patient's injuries may predispose him or her to greater heat loss.

A patient in a litter must have environmental protection both *above and below* the body. In a cold, windy, or wet environment, the patient should have an insulating layer next to the body and a barrier layer on the outside. Blankets or a sleeping bag can serve as an insulating layer. If a sleeping bag is used, it should open all the way around for greater access to the entire body. For even greater convenience, the bag's zipper closure can be replaced with Velcro™. The barrier layer protection should be an impenetrable and tear-resistant material such as a poncho, tarp, or tough plastic.

A reflectorized tarp can be used with the reflecting side toward the patient to help preserve body heat. In hot environments, the tarp can be used with the reflecting side turned to the outside to reflect heat away from the patient.

A patient being transported in a litter should always have adequate eye protection from dirt, debris, and rain. Always keep a pair of goggles or a face shield with the litter as part of the packaging material (Figure 15.3).

The patient should also wear a helmet for head protection unless there are suspected cervical spine or head injuries. The helmet should be designed to avoid hyperextending the patient's neck.

The decision to secure the patient's hands should be made after an evaluation of the patient's mental state and level of consciousness. The hands of a patient who is unconscious must be secured inside the litter, but many conscious patients will not want their hands secured. Patients may think they will be able to keep their hands inside the litter as you instruct them, but a high-angle rescue may cause the patient to become anxious and to grab or hold onto the litter rails. This may result in serious injuries if the hand or fingers are caught between the litter and a hard surface.

FIGURE 15.3

Provide the patient with eye protection from dirt, brush, and rain.

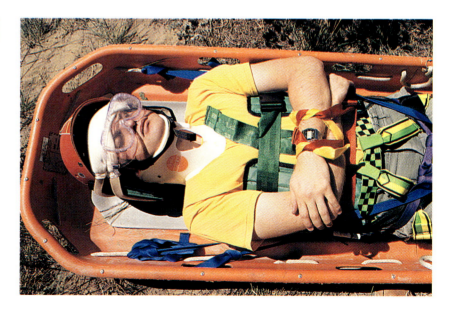

IV Use in Rural Areas

Because intravenous (IV) fluids are both weighty and bulky, the selection of fluids carried by rescuers is extremely important. If IV fluids must be carried into the center of a field or remote area, you must get the most efficient use of them. Blood components, both natural and synthetic, may provide the greatest gain for the weight in the treatment of hypovolemic shock which, in agricultural-rural incidents, commonly results from blood loss. The use of IVs as a line for drug administration is usually a low priority in agricultural-rural incidents.

Weather extremes and patient transport problems may also make it difficult to administer and monitor IV fluids. If a medical team accompanies the rescue team, IVs may be kept with the ambulance and administered once the patient is extricated and transported to the ambulance.

IV Maintenance

In cold weather, it may take a major effort to keep IV solutions warm as they are being administered to the patient and to prevent IV lines from freezing. One possible solution is to pin the bag inside the rescuer's clothing and run the tubing into the litter packaging system. Protect any exposed tubing by insulating with a material such as closed-cell foam pads. Inside the litter, run as much of the tubing as possible close to the patient's skin. Remember, there must be some slack to allow for rescuer and litter movement.

Another option for keeping IVs warm is the adapted heat pack. However, use extreme caution because of the possibility of overheating the fluids, which can cause thermal and chemical burns to both the patient and the rescuer.

CARRYING LITTERS

Carrying litters across difficult terrain requires more personnel and different techniques than those used for conventional, rapid-transport, ambulance-based EMS. These techniques must be practiced before they are used in an actual rescue operation.

The Litter Team

For a short-distance carry (one-fourth mile or less) of a litter, a *minimum* of six rescuers is required—four to carry and two to scout. For a longer carry, a *minimum* of eight rescuers is required—six to carry and two to scout. Additional help is often desirable to provide relief for the six carriers on a regular rotation, particularly if the terrain is rugged or the distances long.

The litter team should be selected so that persons of the same height are across from one another on the litter. This assures that each person carries equal weight and that the litter remains level. Each litter team must have a captain to give directions. The litter team captain is tradi-

FIGURE 15.4

Use a carrying sling made from a 14' to 18' length of 1" tubular webbing to spread the load onto other parts of the body. Create the webbing loop with a water knot.

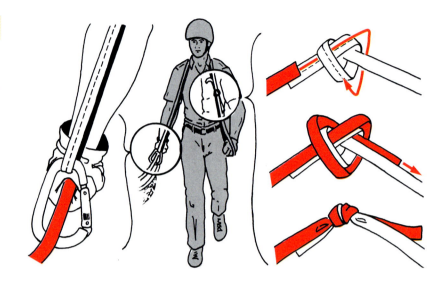

tionally at the patient's right shoulder (front left position on the litter). The scouts walk in front of the litter to point out hazards and remove obstacles from the team's path.

The Load Sling

Carrying a litter with only one hand grasping the litter rail can be extremely tiring. To spread the load onto other parts of the body, create a carrying sling with a 14' to 18' length of 1" tubular webbing (Figure 15.4). Create a continuous loop in the webbing with a water knot. Attach the load sling to the litter rail with a carabiner that will comfortably slip over the rail. Run the tubing over the shoulder away from the litter, and grasp the end of the webbing with the hand that is away from the litter. Adjust the length of the sling to meet individual needs.

BELAYING THE LITTER

While removing a patient from a high-angle environment, such as during a silo rescue, there is the danger that the litter may drop or slide. To avoid this danger, the team must **belay** the litter. To belay a litter, attach a safety or belay rope to the litter and secure it so that if the litter starts to fall, the belay rope supports it. In most cases, the belay rope is controlled by a second rescuer known as the belayer.

During a belay, always grasp the brake side of the rope firmly with your dominant hand (for example, the right hand for right-handed people). This brake hand must never leave the rope until the patient and stretcher are *off belay* and in a secure position.

MOVING A LITTER THROUGH A CONFINED SPACE

Moving a patient in a litter through a confined space can be very demanding on rescuers and extremely difficult for the patient. Confined space litter removal will require more rescuers than usual. Removal to a safe area may require the use of a suitable extrication system. For example, when removing a conscious patient with minor injuries from a silo, a safety harness or sling may be used. If the patient has spinal injuries, a back board or one of the specialized semirigid or body-shaped patient transportation devices may be needed. Figure 8 wraps under the feet of the patient should be used to prevent sliding, even if the board is equipped with a foot rest. Extra straps in a figure 8 should be applied at the groin and shoulders to prevent longitudinal movement or slippage of the patient. Stay alert to sudden changes in patient status, as the patient may need to be turned rapidly to effect proper airway management.

BASIC LOWERING SYSTEMS

Many rescue situations require moving the patient from a higher elevation to a lower one, as when rescuing a patient from a silo, or as when moving a patient down a steep road embankment. The act of moving a patient to a lower elevation in a controlled manner is called **lowering**.

The basic elements of a lowering system are illustrated in Figure 15.5. The patient is secured in the litter to prevent movement or slippage. Litter tenders on the outside ladder guide the litter down, or tag lines can be used to keep the litter from spinning.

A loop of rope is attached to the head of the litter. To help prevent damage to the litter, the rope should not be attached at one point, but wrapped around the litter rail several times before completing the loop (Figure 15.6). The main line is then attached to the loop with a figure 8 overhand knot and locking carabiners.

The rate of lowering is controlled by the **brakeman**. The brakeman does this by grasping the rope and controlling its speed through the lowering device or brake that is attached to a bombproof anchor. A **bombproof anchor** is one that is stronger than any forces that will be placed on the system during the rescue operation. A **rope handler** assists the brakeman by feeding rope and removing kinks in the rope before they can foul the brake. Because of the high angle of a silo rescue, there is great danger to the patient and rescuers if the lowering system fails. Therefore, a belay system should always be used. The belay system is attached to a separate anchor system and attached to the litter.

Lowering Devices

Rescue lowering devices or brakes work on the same principle as rappel devices. The person controlling the device creates friction between the

FIGURE 15.5

A basic lowering system includes litter tenders, a rope handler, a brakeman, and a belayer.

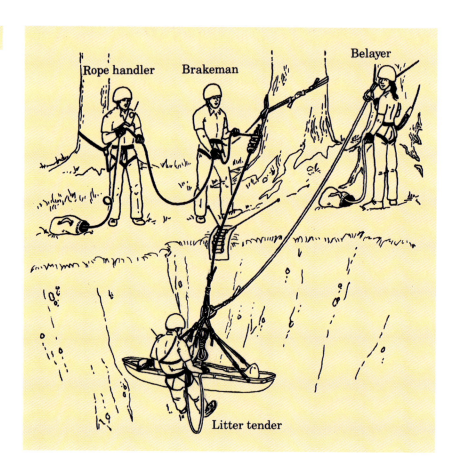

FIGURE 15.6

Wrap a rope around the rail several times to prevent damage to the litter.

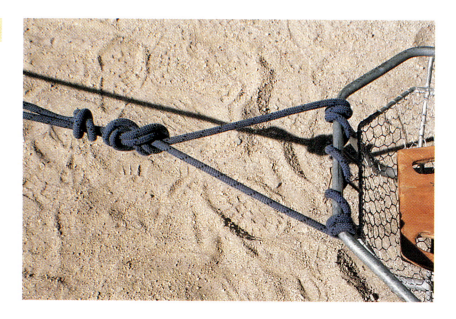

CHAPTER 15 Patient Packaging and Litter Evacuation

rope and the metal surfaces of the device. The difference between using these devices for rappeling and lowering is the relative location of the device.

In rappeling, the load, usually a person, is attached directly to the device that moves with it. The top end of the rope is attached to an anchor and the rope remains fixed during the rappel. In lowering, the device is attached to the anchor and the load is attached to the end of the rope that runs through the device.

The **brake bar rack** provides greater control in rescue lowering for larger loads, such as a patient in a litter. The brake bar rack is also known as a rappel rack or Cole rack. The frame is a stainless steel bar fabricated into a U shape, with one arm of the U longer than the other (Figure 15.7). The end of the longer arm is shaped into an eye that can be attached to an anchor. The eye of a rescue rack should be factory welded and inspected. Using a brake bar rack has several advantages: it is easy to change the friction to adapt to varying loads; it provides greater control for large rescue loads; and it does not twist the rope that runs through it, thus reducing tangles and foul-ups.

HAULING SYSTEMS

In some rescue situations, the patient must be raised from a lower elevation to a higher one, as in a silo rescue. **Hauling systems** are used to raise the patient to a higher elevation.

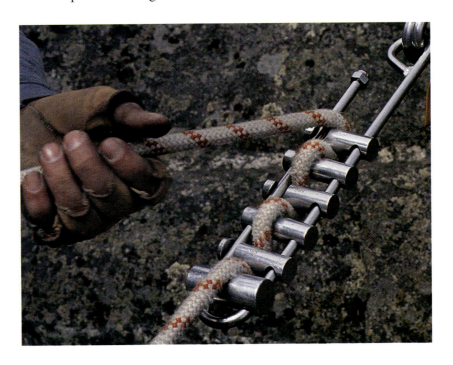

FIGURE 15.7

The brake bar rack is a friction device used in rescue for lowering of larger loads such as a patient in a litter with litter tenders.

Hauling systems are classified according to the mechanical advantage (MA) they provide. Mechanical advantage is the ratio of resistance divided by the effort that it takes to raise the load in a particular hauling system. If, for example, the load weighs 400 lb and it takes 200 lb of effort to move it, then the MA of the system is 2:1. If it takes only 100 lb of effort to move a 400 lb load, then the MA would be 4:1. Figure 15.8 presents diagrams of MA for some basic types of hauling systems.

The higher the MA, the easier it is to raise the load, but such systems will also be more complicated and can place a greater force on rescue system components. A higher MA is created by increasing the distance over which you apply the effort. For example, in a 2:1 MA hauling system, you must pull 200' of rope to move the load 100'. In a 4:1 MA system, you must pull 400' of rope to move the load. Additionally, you never get the full advantage from a hauling system; there is always friction loss in pulleys, abrasion loss on edges, and so forth. The more cautious you are about avoiding friction and other losses, the more efficient the hauling system will be. When using high MA hauling systems, you must be cautious about causing system failure. Keep it simple and use the lowest MA system possible to accomplish the rescue operation.

The simplest hauling system is the 1:1 MA system. In this system, the force needed to move the rescue load is the same as the load. A 1:1 MA system might be used on a steep slope. One of the simplest of the 1:1 MA systems is the **counterbalance system**, which is frequently used in silo rescues because it can both raise and lower the patient effectively.

In this system, one end of the rope is attached to the litter and run up to the top of the silo. There, the rope is run through a pulley and back down the outside of the silo. Rescuers on the outside could rig a second pulley near the silo ladder, and create a hauling system by simply walking away from the silo, raising the litter to the top. Once the litter has cleared the silo, rescuers walk slowly toward the silo, lowering the litter to the ground.

FIGURE 15.8

Hauling systems are classified according to their mechanical advantage (MA).

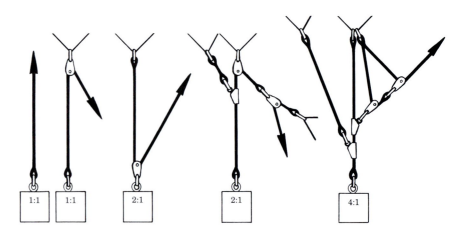

CHAPTER 15 Patient Packaging and Litter Evacuation

SUMMARY

Knowing how to use and move litters is an important aspect of transporting patients in rural areas. The first step is proper patient packaging to prevent shifting or discomfort as the litter is tilted and moved. In addition, patients with suspected spinal injuries must be immobilized to prevent movement of the spinal column.

In rural areas, patients are vulnerable to various environmental hazards, such as temperature extremes, or the risk of falling or being hit by falling objects. Therefore, patients must be packaged with protective clothing to prevent injuries. This includes goggles for eye protection, helmets for head protection, and an insulating/barrier layer for protection from the climate.

The need for administering IV fluids must be considered in the packaging process. Weather extremes and difficulties in patient transport may complicate the use of IVs. Nevertheless, rescuers may be able to administer IV fluids by insulating the tubing in cold weather.

Carrying litters from remote areas requires more personnel and different techniques than those used in conventional, rapid-transport, ambulance-based activities. The number of members required for a litter team depends on the distance of the carry and the ruggedness of the terrain. In general, there should be a minimum of six to carry and two to scout. Persons of the same height should be across from one another on the litter. This enables each person to carry equal weight and helps keep the litter level.

Rescuers should be familiar with the basic litter carrying sequence and understand how to alter the sequence in order to pass the litter across uneven terrain. On a downslope, the litter may need to be belayed to prevent it from sliding during the carry.

Silo rescue operations, especially, require that a patient be raised from a lower elevation to a higher one, and then lowered from a higher elevation to a lower one. Rescuers should understand both hauling systems (to raise the patient) and lowering systems (to lower the patient).

Hauling systems are classified by their mechanical advantage (MA), which is the effort it takes to raise the load. The higher the MA, the easier it is to raise the load. But systems with high MA often place greater force on rescue system components. It is best to use the lowest MA system possible to accomplish the goal.

CHAPTER 16

Vehicles and Transportation

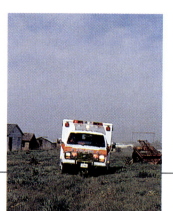

CHAPTER OUTLINE

Overview
Objectives
Ground Vehicle
    Transportation
Air Medical Evacuation
  Landing Zones

Wind Direction, Approach,
    and Departure Paths
Nighttime Landings
Personal Safety
Packaging Considerations
Summary

KEY TERMS

Air medical: method of speeding lifesaving care to patients and of transporting patients with life-threatening injuries or illnesses to definitive medical care.

Fixed-line flyaway: short-distance transport with the stretcher slung under the aircraft.

"Hot" aircraft: term used to describe a helicopter in which the rotors are spinning.

Jump kit: basic life support supplies carried in an ambulance.

CHAPTER 16 Vehicles and Transportation

OVERVIEW

This chapter outlines the vehicle options for ground and air transportation. Because the helicopter is the most common form of air medical evacuation, the chapter contains a discussion of rescue techniques and personal safety when helicopters are used, including issues such as when and where helicopters can be used, landing and departure conditions, nighttime landings, and safety considerations around aircraft.

OBJECTIVES

After reading this chapter, the rescuer should be able to:

- describe how to select the proper vehicle for patient transport.
- explain circumstances in which helicopter evacuation is appropriate.
- identify the limitations associated with helicopter rescue.
- describe how to evaluate operational factors in a helicopter rescue.
- describe how to determine the availability and condition of an airstrip.
- describe how to establish a safe landing zone.
- describe how to prepare a landing zone for nighttime landings.
- explain the appropriate steps to ensure rescuer safety during helicopter evacuations.

GROUND VEHICLE TRANSPORTATION

Transport may be easiest on both rescuers and patients if vehicles can be used. Many of the techniques for transporting patients are similar to conventional, rapid-transport EMS. But weather and terrain may require the rescue vehicle to have special modifications. In rural areas, for example, ambulances may have a four-wheel drive chassis with high ground clearance or other modifications. The distances in rural areas, combined with rugged terrain, mean longer travel times, whether in vehicle or on foot. Many rural roads are unpaved, hilly, winding, and narrow, and require greater care and slower speeds.

In rural areas with a system of mutual aid, the ambulance may come from a hospital, a private company, or a volunteer rescue team. Each ambulance must meet federal regulations, be properly identified, and carry appropriate equipment and supplies. Equipment and supplies should be durable and standardized so that exchanges between ambulances, between ambulances and air medical transport, or between ambulances and emergency departments can be made quickly and easily. Table 16.1 lists minimum equipment and supplies that should be stored on every ambulance.

Under the rural mutual aid system, extrication and rescue may be handled by a separate volunteer rescue team. However, an ambulance should carry some extrication equipment, as shown in Table 16.1. In addition, a rural rescue team should carry basic life support supplies, such as those listed in the **Jump Kit** in Table 16.1.

AIR MEDICAL EVACUATION

The use of air medical evacuation, although expensive and potentially dangerous, is increasing. Air medical transportation is a method of speeding lifesaving care to patients and of transporting patients with life-threatening injuries or illnesses to definitive medical care. The speed and versatility of helicopters in transporting injured individuals increases the chances of patient survival. Helicopters are especially useful in rural areas, where patient injuries are severe and life threatening and where the distance to definitive medical care at a hospital or trauma unit may be hundreds of miles.

Medical indications for use of an air medical helicopter include severe trauma, uncontrollable or internal bleeding, life-threatening burns; profound hypothermia; fractures or dislocations with neurologic or circulatory deficit threatening the limb; life- or limb-threatening snakebite; critical medical conditions such as anaphylaxis; and acute mountain sickness.

In order to use air medical helicopters safely and effectively, rescuers should be familiar with the capabilities, protocols, and methods for accessing the helicopters in their area. Rescue teams should be cross trained by local air medical teams in ground safety when working in and around these aircraft.

If there are medical indications for an air medical evacuation, rescuers must then evaluate operational factors. Will weather, terrain, and altitude conditions permit safe use of a helicopter? Before an air medical rescue mission is attempted, the current and predicted weather conditions for the area must be known. These conditions must be such that the rescue can occur within safe operational guidelines.

TABLE 16.1 Patient Care and Extrication Equipment

Patient Care Equipment

Wheeled litter
Folding litter
Collapsible chair
Litter fasteners
Litter restraints
Oropharyngeal airways for adults, children, and infants
Nasal airways for adults and children
Portable artificial ventilation devices with oxygen supplies and masks in a variety of sizes
Suction equipment (two units, one portable and one installed)
Extra suction tips
Two portable oxygen supply units (300-liter capacity)
One installed oxygen unit (3,000 liters)
Oxygen masks in various sizes
Nasal cannulae
Cardiac compression equipment

Splinting Supplies

One lower-extremity traction splint (telescoping or rigid)
Pediatric-sized traction splint
Upper and lower extremity splints, such as uncomplicated inflatable, vacuum, cardboard, plastic, wire-ladder, canvas-slotted, lace-on, or padded board
Triangular bandages and conforming roller bandages
Short and long spine boards
Cervical collars and accessories
Pneumatic antishock garment with inflation equipment

Patient Care Supplies

Two pillows and pillow cases
Two spare sheets
Four blankets
Four towels
Six disposable emesis bags or basins
Two boxes disposable tissue
Four sandbags
One blood pressure cuff
One stethoscope
One pair trauma shears
One package disposable drinking cups
One package wet wipes
Four cold packs
Four liters irrigation fluid
Two restraining devices
One package plastic bags for waste or severed parts
One sharps container
One set hearing protectors
Two infection control kits (goggles, masks, and waterproof gowns)
Optional:
One bedpan
One urinal
Two disposable thermometers

Dressing Supplies

Sterile universal trauma dressing (10" x 36")
Self-adhering, soft roller bandages (4" x 5 yards and 2" x 5 yards)
Sterile, nonporous, nonadherent dressing
Adhesive tape in several widths
Large safety pins
Sterile gauze dressings (4" x 4")
Sterile laparotomy dressings (6" x 9")

Jump Kit

Disposable gloves
Triangular bandages
Trauma shears
Adhesive tape in various widths
Universal trauma dressings
Self-adhering soft roller bandages, 4" x 5 yards and 2" x 5 yards
Oropharyngeal airways in adult, child, and infant sizes
Bag-valve-mask breathing device with masks for adults, children, and infants
Blood pressure cuff
Stethoscope
Penlight
Portable suction with pharyngeal tips
Sterile gauze dressings (4" x 4")
Sterile laparotomy dressings (6" x 9")
Thermometer
Plastic bandage strips
Sterile, nonporous, nonadherent dressing for occlusion of sucking chest wounds and eviscerations (aluminum foil sterilized in original package)

Acute Poisoning Supplies

Activated charcoal
Syrup of ipecac
Drinkable water
Emesis basins or bags
Equipment and supplies for irrigation of skin and eyes

continued

TABLE 16.1 Patient Care and Extrication Equipment, *continued*		
Childbirth Supplies One pair surgical scissors Three cord clamps or umbilical tapes Five towels Twelve sponges, 4" x 4" Four pairs sterile surgical gloves One infant blanket Two large plastic bags One syringe, rubber-bulb type, for aspiration of infant's mouth and airway **Extrication Equipment** One 12" adjustable, open-end wrench One 12" standard square bar screwdriver One 8" Phillips head screwdriver	Hacksaw with 12" carbide wire blades One pair 10" vise pliers One 5-lb, 15" handle hammer One fire ax, butt, 24" handle One wrecking bar, 24" handle One 51" pinch point crowbar One bolt cutter with 1" to 1 1/4" jaw opening One pointed blade folding shovel Double action tin snips, 8" minimum One pair reinforced leather gauntlets per crew member Rescue blanket Ropes, 5,400-lb tensile strength in 50' lengths in protective bags Mastic knife	Two bale hooks Spring-load center punch Pruning saw Various lengths of heavy duty 2' x 4' and 4' x 4' shoring (cribbing) blocks **Personal Safety Equipment** Reflectorized or flashing warning device Two high-intensity halogen 20,000 candle flashlights, battery powered, stand-up type Fire extinguisher, type BC, dry powder, size 5 Hard hats with face shields and safety goggles Two portable floodlights

A common weather problem is visibility. Another weather constraint relates to a helicopter's vulnerability to winds. Even moderate crosswinds can cause a helicopter to crash while landing, taking off, or hovering. Altitude may be another major restriction. At higher altitudes, the air is less dense so the helicopter rotor blades generate less lift than at lower altitudes. Therefore, the aircraft cannot carry the same weight as it can at lower altitudes.

The pilot is the final authority on the use of the aircraft in a rescue operation, on the aircraft's capabilities, and on landing zones. In making these determinations, the pilot should be unaware of the details of the patient's condition to avoid any pressure to "fudge" the calculations.

Landing Zones

Some ranchers and farmers have their own airstrips. Emergency airstrips are also available in some national forest areas. In any situation, permission should be obtained before using any remote landing airstrip. Always inquire about local restrictions and ensure the airstrip is in shape for landing.

Rescue teams must often create helicopter landing zones. To avoid accidents, follow these three guidelines when establishing a helicopter landing zone:

1. Ensure that the zone is flat, solid, and clear of debris. It should also

CHAPTER 16 Vehicles and Transportation

be free of dust, powdery snow, people, vehicles, poles, trees, and power lines. Power lines are particularly dangerous because they are hard to see. If there are power lines or other hazards present, notify the pilot before the landing approach begins.

2. Make sure the landing zone is large enough for the helicopter (Figure 16.1). The landing zone is usually a square. For a small helicopter, the touchdown area should have 60' sides for daytime landings, and 100' sides for nighttime landings. Medium helicopters require 75' sides for daytime landings, and 125' sides for nighttime landings. Large helicopters need 120' sides for daytime landings, and 200' sides for nighttime landings.

3. Mark each corner of the touchdown area with a low-intensity light that is secured to the ground and can withstand prop wash.

Wind Direction, Approach, and Departure Paths

As with other aircraft, helicopters land and take off into the wind. To indicate wind direction, tie brightly colored plastic tape so it streams out. For nighttime landings, a light can be placed on the side of the touchdown area *from where the wind is coming*. Avoid the use of flares during helicopter operations because of the fire danger.

Approach and departure paths should be free of obstructions, such as power lines, poles, antennas, and trees. Any high obstructions should be described to the helicopter pilot on the initial radio call. A helicopter requires a minimum approach path of approximately 100' and a minimum departure path of 300'.

FIGURE 16.1

The touchdown area should be of a size appropriate to the size of the helicopter.

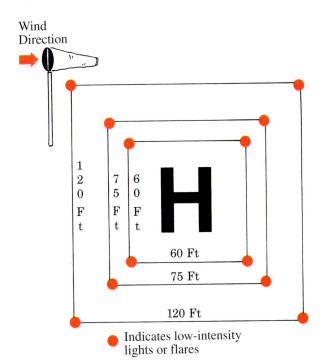

Nighttime Landings

Strobes, emergency lights, and vehicle headlights may be used to orient the pilot to the landing zone from afar. But as the helicopter approaches, all bright lights should be turned off to avoid temporarily blinding the pilot. Low-intensity lights should remain on to outline the landing zone.

Personal Safety

Helicopter safety is nothing more than good common sense, coupled with a constant awareness of the need for personal safety. Rescuers who are familiar with the way helicopters operate and follow the instructions of the pilot will minimize any dangers involved in an air medical operation. The most important rule is to stay a safe distance from the aircraft or helicopter whenever it is on the ground and **hot**, which means that the rotors are spinning.

Keep spectators at least 200' from the touchdown area. The rescue team should remain at least 100' away. There must be no smoking or open flames within 100' of the aircraft. Everyone working near a helicopter should wear eye protection and helmets with securely fastened chin straps. People flying in a helicopter should wear flight helmets, fire-resistant flight suits, and leather boots. Nylon or other flammable or meltable materials should not be worn in helicopter operations. Once the helicopter has landed, no one should approach the helicopter until instructed to do so by a member of the flight crew. The flight crew will also instruct the team on how to load the patient.

Figure 16.2 illustrates helicopter danger zones. Rescuers should only approach a helicopter from within the pilot's line of vision. Because of the tail rotor, never approach a helicopter from the rear, and never go around a helicopter at the rear. If sufficient personnel are available, station a guard outside the prohibited area at the rear of the aircraft to prevent entry into the area.

Since the main rotor may dip in the wind or as it slows, keep low when approaching a helicopter. If the helicopter has landed on a slope, approach and depart the aircraft from the downslope side only (Figure 16.3). Special care must be used when IVs and equipment are carried under the blades. Air turbulence created by the rotor blades can blow off hats and loose equipment, making them a danger to the aircraft and personnel in the area.

Board and depart a helicopter only when told to do so by the pilot or a member of the flight crew. Never attempt to open any aircraft door or move equipment unless instructed to do so by the flight crew. Always hold helicopter doors firmly so they will not slam in the downwash. Seat belts should be fastened securely, low on the pelvis, before a helicopter takes off or lands. Keep the seat belt fastened during the flight, unless you need to move about to care for a patient. Refasten the seat belt when leaving the helicopter.

CHAPTER 16 Vehicles and Transportation

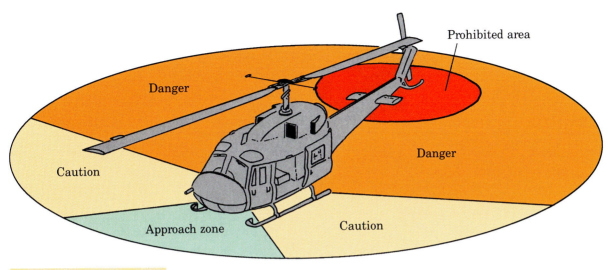

FIGURE 16.2 Never approach a helicopter from the rear and never go around a helicopter at the rear.

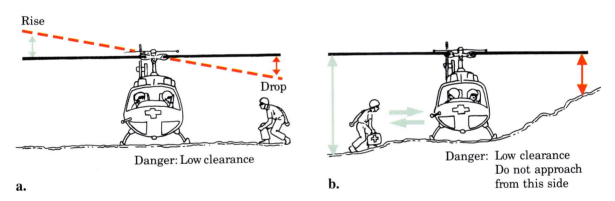

FIGURE 16.3
a. Keep low when approaching a helicopter since the main rotor may drop as it slows or in a wind.
b. Approach and depart the helicopter from the downslope side only.

Packaging Considerations

When packaging for air medical transport, rescuers should be concerned about three things:

1. If the patient is to be transported inside the aircraft, ensure that the patient package does not exceed the aircraft cabin's space limitations.
2. If a **fixed-line flyaway** (a short-distance transport with the stretcher slung under the aircraft) or hoist is to be used, ensure that the patient package will remain structurally sound, despite the stresses associated with helicopter activity.

3. Rescuers involved in air medical operations need to discuss with the flight crew the types of stretchers that are acceptable for use in fixed-line flyaway operations. Certain types of stretchers, such as the solid plastic Stokes, have aerodynamic characteristics that make them unacceptable for such operations because of the high risk of injury or death to the patient.

As with other forms of patient transport, the patient package for helicopter evacuation should always include protection for the head, eyes, respiratory tract, and ears.

SUMMARY

Use of the appropriate vehicle helps both the patient and the rescuer during the transportation phase of a rescue operation. Ground vehicles may need special modifications depending on weather or terrain conditions. Special vehicles may be required in mountainous areas with rugged terrain.

Air medical transportation by helicopter provides rapid transportation of patients. Because helicopters are expensive and potentially hazardous, they should be used only in those special circumstances when medical conditions require rapid transport, or when a helicopter is the only vehicle that can gain access to the patient. Helicopters are also a resource for agricultural-rural incidents. They can bring emergency medical personnel to remote sites and rapidly transport patients to a trauma center.

Oftentimes, the rescue team will have to create a helicopter landing zone. Even if a primitive airstrip exists nearby, rescuers must determine the condition of the landing sites and check to see if there are local restrictions. Landing zones must be flat, solid, and cleared of debris and other obstructions. The touchdown area should be appropriate to the size of the helicopter and marked by a low-intensity light at each corner. There must also be a means of indicating wind direction. At night, strobes or emergency vehicle lights can orient the pilot to the landing zone, but they should not be used during landings to avoid blinding the pilot.

If a helicopter evacuation is indicated, rescuers must consider operational factors, such as the weather, terrain, altitude conditions, and the availability of aircraft and trained pilots. Weather conditions, in particular, are crucial to the safe operation of a helicopter.

Altitude is another major restriction on helicopter operations. Helicopters cannot function safely and efficiently at higher altitudes where the air is less dense. Problems can also occur if the air is warm and humid, or if the helicopter must hover over water or snow.

CHAPTER 16 Vehicles and Transportation

Personal safety is a major consideration in air medical evacuation, as in any rescue operation. Rescuers must stay clear of the touchdown area and refrain from smoking. Everyone working near or in a helicopter must wear appropriate protective clothing and gear. Do not wear flammable or meltable material while involved in air medical operations.

There are definite danger zones when approaching a helicopter. Rescuers must know these zones and avoid them. Rescuers must also remember that no one should board or depart a helicopter unless the pilot or a member of the flight crew gives permission.

CHAPTER 17
Crisis Intervention

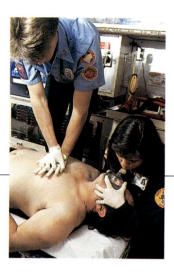

CHAPTER OUTLINE

Overview
Objectives
Crises in Agricultural-Rural Settings
Emotional Reactions to a Crisis
   High Anxiety or Emotional Shock
   Denial
   Anger
   Remorse
   Grief
Crisis Management
   Communicating With the Patient
   Communicating With Others
Management of Sudden Death
   Legal Determination of Death
Stress
   Immediate Stress Reactions
   Delayed Stress Reactions
   Effects of Excessive Stress
   Recognizing Excessive Stress
Critical Incident Stress Debriefing (CISD)
Summary

KEY TERMS

Critical Incident Stress Debriefing (CISD): program, composed of peer support and mental health professionals, designed to help rescuers deal with major stresses that may occur as a result of a critical incident.

CHAPTER 17 Crisis Intervention

Delayed stress reaction: emotional effects of a critical incident or traumatic stress that may occur either long term or short term.

Dependent lividity: discoloration of the skin due to pooling of blood.

Immediate stress reaction: response that often occurs at the scene or shortly after leaving the scene. Symptoms vary widely, depending on the individual.

Rigor mortis: stiffening of the body after death.

Situational crisis: state of emotional upset or turmoil caused by a sudden, disruptive event, such as an unexpected illness, traumatic injury, or death of a loved one.

OVERVIEW

In many agricultural-rural incidents, the rescue team is called only as a last resort, usually only after friends, co-workers, and family members have attempted a rescue themselves. Oftentimes, rural rescue teams may be called to situations involving friends, neighbors, or even family members. These are perhaps the most difficult and most traumatic of all agricultural-rural incidents.

This chapter reviews common emotional and psychological responses to situational crises. It reviews specific aspects of stress common to rescuers, and then presents methods for coping and techniques for managing stressful situations. The importance of Critical Incident Stress Debriefing (CISD) for rescue teams is also discussed.

OBJECTIVES

After reading this chapter, the rescuer should be able to:

- identify the emotional phases experienced by an individual in a situational crisis.
- describe effective crisis management techniques.
- describe responses to sudden death and how to deal with them.
- identify the stresses placed on rescuers, indications of excessive stress, and coping techniques.
- explain the importance of Critical Incident Stress Debriefing for rescue teams.

CRISES IN AGRICULTURAL-RURAL SETTINGS

Life-and-death crises occur almost daily, and sometimes rescuers can do very little to alter the effects of serious illness or traumatic injury. A **situational crisis** is a state of emotional upset or turmoil caused by a sudden, disruptive event such as an unexpected illness, traumatic injury, or death of a loved one. Situational crises usually last for only a short time. For example, a rescue team is called to an incident in which a child has fallen into a tub grinder. By the time the team arrives at the scene, the child is dead, the family is in shock, and the team has to hold the situation together until the body can be recovered. Such an operation may last only an hour or two, but the intense nature of the incident is likely to stay with the team for days or even months. Some incidents are never forgotten.

In many agricultural-rural incidents, the rescue team is called only as a last resort. Friends, co-workers, and family members will oftentimes attempt a rescue themselves first. But if the entanglement and/or the injuries are too severe for the family to handle, the rescue team will be summoned. Because amputations, massive crushing injuries, severe lacerations, and/or whole body destruction are common, family and friends at the scene are likely to experience stress reactions and emotional trauma in response to the incident.

The intense nature of agricultural-rural incidents affects all individuals at the scene. Rescuers must extricate and provide emergency medical care to a patient with severe, often disfiguring, injuries. Rescuers may also be called upon to provide psychological support to the friends and family members. Rescuers must also take care of themselves emotionally during and after the incident. The first step in this process is to recognize the emotional phases associated with a crisis.

EMOTIONAL REACTIONS TO A CRISIS

A person experiencing a crisis goes through some or all of the following emotional phases: high anxiety or emotional shock; denial; anger; remorse; and grief. Rescuers who understand these emotional reactions and why they occur will better understand how to help people experiencing a crisis.

High Anxiety or Emotional Shock

In the first phase of a crisis, a person experiences high anxiety or emotional shock. High anxiety is characterized by easily identified signs and symptoms: flushed, red face; rapid breathing; rapid speech; increased activity; loud or screaming voice; and general agitation. Emotional shock is often the result of sudden illness, accident, or sudden death of a loved one. It is characterized by cool, clammy skin; a rapid, weak pulse; vomiting and nausea; and general inactivity and weakness. Talk with a patient or bystanders experiencing these signs and symptoms to let them know someone cares. Also, if appropriate, place a hand on the shoulder or arm of an anxious person to show you care.

Denial

The next phase of a crisis may be denial—refusal to accept the fact that an event has occurred. In an attempt to block the memory of the incident, an individual may insist that it did not happen. Allow the individual to express denial. Do not argue, but try to understand the emotional and psychological trauma that he or she is experiencing. However, rescuers should avoid agreeing with someone who is denying what has actually occurred.

Anger

Anger may precede or follow denial. For example, a patient's spouse may, for no apparent reason, begin screaming at members of the rescue team, calling them incompetent, or using foul language. Remember that anger is a normal human response to emotional overload or frustration. Do not take a person's anger personally, but acknowledge it is a reaction to stress.

Frustration can also result in anger. If not released, anger can develop into violent behavior. For example, in an incident involving a child entangled around a PTO shaft, rescuers must attempt to show the family and bystanders that they are making progress. This may be done through constant communication with the family, explaining the steps of extrication as they are done. If bystanders perceive that little or no progress is being made, they may become angry, hostile, overly critical, and perhaps violent. In such situations, show confidence and be professional. Ensure that a member of the rescue team or a law enforcement officer is assigned to communicate with the family. Do not react to anger by becoming angry or hostile. Avoid "sick" humor in the presence of the patient's family and friends, even though it may relieve stress and frustration in rescuers.

Remorse

Remorse may follow anger. Feelings of remorse are generally a mixed bag, including sadness and guilt.

Grief

Grief is a sense of mourning and loss. People are distressed about being around others in grief, because grief makes people feel vulnerable to their own losses. Except in rare instances, repeated and prolonged contact with grieving people may actually "rub off" onto rescuers. Be calm and professional when dealing with the patient's family and with other bystanders.

Communicating With the Patient

CRISIS MANAGEMENT

Verbal Communication The first, most important step in crisis management is to talk with the patient. Talking lets the patient know that there is someone who cares. Be honest, warm, caring, and empathetic when communicating with the patient. Always speak slowly, clearly, and distinctly. Select words that the patient uses. For example, if the patient states that he has "burning" pain in the area of an impalement injury, refer to the pain in that way. Do not suddenly change how the patient refers to the pain. Do not "talk up" or "talk down" to the patient in any way.

Avoid making false statements or giving false assurances. A patient does not want to be told that everything is all right when it obviously is not. Telling an "untruth" destroys patient trust and ultimately decreases a rescuer's self-confidence.

Use the patient's proper name. Do not use terms such as "old man," "lady," "kid," or "the farmer." Except with children, try to avoid using a patient's first name, unless he or she asks you to. Rather, use the patient's last name, preceded by the proper courtesy title, such as Mr., Ms., Mrs.

Do not assume an elderly patient is deaf or otherwise unable to understand you. Never use "baby talk" with an elderly patient. If the patient is hearing impaired, speak clearly and face the patient so that he or she can read your lips. Never shout at the patient.

Communicating with children presents a variety of challenges for the rescuer. Children will likely be frightened about what is happening around them. And even though a frightened child says very little, the child will be very much aware of what is happening. In a calm, reassuring voice, constantly explain to the child what is happening and why certain things are happening. A parent or relative who is calm, even in the event of a serious injury to the child, may help reduce the child's fear and anxiety.

Nonverbal Communication A second important step is to understand the importance of nonverbal communication or "body language" when caring for a patient. Be particularly careful to avoid assuming a threatening posture; instead, maintain a calm, professional stance. If the patient is lying down, kneel beside him or her. If the person is sitting, move down to his or her level (Figure 17.1).

Establish and maintain eye contact. This will not only establish rapport with the patient, it will help reassure a patient that he or she is your main interest.

Remember to use the following crisis intervention techniques to help calm the patient so extrication, if necessary, can proceed smoothly and emergency medical care can be administered:

FIGURE 17.1

Assume a calm, professional manner when interacting with patients. Establish eye contact to reassure them that they are of concern to you.

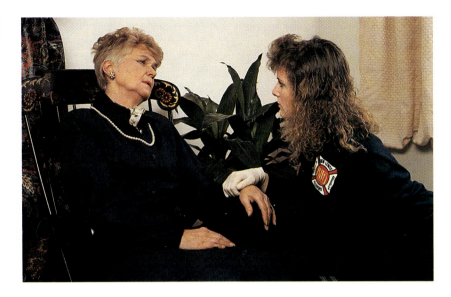

1. Remain calm.
2. Reassure the patient.
3. Take your time.
4. Establish and maintain eye contact.
5. Touch the patient.
6. Speak in a calm, steady voice.
7. Be professional and confident at all times.
8. Do not take the patient's comments personally.
9. Remember to keep your sense of humor.

Communicating With Others

Once the rescue team has done everything possible to treat a patient medically, the patient's and the family's psychological needs must be considered. The mere presence of the team will be helpful. Putting an arm around a shoulder, or holding the hand of the patient or a member of the patient's family helps everyone.

While rescuers should not make false statements about the situation, they should be careful to not destroy hope. Even if the situation seems hopeless, try to give comfort by making such positive statements as, "We are here to help you, and we are doing everything we can." In every case, the rescue team must do whatever is possible to attend to the patient's medical needs.

In a crisis situation, rescuers should communicate with the family with the following six considerations in mind:

1. Answer questions as truthfully as possible. If you do not know the answer to a question, simply say so.
2. Give straight answers to all questions. Do not hide unpleasant facts.
3. Report all information that you know to be true.

4. Do not guess about the unknown.
5. Do not try to argue with someone who is in denial. Denial is sometimes a useful protective reaction to give someone time to adjust to what has happened. At the same time, avoid agreeing with someone who is denying what actually occurred.
6. Maintain a professional attitude at all times. Control your own feelings, demonstrate caring and concern for the patient and the family, and perform your duties calmly and effectively. If anger is directed at you or the team, do not take it personally or fight back. However, if you are in danger, back away to avoid further confrontation. Wait for more help and allow time for the situation to calm down.

MANAGEMENT OF SUDDEN DEATH

Frequently, agricultural-rural incidents result in sudden, unexpected death. The rescue team must be prepared for any number of reactions from the deceased's family and friends, ranging from severe anxiety to agitation to withdrawal. Some of the more common emotional responses to sudden death include denial, guilt, grief, and hostility and anger.

At times, these emotional responses will come rapidly, one after another; other times, the only response will be withdrawal and an intense desire for solitude. A person who withdraws might experience a delayed response, particularly if he or she appears unusually calm.

Responses to sudden death are sometimes physical; that is, a person may feel faint, dizzy, nauseated, or even have the urge to vomit. Regardless of the type of response, it is important for rescuers to remember that a physical or emotional response is a normal part of grief that follows sudden, unexpected death.

Dealing with death is an unfortunate, yet routine, part of a rescuer's job. It is not, however, routine for the deceased's family and friends. Therefore, rescuers must not allow "sick humor" or any callousness to enter their interactions with family and friends.

Even though rescuers must deal with death as part of their jobs, all human beings are afraid of dying. Witnessing death, no matter how often, catapults this fear to the forefront, if only for a brief time. Rescuers must work through their personal feelings about death in order to confront it on the job. Some rescuers may attempt to act "tough" when dealing with death, while others seem hostile or callous, or withdrawn, hoping their feelings will go away.

In an attempt to avoid the emotional impact of a particularly stressful incident in which, for example, a child has died unexpectedly, some rescuers may become "hyperclinical." They tend to focus specifically on the medical and/or technical aspects of the operation. Sometimes rescuers have recurring memories of tragic events surrounding death and have nightmares or difficulty sleeping. All of these responses are normal and should lessen and end with time.

Although the subject of death and dealing with death may be uncomfortable, it helps to discuss feelings associated with death with others on the team. If you are uncomfortable speaking with other members of the rescue team, contact a member of the emergency department staff or a specialist on a Critical Incident Stress Debriefing (CISD) team.

Legal Determination of Death

In most jurisdictions, only a licensed physician can legally pronounce a person dead; members of the rescue team cannot. There are four presumptive signs of death: **dependent lividity** (discoloration of the skin due to pooling of blood), **rigor mortis** (stiffening of the body after death), decapitation, and decomposition. If there is any doubt that a patient is dead, rescuers should initiate full resuscitation. Family members will often insist that "something be done," even when the rescue team is certain that the patient is dead. In these situations, initiate resuscitation. However, do not raise false hopes by telling the family that everything will be all right.

If the patient is obviously dead, rescuers should attend to family members, friends, and co-workers at the scene. Expect a wide range of emotions and reactions to the patient's death. Ensure that the family is kept informed about what is happening at all times. Respect the family's need for sympathy and solitude. If the family wishes to see the body, try to follow their wishes.

A patient may have a living will. It is a legal document in most states with specific instructions that the patient does not want to be resuscitated—a DNR (do not resuscitate) order—or to be kept alive by mechanical life support systems. The patient's wishes expressed in a living will should be respected. On occasion, a serious conflict or problem with a living will may arise. A family member may disagree with the will's intent ("Grandpa was senile when he wrote that will. We want you to give him mouth-to-mouth resuscitation"); or the will itself may not be available. In such situations, you should contact medical control for advice. Be familiar with your local and state laws, and ensure that each member of the rescue team is familiar with your system's pre-arranged protocols to deal with a living will. In general, you will be directed to follow the patient's wishes.

STRESS

The types of traumatic injuries common in agricultural-rural incidents, coupled with the feeling of community inherent in these areas, can result in intense stress on rescuers. Reactions to critical incidents or traumatic stress may appear immediately, or they may not appear until long after the incident.

Immediate Stress Reactions

Immediate stress reactions may vary from mild to moderate to severe. An immediate stress reaction may manifest itself as irritability, apathy, or in more severe cases, intense weeping, panic, or loss of control. Some individuals may appear subdued or depressed; they may sit and stare or wander aimlessly, and may seem to be mentally confused or disoriented. Individuals with severe symptoms, regardless of whether they are bystanders or members of the rescue team, should be removed from the scene as quickly as possible. If they cannot be removed from the scene, they should be taken to an area where their view of the incident is blocked. Do not leave the patient alone, if possible, in these circumstances. Oftentimes a calm bystander may be of assistance.

Delayed Stress Reactions

Delayed stress reactions can be short term or long term following a critical incident or traumatic stress. As with immediate stress reactions, delayed stress reactions can affect both patients and rescuers. Manifestations of this type of reaction include sleep disturbances, loss of appetite, alcohol and substance abuse, sexual dysfunction, feelings of guilt for surviving, and family problems. The extent and depth of patients' emotional problems following a critical incident may depend on the rescue team's initial response to the incident.

Delayed stress reactions can also affect rescuers. Repeated exposure to patient suffering, sudden death, and traumatic, disfiguring injuries places extraordinary demands on a rescuer's coping mechanisms. But rather than maintaining a "stiff upper lip," rescuers should support one another by openly discussing the emotional impact of a critical incident. This may mean discussing fears about death, the pain and guilt of feeling helpless to save a patient, or it may mean venting anger and frustration about procedures or techniques that failed to work. Because emotions will vary widely after a critical incident, it is important that the team have access to postincident counseling or Critical Incident Stress Debriefing, which is described later in this chapter.

Effects of Excessive Stress

The very nature of a rescuer's work is stress related. Rescuers face life-and-death crises almost daily, which is both physically and emotionally demanding.

The work is physically demanding in that it often interrupts sleep and routine life activities, particularly for volunteer rescue teams. Rescuers must be in good physical condition in order to perform effectively in extended incidents where, for example, a patient trapped in a rear overturn requires extrication. Changing weather conditions and altitude also affect a rescuer's physical well-being. Rescuers have the means and resources to protect themselves from these physical demands by wearing appropriate protective gear and ensuring they eat and drink during the operation to maintain their strength.

The work is emotionally demanding in that rescuers take pride in their work and care about the people they are helping. While it is natural and appropriate to care about patients, rescuers must strive to keep a balance between sympathetic concern and excessive emotional involvement. Excessive emotional involvement may hinder a rescuer's ability to perform effectively and efficiently.

Another problem rescuers face following a crisis is unfair and sometimes widely publicized criticism by a patient, the patient's family, the community, the media, or even by co-workers. Responding to criticism that is based on inaccurate information or sensationalism is often frustrating.

Perhaps the most difficult problem for rescuers is coping with grief. Except in rare instances, repeated and prolonged contacts with grieving people will have an effect on rescuers. The responsibilities of the rescue team to care for the sick and injured prevent them from showing their true emotions; rescuers must remain calm and professional during a crisis. As a result, rescuers' feelings of grief and despair are often left unresolved.

Recognizing Excessive Stress

It is important for rescuers to learn to recognize the common signs and symptoms of stress, so that it does not begin to interfere with their work or their life away from work, including family life. The signs and symptoms of chronic stress may not be obvious at first; they may be subtle and not present all of the time. The following 12 signs and symptoms may indicate a delayed stress reaction or the presence of excessive stress:

1. Increased headaches, gastrointestinal complaints, unexplained aches and pains, and increased blood pressure
2. Anger and hostility toward family, friends, supervisors, the system, and even patients
3. Feelings that life has lost its meaning; apathy, despair, or sadness; lack of enthusiasm toward work and life in general
4. Feelings characteristic of depression: chronic fatigue; difficulty sleeping; loss of appetite; or even bouts of uncontrollable weeping
5. Lack of concentration, which increases the number of mistakes made on the job
6. Periods of intense anxiety, even panic
7. Suicidal thoughts
8. Repeated thoughts about death, suffering, or pain
9. Nightmares
10. Alcohol and/or other substance abuse

11. Flashbacks of severe, disfiguring injuries, tragedies, or other incidents on the job
12. Desire to quit work

Any of these signs or symptoms may indicate chronic stress or delayed grieving; they are normal responses to the many daily stresses under which rescuers work. Learn to recognize them as such and take steps to relieve their cause(s). Rescue teams should discuss and support openness when dealing with these signs of stress. Discuss any of these feelings with co-workers, as many of them will have had similar experiences. The result may be a realization that these are normal, common feelings and the symptoms may resolve spontaneously.

However, persistent and severe symptoms may require professional guidance from a counselor within the EMS system who is trained in this type of stress management. This type of counseling should be confidential and easily available to anyone who needs it.

CRITICAL INCIDENT STRESS DEBRIEFING (CISD)

The types of critical incidents encountered in agricultural-rural settings often involve traumatic, disfiguring injuries, sudden death, and tragedies involving children. Traumatic stress, when added to the typical stresses rescuers face as part of the job, as well as the stresses associated with daily living, can be debilitating for the rescuer and devastating for the rescue team. This type of stress, as stated earlier in the chapter, is a normal response to what is often a devastating event.

Rescue teams in rural areas may be staffed with volunteers from the community; therefore, it is particularly important to have a mechanism in place for dealing with traumatic stress. These volunteers may not be called for several days or even weeks between incidents, so they may not have the opportunity as a team to discuss their feelings about a critical incident.

A **Critical Incident Stress Debriefing (CISD)** program, composed of peer support and mental health professionals, should be in place to help rescuers deal with the major stresses that may occur as a result of a critical incident. The key to an effective CISD program is twofold: early intervention and a committed team of professionals trained to deal with critical incident stresses. A CISD program is usually started within 24 hours of the event and involves several steps to relieve the major stresses rescuers have experienced as a result of the incident. A CISD session will help rescuers put a critical incident into perspective; it helps rescuers see themselves as normal people thrust into a painfully abnormal event. The environment of a CISD session allows rescuers to vent their own frustrations about an incident, and to listen to the responses of other members of the team. CISD also helps rescuers recognize the signs and symptoms of stress and encourages them to seek professional help, if needed.

SUMMARY

Emergencies are crisis situations. Everyone involved—patients, family members, bystanders, and rescuers—responds to a crisis differently. Rescuers must recognize reactions to stress placed on all individuals involved in a crisis, and they must be prepared to cope with these various responses.

Agricultural-rural incidents commonly result in massive traumatic injuries or sudden death. Rescuers may need to provide psychological support to both the patient and the patient's family. Constant communication and honest reassurance are effective techniques. Both immediate and delayed responses to sudden death are common. Physical responses include nausea, vomiting, and/or dizziness. Common emotional responses include denial, guilt, hostility, and anger. Complicating matters in agricultural-rural incidents is the fact that rescuers are likely to know patients as friends, neighbors, or relatives.

Rescuers must also be aware of their own responses to stress, their personal feelings about death, and their need for support. The very nature of the work is stress related, so rescuers must strive to maintain a balance in their lives. Stress reactions are normal, natural responses. Recognizing this fact will help rescuers take control of it. Discussing concerns with co-workers or with professionals trained in handling this type of stress can be helpful.

Most agencies have established Critical Incident Stress Debriefing (CISD) teams to help rescuers cope with the aftermath of a critical or particularly tragic incident. A CISD session within the first 24 hours of an incident can be especially helpful in relieving stress and preventing long-term problems.

Appendix
Selection, Storage, and Maintenance of Extrication Tools

Rescue teams need a considerable amount of heavy rescue equipment that must be properly selected, stored, and maintained in order to be readily available and in good, safe working condition. The information presented in this appendix may assist rescuers responsible for buying and maintaining equipment.

SLINGS

Slings are generally manufactured in one of five materials: chain, wire rope, wire mesh, synthetic roundslings, and synthetic web slings. The synthetic roundslings and web slings are more commonly used in rescue work for quick setup of anchors and attachments for lifting, stabilizing, pulling, and moving operations.

Nylon and polyester are used for synthetic slings. Nylon has greater elongation than polyester, but polyester is more resistant to acids and absorbs less water than nylon. Neither material is very resistant to high temperatures. Most manufacturers state that there is significant deterioration of the synthetic slings at temperatures exceeding 200°F.

Roundslings

A roundsling is a synthetic sling made from a continuous loop or hank of yarn and then covered with a jacket. The most common roundslings used today are made of polyester fibers twisted into yarn bundles. The yarn bundles are then twisted into multiple, continuous strands. These strands are the load-bearing members of the sling. It is the number of strands that determines the strength. The load-bearing strands are covered with a polyester jacket, which is independent of the interior strands. The jacket does not contribute to the load capacity but serves as a protective covering that reduces mechanical or physical damage to the interior strands. Metal fittings can be attached by the manufacturer to enhance the rigging potential of the roundslings while reducing sling wear.

Web Sling Configurations

Three types of web slings are commonly available: the endless sling, the standard eye and eye sling, and the twisted eye sling. With the endless sling, both ends of one piece of webbing are lapped and sewn together to form a continuous piece. The standard eye and eye sling is a single piece of webbing sewn with an eye at either end in the same plane as the sling body. The eyes may be the same width as the web body or tapered so that the eye is narrower than the web body. The twisted eye sling is a single piece of webbing with an eye at either end sewn at 90° to the plane (tapered or full width) of the sling. The twist allows for better rigging of choker slings.

Protection, Maintenance, and Storage of Slings

Despite the inherent toughness of synthetic slings, they can be cut by repeated use or by use without proper barrier protection. Manufacturers provide several types of barrier protection to help reduce tears, cuts, or punctures. There are edge guards, movable sleeves, reinforcement strips sewn to the sling, coatings, and loose buffer strips or pads. All synthetic slings used for heavy equipment extrication should have one or more protective barriers. These protective barriers should be placed at all actual or potential sharp edges and anywhere the sling is not visible, such as when anchoring a sling to the underside of an upright vehicle.

Synthetic slings should be inspected every 30 days and after each incident. The inspection should take place in a well-lighted room. The entire sling should be inspected on both sides. Pay particular attention to the stitching and to the ends for wear. Check the body of the sling for cuts, tensile damage, abrasion, punctures, snags, chemical damage, and heat damage. The sling should be removed from service and destroyed if there are any cuts, chemical damage, heat damage, discoloration, welded fibers (sling areas with a glossy, smooth look) or interior fibers (roundslings) showing through the jacket.

Store synthetic slings in a labeled bag. The bag should be stored on the rescue vehicle so that there is minimal potential for exposure to moisture, high temperatures, chemicals (like battery acid), or mechanical damage from other tools rubbing or falling against the sling.

MANUAL EFFORT TOOLS

The most important aspect of maintaining manual effort tools is to keep an active inventory list in the station and on the rescue vehicle. Each month, manual effort tools, as well as most other rescue tools, should be inventoried, cleaned, and coated with a nonoily film as specified by the manufacturer. The hand tools used for cutting need to be checked for sharpness and integrity of the cutting surfaces. Tools with moving parts need to be checked to ensure that all parts are present, intact, and functioning properly.

Hand tools should not be carried loose. Pry bars should be mounted in brackets. Come-alongs should be boxed, hung from hooks, or secured so as not to move around the compartment. Come-alongs should be stored in a ready-to-use configuration.

Loose tools are lost tools. Having a place for each tool ensures that equipment is available when needed. Inventory all tools before leaving any incident or training session.

WIRE ROPE

Selecting Wire Rope

The strength, size, length, grade, construction, and types of wire rope selected depend on how it will be used and the environmental conditions to which it will be exposed.

Before selecting a specific wire rope, the rescue team should evaluate the following features to determine which rope will best meet their needs.

- Rated load—the maximum recommended load that should be exerted on the wire rope (also called the working load)
- Proof load—the average load to which a wire rope may be subjected before visible deformation occurs
- Proof test—a tensile strength test (a quality control test used by manufacturers) used to detect defects in the material or in the manufacturing process
- Ultimate load—the average load at which the wire rope fails or no longer supports the load
- Shock load—a load resulting from a rapid change of movement of a static load (a shock load is generally significantly greater than the static load)
- Safety factor—the theoretical reserve capacity of the wire rope

Rope Strand There are four basic types of strands used in wire ropes: round strand, flattened strand, locked coil, and concentric strand ropes. For rigging and extrication work, round strand is the most commonly used.

Round strand ropes are described by the number of wires in each strand. If the rope diameter remains the same but the number of wires per strand increases, the wire rope becomes more flexible but less resistant to abrasion. The opposite is true concerning fatigue resistance. Given two wire ropes of the same diameter, the one with fewer wires per strand will be more fatigue-resistant but less flexible. Two of the most popular styles of wire rope are the 6 x 19 (6 strands with 19 wires per strand) and the 6 x 37 (6 strands with 37 wires per strand).

There are four patterns of combining wires in strands:

1. Ordinary, in which all wires are the same size

2. Seale, in which there are smaller wires inside the strand with larger wires on the outside to provide better abrasion resistance
3. Warrington, in which large wires alternate with small wires to provide good abrasion resistance and flexibility
4. Filler, in which there are very small wires filling in the valleys between larger wires for good abrasion and fatigue resistance

Rope Lay Rope lay refers to the direction or rotation of the wires and the strands made during the construction of the wire rope. An easy way to determine a right lay from a left lay of the strands is to grasp the wire rope with your right hand, thumb up. If the strands rotate in the direction of your fingers, it is a right lay. If the strands rotate in the direction of your thumb, it is a left lay. The wires in the strand may have the opposite or the same direction of rotation as the strand.

Manufacturers use the term regular lay to mean that the wires of the strand rotate in the opposite direction from the strand. A rope with wires rotating in the same direction as the strand is said to have lang lay. The lang lay wire rope is more flexible than the regular lay wire rope, but the lang lay rope is more easily damaged and often wears out faster than the regular lay wire rope.

The term lay length means the distance along the wire rope for a single strand to make one complete rotation. The most commonly used wire rope is a right regular lay that has all wires rotating in one direction while all of the strands (6 strands made up of 19 or 37 wires) rotate in the opposite direction. This type of wire rope has good resistance to abrasion, kinking, and twisting. It is also able to withstand significant distortion and crushing.

Preforming a wire rope means the wires and strands are shaped to fit their respective positions in the finished rope. This preshaping or preforming of the wire reduces the tendency for the wire rope to unwind. Preformed wire rope has increased resistance to bending fatigue, and broken ends do not unravel. Each strand in this configuration when used on a winch drum (like a come-along or winch) or run through a pulley carries an equal share of the load, reducing wear.

Wire Grade The term plow is used by the wire rope industry to designate the grade of the wire. Extra-extra improved plow or special improved plow type II is used when maximum rope strength is needed because it is 10% stronger than the extra improved plow. Extra improved plow or special improved plow type I is 15% stronger than the next lower grade of wire called improved plow type I. Improved plow type I does not wear as well as special improved plow type I when placed in adverse conditions.

Wire Type The common types of wire used in wire rope include bright wire, stainless steel wire, aircraft wire, and galvanized wire. Most wire ropes are made of bright wire, which is an uncoated, high-carbon steel wire. Stainless steel wire is a corrosion-resistant alloy used in yachting and aircraft control cables. Aircraft wire is a specially drawn steel with high tensile strength and high fatigue resistance. It is zinc- or tin-coated before being stranded. It may also be used in aircraft control cables. Galvanized steel wire is used to improve the corrosion resistance of bright wire ropes.

Aircraft wire is a good choice for extrication work because it provides a low weight to high strength ratio, and it has excellent wearing qualities. Stainless steel wire also has qualities that make it good for extrication. The initial cost of these two types of wires will likely be higher than that of bright or galvanized wire, but their durability and high strength may offset the initial higher cost.

Wire Core The core of the wire rope supports the strands and provides the rope's shape. The core also prevents the strands from rubbing together during normal loading and unloading while supplying a mechanism for storage and distribution of lubricating oil to the wires. A fiber center core, made of natural fibers such as sisal or manila or synthetic fibers such polypropylene or nylon, is more flexible than a steel core rope. But because fiber core wire rope is subject to crushing and separation, it is not commonly used where there are to be multiple layers of wire rope on a drum.

Independent wire core uses wire strands the same as the main wire rope for a core. This type of wire rope does not crush easily. Independent wire cores tend to preserve the circular shape of the wire rope when it is bent.

The steel stranded rope core consists of strands with no core. In general, it is not as flexible as independent wire core rope.

Protection, Maintenance, and Storage of Wire Rope

All wire rope should be exercised and inspected monthly. Inspect the full length of the wire rope as it is pulled off the spool under a light load for the following: abrasion; wear (loose strands); fatigue (broken wires); corrosion (discoloration); bird's cage (strands or partial strands that balloon out to form a hollow "bird's cage" along the wire rope); and flattened areas.

Remove broken wires by using a gentle rocking motion. The rocking motion will cause the broken wire to tuck between the strands. If there are six or more broken wires, or if one strand is badly damaged, take the rope out of service immediately and destroy it. Replace it as soon as possible with a new wire rope.

Rope should be replaced if any of the following signs of damage appear on inspection:

- Visible corrosion
- Excessive rope stretch (reduction in rope diameter is one sign)
- Damaged splices
- Corroded, cracked, worn, or bent end connections
- Crushed, flattened, or jammed strands
- Bird's cages
- Bulges or gaps in the rope
- Core protrusions
- Unbalanced or worn areas
- Heat damage

Regular maintenance of wire rope should include lubricating the rope in order to reduce wear, corrosion, and potential damage from moisture. The rope must be dry before the lubrication process begins. Follow the manufacturer's instructions for specific instructions. If the instructions are not available, apply light oils using a dip or spray. Do not use crankcase oil for lubrication because it is acidic and contains tiny metal fragments that are harmful to the wire rope. Apply the lubricant where the rope tends to spread apart. The lubrication works best if done in a warm area. Use a light, penetrating cleaner other than gasoline or kerosene as they have a tendency to remove too much of the internal lubricant.

When storing wire rope on a drum, ensure that the first few turns on the drum are tight and true. Do not jam the rope and interlock the strands. Try to put no more than three layers of wire rope on the drum because more layers will cause crushing and excessive wear.

When the wire rope is pulled off the drum, leave a minimum of two or three full turns of rope on the drum (do not pull all of the rope off). When the wire rope is fully retracted, there should be a space left at the top that is at least twice the diameter of the rope. Do not overfill the drum.

CHAINS AND HOOKS

Chains

Before selecting a particular type of chain, the rescue team should evaluate the following features to determine which type of chain will best meet their needs.

- Safe working load or working load limit—the maximum load in pounds that should ever be applied to a chain when it is new or in as-new condition. This rating is used only when the load is uniformly applied to a straight length of chain.
- Proof test—a quality control tensile test applied to the product during or subsequent to the manufacturing process to detect defects. It is the minimum force in pounds that the chain withstood in the condition

and at the time it left the factory. The proof test rating is twice the safe working load.
- Minimum ultimate load (breaking strength)—the minimum load at which a new chain will break. The test is performed by applying direct tension to a straight length of chain at a uniform rate of speed. The minimum ultimate load rating is normally four times the working load.

Grades of Chain The National Association of Chain Manufacturers (NACM) has agreed on a grading system for welded chain that makes it easier to evaluate and select chain. The grading system uses grades 30, 40, 70, and 80. The actual markings in use by manufacturers may be one, two, three, or four digits that are embossed onto the links of chain. This system is used by manufacturers who are members of NACM and does not apply to light welded chain.

Grade 30. A low-carbon steel, general utility chain that was once called proof coil. This is the poorest grade of chain that is normally available. It is very soft, non-heat-treated chain and should not be used in extrication work.

Grade 40. This is a higher carbon steel, also called high-test chain, and stronger than the grade 30. However, it is not heat treated and is not recommended for extrication work.

Grade 70. A high-strength, low-weight chain, also called transport/binder chain, made of boron manganese steel. This chain is designed for binding applications such as those in the trucking industry and is generally marked on the links with a G7, 70, or 700. Grade 70 is not recommended for use in extrication work.

Grade 80. This is a heat-treated, high-strength alloy chain that has a high strength to weight ratio. It provides good wear and strength. The chain should be marked on the links with an A, 8, 80, or 800 and should have a metal tag attached that certifies the strength rating and the grade of the chain. High-strength alloy chain is the only type of chain that should be used in extrication work.

Protection, Maintenance, and Storage of Chains

All chains used for rescue work should be inspected on a monthly basis and immediately after each incident. Chains should be cleaned before they are inspected because dirt or excessive oil can hide cracks and nicks. Clean chains with a mild solvent, and dry as instructed by the manufacturer. Inspect chains by hanging or laying them in a well-lighted area. At purchase and with each inspection chains should be remeasured, and the data recorded on an inspection sheet. If the measurement indicates more than 3% elongation, remove the chain from service and destroy it. Next, make a link-by-link inspection looking for wear (particularly at the interior ends of the links), nicks, gouges, cracks, elongation (the link opening gets narrower when elongated), bending, twisting, and arc burns. All chains should be inspected by a competent supplier for matched components and proper grade (grade 8) before being placed in service. All chains and their components should have a metal tag attached stating certification of the unit for grade and strength rating.

All chains used for rescue work should be stored in containers that are labeled with type of chain, configuration, and intended use. The container should be stored on the rescue vehicle to minimize exposure to moisture and other contaminants. A coating of light oil may help minimize deterioration during prolonged storage. Chains should be stored free of knots. Chains should not be stored on the rescue vehicle so that they can swing free, banging against the side or door of the compartment. This type of storage creates unnecessary wear on the chains and the compartment interior.

Hooks

Hooks should be made of forged alloy steel with the safety rating stamped on the hook. A chain configured with hooks and/or master links should have a metal tag certifying the strength rating of the chain and its attached components. The minimum ultimate load rating on hooks is normally four times the safe working load (the same as the chain).

Protection, Maintenance, and Storage of Hooks

All hooks should be inspected at the same time as chains. Hooks should be cleaned before inspection and placed on a flat surface or hung at eye level in a well-lighted area. Check for wear or cracks at the top and bottom of the ring or clevis and in the outer and inner bend. Test the safety catch for ease of opening and closing. Inspect all hooks and rigging when chains are inspected. Examine the hook opening to see if there is any twisting or expansion of the metal. Next look at the throat, saddle, and the neck of the hook for cracks and wear.

PNEUMATIC TOOLS

Both pneumatic and hydraulic systems are fluid-powered systems that transmit energy through fluid. Pneumatic systems use a highly compressible gaseous fluid, while hydraulic systems use liquid fluid.

Before selecting a particular type of pneumatic air chisel, the rescue team should evaluate the following features to determine which type of chisel will best meet their needs.

- Cubic feet per minute of air usage (cfm)—4 to 8 cfm is the average range
- Number of blows per minute—from 1,800 to 3,500/minute at 90 psi
- Range of recommended working pressures—90 to 110 psi is the average range
- Diameter of air inlet—1/4" is common
- Minimum diameter of supplying air hose—3/8" is the often stated minimum
- Diameter of the shank of the bits accepted—0.401" (10.2 mm) is most common
- Type of chisel retainer assembly accepted

Protection, Maintenance, and Storage of Pneumatic Tools

Pneumatic tools should be exercised every 30 to 60 days, at which time they should be oiled and checked for air leaks and proper function. Follow the specific instructions for maintenance, cleaning, and storage provided in the operator's manual. If the operator's manual is not readily available, the checklist below specifying general maintenance functions may be useful.

1. Oil the tool according to the operator's manual. If the system has an in-line oiler, ensure that the oiler is filled properly.
2. Connect the air regulator to the air source, and then connect the air hose and tool. Check the pressure regulator to see whether the gauge is intact and that it is registering no pressure. Before connecting the air fittings, check for dirt, corrosion, and ease of connecting and disconnecting the fittings. Check along the length of the air hoses for cuts, abrasions, and other signs of weakness or damage.
3. Slowly open the control valve from the compressed air source. Check for leaks in the regulator and fittings between the air source and the regulator. If the air source and the regulator have gauges, compare the two to see if they match.
4. If the regulator is adjustable, set the regulator to the tool's recommended pressure during its normal operation. Check the fittings between the regulator and the tool for leaks. Check the tool itself for leaks before testing its operation.
5. Operate the tool according to manufacturer's recommendations. Air hammers must be operated with a chisel and chisel retainer in place and resistance put against the chisel. Point the tool toward the ground, and wear appropriate protective clothing including gloves, helmet, eye, and ear protection.
6. Check the entire system for air leaks, bulges, or cuts in the hoses or other noticeable abnormalities while the system is under pressure.
7. Shut down the system, and oil the tool according to the operator's manual.
8. Check all chisels and blades after every incident. Check the chisel

shank for damage. It should not have any major chips or be bent. If the chisel shank appears to be damaged, remove it from service and destroy it. Blades should be sharp and intact, not bent or distorted. Chisels can be sharpened with a hand file, belt sander, or a bench grinder. When using a belt sander or a bench grinder be careful not to heat the chisel during the sharpening. Heating the chisel softens the metal and reduces its ability to hold a cutting edge.

Follow the specific instructions for storage in the operator's manual. If the operator's manual is not readily available, the checklist below specifying general guidelines for storage may be useful.

1. Place all components of the pneumatic system in labeled containers that provide secure holders for all parts. Place the containers in a compartment where the exposure to moisture, road salt, fuel, and battery acid will be kept to a minimum.
2. Turn all adjustable valves and regulators to a neutral position.
3. Ensure all tools in the compartment are secured to reduce the chances of damage. Allowing tools to bounce around during transport will significantly increase the wear and the chances for damage.
4. Store hoses bound in coils or secured to protect them from cuts and mechanical damage.
5. Ensure that fittings, blades, hoses, and chisels do not touch diamond plate compartment walls. Also ensure that doors cannot close on hoses, fittings, and chisels.

Follow the specific instructions for cleaning as outlined in the operator's manual. If the operator's manual is not readily available, the checklist below specifying general guidelines for cleaning pneumatic tools may be useful.

1. Use a mild soap and brush to clean off mud and grease, followed by thorough rinsing and drying.
2. Protect all metal components with a light oil or silicone. Equipment that is put away wet can become moldy, rusty, or corroded.
3. Check for corrosion on all hose couplings and air hammers. Keep them properly lubricated and coated according to manufacturers's recommendations.

AIR BAGS

Protection, Maintenance, and Storage of High-Pressure Air Bags

High-pressure air bags should be exercised at least once every 30 days, according to the specific instructions in the operator's manual. All high-pressure air bags should be tested in this same systematic manner. This is good for equipment maintenance and also keeps rescue skills sharp.

The system for exercising high-pressure air bags may include the following steps:

1. Connect the regulator to an air source and attach the air hoses, air bag control valve and relief valve, and the air bag.
2. Check the pressure regulator to ensure that the gauge is intact and registering no pressure; if a pressure gauge is available on the air bag control assembly, check it as well to make sure that it is registering no pressure.
3. Check the air fittings for dirt, corrosion, and ease of connecting and disconnecting.
4. Check the air hoses for cuts, abrasions, and other signs of weakness or damage.
5. Close the shut-off valve on the regulator, if available, to the hose line leading to the air bag control valve assembly, and slowly open the valve to the pressurized air source. Check the regulator and any connecting hose lines/fittings for leaks.
6. Ensure that the control valve (if manual) to the air bag is closed, and charge the system slowly by opening the regulator shut-off or the air source shut-off valve. If the regulator is adjustable, slowly raise the system to the operating pressure recommended by the manufacturer.
7. Check for air leaks. Also, recheck the full length of the air hose for air leaks, bulges, weak spots, cuts, or other visible damage.
8. Slowly open the control valve to the air bag, and raise the pressure to fill the bag to at least half its capacity. Check the air bag pressure gauge (if available) for a pressure reading. The air pressure reading (if a gauge is available to indicate the air bag pressure) should be checked periodically during the physical examination to determine if there is any drop in air pressure.
9. Recheck the air hose, air hose fittings, and the air bag for leaks, cuts, tears, abrasions, and other visible damage. Some high-pressure air bag manufacturers suggest that most cuts and nicks that are not leaking are not a problem unless the fabric or steel cords are exposed. If the cords are exposed, mark the air bag as unusable, and remove it from service.
10. Follow the manufacturers's guidelines to test the relief valve in the air bag control valve assembly. The relief valve may stick if the valve has been stored in the closed position. Manually opening and closing the relief valve will usually free it up.

Follow the specific instructions for storing air bags in the operator's manual. If the operator's manual is not readily available, the checklist below specifying general guidelines for storage may be useful.

1. Store all components away from road salt, batteries, fuels, high-moisture areas, and other possible contaminants.

2. Turn all valves and regulators to the neutral position so that there is reduced pressure on valve components.
3. Secure all components so that they will not slide around in the compartment or the storage box. Make sure that all other equipment in the area is also secured. Loose equipment in a compartment or storage box will very likely damage rescue equipment.
4. Store the hoses in a bound coil, and keep heavy objects from crushing the hose and hose fittings against the side walls.
5. Ensure that the air bag fittings do not touch the compartment walls, floors, ceiling, or doors. Also ensure that the doors do not slam against the air bag fittings when closing the compartment doors. Store the air bags with the fittings visible to the rescuers so that the fittings can be easily inspected and protected during removal and replacement in the vehicle compartment. A short piece of rubber tubing placed over the fitting may help keep the air bag fitting in good shape.

Follow the specific instructions for cleaning as outlined in the operator's manual, including using a mild soap and medium bristle brush to clean off mud, grease, and oil residue on the surface of the air bag. Rinse thoroughly, and let air dry before storing the air bags back on the vehicle. The use of rubber preservatives and paint is not recommended for high-pressure air bags.

Protection, Maintenance, and Storage of Low-Pressure Air Bags

Low-pressure air bags should be exercised every 30 days, if possible, in order to detect problems and make adjustments or repairs before serious damage occurs to the system.

A special note about the side walls on low-pressure air bags: the side walls should be kept tucked toward the middle of the air bag to reduce the chances of abrasion during storage and transport.

For specific details regarding the maintenance and storage of low-pressure air bags, consult the operator's manual.

TYPES OF HYDRAULIC FLUIDS

Petroleum Oils

Petroleum oils are one of the most commonly used bases for hydraulic fluids. Most of the desirable characteristics for hydraulic fluids can be incorporated into petroleum oils using additives and refining techniques. Petroleum-based hydraulic fluids possess good lubricating/anti-wear qualities, protect against rust, dissipate heat easily, resist oxidation at higher temperatures, and can be formulated to meet viscosity requirements of many hydraulic systems. The major disadvantage of petroleum-based hydraulic fluids is that they will burn. Petroleum-based hydraulic fluids are not suitable for situations in which a fire could occur.

Fire-Resistant Fluids

It is important to remember that fire-resistant fluids (FR fluids) are not fireproof; most of these fluids will burn under certain conditions. However, the fire-resistant fluids will not ignite easily; the fire is not as hot as that of petroleum-based hydraulic fluids, and is usually easier to put out.

There are six major types of fire-resistant hydraulic fluids, but there are only three basic fire-resistant hydraulic fluids: synthetic, water-oil emulsions, and water glycols.

Synthetic Hydraulic Fluids Synthetic fire-resistant fluids are developed from chemicals that are less flammable than oils. The synthetic fluids include phosphate esters, chlorinated (halogenated) hydrocarbons, or a combination with other additives. Synthetics do not contain water or volatile material. They are formulated to operate at high temperatures and at high pressures. They do not function well at lower temperatures. Synthetic hydraulic fluids are the most costly fluids on the market today.

Synthetic fluids are not compatible with commonly used hydraulic system seals such as nitrile (buna) or neoprene. To change over to a synthetic hydraulic fluid from hydraulic fluids such as petroleum oils, water glycol, or water-oil emulsions normally requires a complete system breakdown with cleaning and seal replacement.

Water-Oil Emulsions The emulsion-type hydraulic fluids are generally the least expensive type of fire-resistant fluid. The fire resistance depends upon the water emulsion to reduce the fire hazard. These hydraulic fluids contain oil, water, stabilizers, and other additives to hold the fluids together. Emulsion-type hydraulic fluids must be kept at low operating temperatures to avoid oxidation and water evaporation. Care must be taken to avoid freezing, which separates the fluids, and to ensure that the ratio of oil to water is kept constant. Changes in this ratio create problems with lubrication and viscosity of the hydraulic fluid. Neoprene and nitrile (buna) are two common types of seals used in these hydraulic systems.

Water Glycol The water glycol hydraulic fluid compounds include water-soluble thickeners to improve viscosity, a synthetic chemical such as glycol, and approximately 40% water for fire resistance. These fluids have good wear resistance and a higher specific gravity rating than oils. When using this type of hydraulic fluid, make sure that the water content stays constant to maintain the operating characteristics at a high level. This type of hydraulic fluid uses the more common types of seals such as nitrile (buna) and neoprene.

Protection, Maintenance, and Storage of Hydraulic Systems and Tools

All rescue hydraulic tools systems should be exercised monthly to lubricate the system seals and cylinders, allow for basic system maintenance, expose potential or actual defects, and permit the rescuer to practice assembly and disassembly of the hydraulic system. It is important to remember that all hydraulic rescue systems are intended to be closed systems. These monthly exercise periods will help keep the hydraulic system intact and fully operational.

Follow the specific instructions for exercising hydraulic rescue equipment outlined in the operator's manual. If the operator's manual is not readily available, the checklist below specifying general guidelines may be useful.

1. Remove the hydraulic equipment from storage. Check for oil leaks (check the storage compartment), hose line cuts, abrasions or visible damage, coupling damage, adapter damage, and tool integrity. Lay out all the system components and make an inventory list of all system items.
2. Check fluid levels in the hydraulic fluid reservoirs, engine oil level, fuel level or battery charge and fluid.
3. Connect the system including the pump/power unit, the hydraulic lines, and one of the hydraulic rescue tools. Closely inspect the hose and the tool couplings when making connections. If the couplings are dirty, dip in a compatible hydraulic fluid, brush clean, and dry with a lint-free rag. The couplings should fit together smoothly with little difficulty. The hose immediately next to the coupling should be checked for signs of wear or fatigue.
4. Put all hydraulic valves into a neutral position (dump valves should be positioned to return fluid directly into the reservoir), and activate the pump. Gasoline or diesel motors start more easily when there is little resistance on the hydraulic pump. Check the system for problems around the pump and the fluid reservoir.
5. Open the necessary valve to put pressure on the hose lines to the tool. Check the entire system for leaks or signs of damage or malfunction. A qualified technician should check the hydraulic pump pressure with a gauge at least once a year.
6. Activate the tool. Check the speed of the opening and closing. Look for rust, pitting, or scoring of the tool cylinders, rams, or rods. Check the linkage to the arms and alignment of the blades or arms. Check the responsiveness of the tool directional valve.
7. If possible, put the tool under a load. This will permit the system to develop higher working pressures that will indicate system integrity, motor performance, electrical power output, and pump output.
8. Operate all tools to their fullest extension and retraction several

times to lubricate the system. Hydraulic tools such as the Porta-power spreader have spring-return mechanisms. If the seals are dry or the rod/ram becomes rusty, the spring may not be able to retract or close the tool.
9. Put all valves back into the neutral position, and shut the pump down.
10. Disassemble the system, checking for visible damage. Once again check the fluid levels of the motor and the hydraulic reservoir.

Follow the specific instructions for storing hydraulic systems and tools outlined in the operator's manual. In general, all components of hydraulic systems should be stored in compartments, racks, reels, or containers that reduce or eliminate exposure to road salt, water, battery acid, and high or extremely low temperatures. Store all valves in neutral positions. Secure all loose items in containers or on racks to prevent them from sliding or bouncing around. Make sure that other equipment stored in the same area is secure so they cannot cause damage to the hydraulic system components. Hose and hose couplings are particularly easy to damage in apparatus compartments, if not properly secured away from doors and hinges.

Follow the specific instructions for cleaning outlined in the operator's manual. In general, use compatible hydraulic fluid to clean hose coupling or fittings. Exposure of some hydraulic system components such as seals to diesel fuel or other cleaning agents may damage the hydraulic components. Metal system components and hose lines should be kept clean using a mild soap and brush to remove mud, grease, and other external contaminants. This washing should be followed by a thorough rinse and dry process. All external metal components need to be protected from rust and corrosion. Check the manufacturers' recommendations for suggestions.

GLOSSARY

Agricultural-rural incident: incident involving farm equipment, animals, electricity, falls, fires, chemicals or pesticides, confined spaces, or natural events. These incidents may occur in isolated locations and may not be discovered for several hours.

Air medical: method of speeding lifesaving care to patients and of transporting patients with life-threatening injuries or illnesses to definitive medical care.

Ammonium hydroxide: a highly caustic solution that corrodes metals and causes progressive chemical burns to soft tissue.

AMPLE: acronym used for recording a patient's history (Allergies, Medication, Pertinent medical history, Last meal, Events).

Anhydrous ammonia: fertilizer used to supply nitrogen to grain crops; it contains no moisture, but when combined with water forms the highly corrosive alkali ammonium hydroxide.

Articulated tractor: four-wheel drive tractor divided into two sections and steered by the articulation of the two sections.

Auger: implement that applies the screw theory to move material from one point to another.

Autonomic stress reaction (ASR): temporary reduction in perfusion of the brain in response to extreme emotional situations, such as fear and bad news.

AVPU scale: method by which to measure level of consciousness based on four factors: Alert, Verbal, Pain, Unresponsive.

Ballast: weight added to the tractor tires, usually in liquid form, to increase traction.

Belay: system of safety ropes attached to a litter that acts to support the litter in the event the litter starts to slip or fall during evacuation.

Big net principle: method of anticipating the worst case scenario to avoid overlooking injuries or complications.

Bipyridyls: a common class of herbicide.

Block and tackle rigging: a configuration of rope and pulleys used to gain mechanical advantage for lifting, pulling, or moving a load.

Boiling liquid expanding vapor explosion (BLEVE): an explosion of liquified compressed gas in which the compression heats the liquid in the tank, increasing vapor pressure until the tank ruptures.

Bombproof anchor: one that is stronger than any forces that will be placed on the system during the rescue operation.

Brake bar rack: U-shaped frame in which one arm of the U is longer than the other. This rack helps control lowering large loads.

Brakeman: rescuer who controls the rate of lowering.

Callout information sheet: document that provides the dispatcher with the information necessary to brief resources properly when they are requested to respond.

Center of gravity: the point in any body at which all of the body's weight is said to be concentrated.

Come-along: commonly used manual effort pulling tool consisting of rope, hooks, blocks, and pulleys.

Confined space: any space not intended for continuous occupancy, with limited or no ventilation, and limited entrance and exit.

Counterbalance system: a simple 1:1 MA system commonly used in silo rescues.

Critical Incident Stress Debriefing (CISD): program, composed of peer support and mental health professionals, designed to help rescuers deal with major stresses that may occur as a result of a critical incident.

Decontamination: the process of removing toxic and other harmful materials and properly disposing of them.

Delayed stress reaction: emotional effects of a critical incident or traumatic stress that may occur either long term or short term.

Dependent lividity: discoloration of the skin due to pooling of blood.

Disaster: any event that exceeds the capacity of local resources to respond effectively in an appropriate time frame.

Dogs: two catch levers on the come-along.

Drawbar pull: the force produced by the equipment pulled behind the tractor.

Equilibrium: when objects are balanced or at rest.

Extended incident: situation in which the time from the initial injury to definitive medical care is longer than 2 hours.

Field speed: speed of under 10 mph.

Fixed-line flyaway: short-distance transport with the stretcher slung under the aircraft.

Flighting: large, fluted blades on a turning shaft that moves grain or some other product from one point to another.

Friction: the force resisting the relative motion between two surfaces.

Front-end loader: hydraulically powered implement mounted to the front end of a tractor and equipped with a bucket for hauling a variety of materials.

Fumigants: insecticides used to treat and protect stored grain, greenhouse crops, and stored fruits and vegetables.

Golden hour: the period after an injury in which the patient's body is able to compensate for the injury and remain relatively stable.

Hauling system: system used to raise a patient to a higher elevation.

Hazardous material: product or material that can cause damage or injury when released from its normal container or environment, or when exposed to another agent or environment.

Header: part of the combine that cuts the grain.

"Hot" aircraft: term used to describe a helicopter in which the rotors are spinning.

Hydraulic power: type of energy transmission that uses a closed fluid system to transform energy to work.

IDLH: immediately dangerous to life and health.

Immediate stress reaction: response that often occurs at the scene or shortly after leaving the scene. Symptoms vary widely, depending on the individual.

Implement input shaft: shaft that connects the implement to the intermediate shaft.

Incident Command System (ICS): standardized emergency management system developed to organize and manage all functions required to handle an emergency situation.

Incident commander: the individual in charge of the rescue operation.

Inclined plane: simple machine consisting of a ramp, wooden wedge, or screw thread.

Inertia: a body at rest remains at rest until acted upon by a force.

Intermediate shaft: shaft that transfers the tractor power to the attached implement.

Joule (J): unit of measure of work.

Jump kit: basic life support supplies carried in an ambulance.

Kernmantle: rope design consisting of a tightly woven outer sheath that helps protect the inner core that supports most of the load.

LAST: acronym that presents the four separate phases of rescue (Locate, Access, Stabilize, Transport).

Lever: simple machine consisting of a rigid bar that rotates about an axis.

Lifting force: the amount of air pressure in the bag multiplied by the number of square inches of bag surface contact area.

Lockout: a process by which all power sources are shut off and secured.

Lower explosive limit (LEL): the point at which a gas mixes with just the proper amount of oxygen to burn.

Lowering: controlled movement in which a patient is moved from higher elevation to lower elevation.

Machine: device that converts energy into work by transferring energy to a body or an object.

Maillard reaction: chemical reaction responsible for silo fires.

Mechanical advantage (MA): the ratio of effort applied to move a given load.

Moment of force (torque): Special type of work when a force rotates around a pivot point or fulcrum.

Momentum: a body in motion remains in motion until it is acted upon by an outside force.

Multiple trauma: incident in which there are two or more patients.

Mutual aid: system in which different agencies or organizations may be preassigned to various functional areas during a rescue operation.

Omnivorous: characteristic of some animals that will eat anything, plant or animal flesh, including human flesh.

Outer layer: a shell of windproof, waterproof material that resists wind and precipitation.

Patient Assessment System (PAS): seven-step assessment system based on the widely used SOAP format.

Perfusion: the circulation of blood within an organ or tissue.

Polytrauma: injuries that involve multiple body systems.

Power: the rate at which work is done.

Power take-off (PTO): a shaft or shafts that transmit power from a mechanism to an accompanying machine.

Primary driveline: transfers power from the engine or tractor to a gearbox.

Primary survey: examination that covers immediate life-threatening conditions, commonly known as ABCD (airway, breathing, circulation, disability).

Pulley: specialized wheel that uses the mechanical advantage of the lever.

Purchase point: point at which rescuers can apply a tool or insert air bags.

Rigor mortis: stiffening of the body after death.

Rodenticides: agents that kill, repel, or control rodents.

Rollover protective structure (ROPS): a heavy steel frame mounted to the rear axle and the tractor frame designed to support the maximum weight of the tractor without breaking or collapsing.

Rope handler: rescuer who assists brakeman by feeding rope and removing kinks in rope before they foul the brake.

Rule of Nines: method used to determine the percentage of the total body surface area burned.

Safety zone: area that encompasses at least 50' in all directions from the equipment in which rescuers extricate the patient and provide medical treatment. Bystanders are to be escorted out of the safety zone.

Secondary driveline: connects the gearbox with the equipment.

Secondary survey: complete head-to-toe examination of the patient, to be completed before beginning any treatment other than basic life support (BLS) or advanced life support (ALS).

Shielding: all protective equipment used by the rescuer during a hazardous materials incident.

Shock: a condition of acute peripheral circulatory failure causing inadequate and progressively failing perfusion of tissues.

Shock load: a load resulting from a rapid change of movement of a static load.

Silo gas: nitrogen dioxide that tends to collect at the surface of silage and flows down the silo chute to low areas around the base of the silo. The gas may appear yellow or reddish-brown.

Situational crisis: state of emotional upset or turmoil caused by a sudden, disruptive event, such as an unexpected illness, traumatic injury, or death of a loved one.

Sling: a length of synthetic rope, wire rope, chain, or webbing that attaches to a load or anchor for the purpose of stabilizing, lifting, pulling, or moving objects.

Snapping rolls: paired rollers that are part of the row unit of a combine.

SOAP: acronym that represents a method of relaying patient information commonly used by medical personnel (Subjective, Objective, Assessment, Plan).

Span of control: the optimum number of resources that can be effectively supervised by one person.

Squeezing: incident in which an animal pushes a person against a wall or fence that may result in serious injury.

Step-up plan: plan that defines responsibilities for determining the need for and requesting additional resources.

Straw walkers: part of the combine that separates threshed grain from the straw, consisting of several longitudinal sections that move in an alternating rise and fall motion.

Stress: distorting forces within a body, such as compression, tension, and shear.

Strike zone: an area of potential injury from a moving tool or object.

Thermal layer: a second layer of clothing worn on the outside of the transport layer to provide insulation.

Torque: force that produces rotation or torsion.

Toxicity: the level of poison in a pesticide.

Tractor output shaft: shaft that delivers power from the engine and protrudes from the rear of the tractor.

Transport layer: a thin layer of clothing worn next to the skin that wicks moisture away from the skin to keep the wearer dry and warm.

Trauma: the transfer of the energy of movement to the body tissues, resulting in injury.

Turnout gear: protective clothing garments designed for use in structural fire-fighting environments.

Universal gravitation: another term for the law of gravity.

Universal joint: joints at the ends of the PTO drivelines that connect the tractor to the implement, and allow the driveline to change angles.

Universal precautions: protective measures that emphasize infection control and urge caution when dealing with equipment subject to breakage or accidental puncture of the skin.

Venturi effect: increased volume of air created by pressurized air stream.

Windrow: crop that has been cut and raked into a row.

Work: the application of a force over a distance.

INDEX

ABCD elements of a primary survey, 255–256
   in auger incidents, 154
   in burns, 297
   in combine incidents, 126
   in tractor incidents, 114
abrasions, 293
   protecting rope from, 68
absorbents, 237
acid, 183
action plan, developing, 55
advanced life support (ALS), 246, 255, 273
agricultural equipment. *See specific piece of equipment*
agricultural gases, 181
   ammonia, 184
   carbon dioxide, 181–182
   carbon monoxide, 182–183
   hydrogen sulfide, 184
   methane, 183–184
   nitric oxide, 183
   nitrogen dioxide, 183
   nitrogen tetroxide, 183
agricultural-rural incidents, 7
   air medical evacuation, 23
   big net principle, 271–272
   communications in, 20
   crisis intervention in, 328
   definition of, 6, 7
   determining urgency, 17
   disasters and mass casualties, 24
   extended, 23
   incident command system in, 19–20
   injured or deceased rescuers in, 28
   injury to patient caused by rescuers, 28
   lighting in, 42
   managing, 14–15
   multi-jurisdictional/multi-agency incident management, 20
   notification, 18
   obstacles to overall coordination and leadership, 24–25
      breakdown in information flow, 26
      change in nature of incident, 27
      disruption in logistical support, 26
      equipment failure, 27
      inadequate leadership, 26–27
      loss of communication, 25–26
      loss of span of control, 27
      personality conflicts, 27
   overwhelmed rescuers, 28–29
   polytrauma, 266
   problems with initial strategy and tactics, 28
   resource tracking system, 18–19
   terminology for, 21–22
   traumatic injuries, 262
      anticipating problems, 264–265
      associated conditions, 265–266
      types of, 262–264
      understanding, 262–264
   using specialists untrained in rescue, 20, 23
agricultural-rural rescue, 7–8. *See also* rescue operations
   comparisons to other rescues, 7
   extrication considerations, 9–10
      assistance resources, 10
      scene accessibility, 10
   mutual aid in, 19–20
   personal safety of rescuers in, 10
   preincident planning in, 11, 15–17
   safety considerations at scene, 8–9
   specialized resources for, 18
agriculture, as dangerous occupation, 8
AIDS exposure, 33–35
air bags, 76–77
   high-pressure, 77–79
      advantages of, 78
      in baler incidents, 164
      barrier protection for, 80–81
      disadvantages of, 78–79
      in ensilage cutter incidents, 168–169
      in lifting combines, 125–126
      in lifting front-end loaders, 118
      lifting and lowering considerations, 81
      in lifting tractors, 112–113
      protection, maintenance, and storage of, 347–349
      safety considerations, 80–81
      stability considerations, 80
      stacking, 79–80
   low-pressure, 81–82
      advantages of, 82–83
      barrier protection for, 84
      components of, 82–84

357

disadvantages of, 83–84
protection, maintenance, and storage of, 349
safety considerations, 84
stability considerations, 84
air chisel, 155
air medical evacuation, 23, 316, 318, 320
landing zones, 320–321
nighttime landings, 322
packaging considerations, 323–324
personal safety, 322–323
wind direction, approach, and departure paths, 321
air splints, in litter transport, 42
aircraft wire, 342
airway management, and litter transport, 307
aluminum phosphide, 228
ambulances, 317–318
in transporting contaminated patients, 240
ammonia, 183, 184
anhydrous, 220–223
ammonium hydroxide, 215, 220
AMPLE, 252, 259
amputations, 294
anaphylactic shock, 274
treating, 277
anger, as crisis reaction, 329
anhydrous ammonia
definition of, 215, 217
management of exposure, 222–223
mechanisms of injury, 221, 271
personal safety with, 222, 239
physical properties of, 220
storage requirements of, 220–221
animal incidents, 207–208
cattle, 210–211
common injuries involving, 212, 270
horses, 208–210
pigs, 211–212
traps for, 212–213
ankle hitch, 306
aortic tear, 263
articulated tractor, 94, 99
atmospheric hazards, 32
ammonia in, 184
carbon dioxide in, 181–182
carbon monoxide in, 182–183
combating, 184–187
in confined spaces, 180–187
hydrogen sulfide in, 181, 184
methane in, 183–184
nitric oxide in, 183
nitrogen dioxide in, 183
nitrogen tetroxide in, 183
augers
definition of, 138, 150
grain tank, 128–129
extrication technique for, 129–130
open, 150–151
open auger entanglement, 156–157

extrication technique for, 158
portable, 150
portable auger entanglement, 151–152
common injuries involving, 154, 268
extrication technique for, 153–154
minor entanglement, 154–156
autonomic stress reaction (ASR), 260, 266, 277–278
AVPU scale, 252, 257, 279
avulsions, 293, 296

back board, 129
backup equipment, need for, 27
balers, 158–159
conventional
common injuries involving, 161, 269
extrication technique for, 160–161
types of entanglement, 160
large round
common injuries involving, 164, 269
extrication technique for, 163–164
types of entanglement, 161–163
ballast, 94, 104
barrier protection. *See also* environmental protection
for air bags, 80–81, 84
for slings, 339
basic life support (BLS), 255, 273
basic rigging, 60
pulleys, 60
slings, 61–62
basket hitch, 61
belay system, 302, 310
and litter transport, 306
big net principle, 261, 271–272
bipyridyls, 215, 231
bleeding
controlling
in auger incidents, 154
in combine incidents, 126, 130, 132, 133
in PTO entanglement, 146
in tractor incidents, 114
block and tackle rigging, 58, 60
blood-borne pathogens
OSHA requirements for, 37
rescuer exposure to, 33–35, 39, 40
blood pressure, 256–257
boiling liquid expanding vapor explosion (BLEVE), 215, 220–221
bombproof anchor, 302, 311
brake bar rack, 302, 313
brakeman, 303, 311
bridle hitch, 61–62
bright wire, 342
buddy rescuer system, in confined space rescue, 179
bunker gear, 37
bunker jacket, 38
burns, 297
assessment of, 297–300
chemical, 221, 222

Index

electrical, 170
first-degree, 298, 300
respiratory, 297
second-degree, 298, 300
third-degree, 298, 300
treatment of, 300
    extended transport, 300
    IV volume replacement, 300–301
bursting pressure, 88
bystanders, need to escort from safety zone, 8–9

calcium hypochlorite, 237
callout information sheet, 13, 18
carabiners, 70–71
carbamates, 227–228
carbon dioxide, 181–182, 221
carbon monoxide, 182–183, 221
cardiac arrest, 272–273
cardiogenic shock, 273, 274
    treating, 276–277
cardiopulmonary resuscitation (CPR), 239
cardiovascular accidents, 278
cattle, 210–211
center of gravity
    definition of, 46, 51, 52, 94, 103
    estimating, and use of air bags, 84
    and tractor stability, 102, 103
center pivot irrigation systems, 169–170
Centers for Disease Control (CDC) universal precautions, 33–35
cerebrospinal fluid (CSF), 281
cervical spine injuries, 285
chains, 71–72, 343–344
    grades of, 344
    protection, maintenance, and storage of, 344–345
chain-type come-along, 64
chemical burns, 221, 222
chemical release, 24
chemical washes, 237
CHEMTREC, 216
children, communicating with, in crisis intervention, 330
chisel shank/threaded collar, 74
chisels, pneumatic, 74–75
chronic heart disease, 265
circulation, sensation, and movement (CSM), 290
closed soft tissue injuries, 282–283
cold chisel, 75
cold water, protective clothing for, 38
cold weather, protective clothing for, 35–36, 37
cole rack, 313
combine
    common injuries involving, 134, 267
    drive belts or chains, 126
        extrication technique for, 128
    entanglements, 126
    grain tank augers, 128–129
        extrication technique for, 129–130
    header collapse, 134–136
    history of design, 121–123
    lifting, 125–126
    overturns, 123
        extrication technique for, 124–126
    safety features of, 123
    securing, 124–125
    snapping rolls, 130–131
        extrication technique for, 131–132
    straw walkers, 132–133
        extrication technique for, 133
    turning engine off, 124
come-along, 339–340
    chain-type, 64
    definition of, 59, 63–64
    dogs on, 59, 64–65
    wire rope, 64–65
command, 21
command staff, 21
committed resource, 21
communication, 248–249
    in agricultural-rural rescues, 20
    in confined spaces, 179, 198–199
    in crisis management, 329
        with others, 331–332
        with patient, 330–331
    in silo rescues, 198–199
    loss of, and emergency responses, 25–26
compression chamber, entanglement in, 160
compression injuries, 262, 263
concussions, 280
confined space
    common injuries involving, 197, 270
    definition of, 176, 178
    flowing grain
        entrapment in, 189–193
        extrication from, 193–196
    hazards in, 180
        atmospheric, 180–187
        physical, 187–188
        psychological, 188–189
    moving litter through, 311
    preincident planning for, 178–179
    silos as, 196–199
contaminants, protection of rescuers from, 39
contusions, 280
coordinated steering, 101
cotton picker
    entanglement in, 165, 175, 269
    extrication from, 165
counterbalance system, 303, 314
coupling links, 72
crab steering, 101
cribbing
    in lifting tractor, 113–114
    support of air bags with, 81
crisis intervention
    in agricultural-rural settings, 328
    communication in, 329, 331–332

critical incident stress debriefing (CISD) in, 336–337
emotional reactions in, 328–329
patient communication in
    nonverbal, 330–331
    verbal, 330
stress in, 333–334
    delayed reactions, 334
    effects of excessive, 334–335
    immediate reactions, 334
    recognizing excessive, 335–336
sudden death in, 332–333
critical incident stress debriefing (CISD), 28, 326, 334, 336–337
critical incident stress debriefing (CISD) team, 333
cutting tools, 62
cyanide, 221

deadman valve, 86
death
    crisis management of sudden, 332–333
    legal determination of, 333
    of rescuer, 28
deceased persons, 249–250
deceleration injuries, 262, 263
decontamination, 215, 236–238
dehydration, as physical threat to rescuer, 32
delayed stress reaction, 327, 334
denial, as crisis reaction, 329
dependent lividity, 327, 333
dermal exposure to pesticides, 225
dilutional decontamination, 236
diquat, 231
direct injury, 292
disassembly tools, 65
disaster, 13, 24
dislocations, 291–292
    assessment, 292
    mechanisms of injury, 292
    treatment, 292
dispatch, 21
DNR (do not resuscitate) order, 333
dogs, 59, 64–65
double-acting hydraulic cylinders, 85
double basket hitch, 61
double choker hitch, 61
double panel cutter, 75
down-filled clothing, 36
drawbar pull, 94, 104
drive belts and chains, entanglement in, 175, 269
dump valve, 86
dust, protection of rescuers from, 39

ear protection, 39
earplugs, 39
edge rollers, 68

elasticity of solids, 56–57
electrical hazards, 38, 169–170
electrical injuries from elevated augers, 152
electrocution, 170
    as danger from center pivot irrigation systems, 169
endless sling, 338–339
engine, turning off, in extrication technique for, 9
ensilage cutters, 166–168
    entanglement in, 175, 269
    extrication technique for, 168–169
environmental extremes, 264
Environmental Protection Agency (EPA)
    banning of organochlorines by, 230
    classifications of protective equipment, 235
environmental protection for litter transport, 42–43, 307–308
equilibrium, 46, 52
equipment failure, in incident command system, 27
exercise, as physical threat to rescuer, 33
extended incidents, 23–24, 245–247
    definition of, 242, 245
    patient care during, 301
    rescuers involved in, 255–256
extended transport, 245–247
    burn treatment in, 300
external forces, estimating, 55
extremity fractures, 287
    assessment of, 288–289
    treatment of, 289–291
extrication
    from conventional balers, 160–161
    from cotton picker entanglement, 165
    from drive belt entanglement, 128
    from ensilage cutters, 168–169
    from farm equipment, 9–10, 11
    from flowing grain entrapment, 193–196
    from large round balers, 163–164
    from mixing wagons, 170–171
    from open auger entanglement, 158
    from overturned combines, 124–126
    from portable augers, 153–154
    from potato diggers, 173
    from PTO entanglement, 144–146
    from rear overturn of tractor, 106–114
    from silos, 199–201
    from snapping rolls, 131–132
    from straw walkers, 133
    from sugar beet harvesters, 173
extrication tools
    air bags, 76–77
        high-pressure air bags, 77–81, 347–349
        low-pressure air bags, 81–85, 349
    basic rigging, 60
        loading effects, 62
        pulleys, 60
        slings, 61–62
    chains, 71–72, 343–344
    hooks, 72, 345
    hydraulic cylinders, 85

hydraulic fluids, 86–87, 349–352
hydraulic hoses and couplings, 87–88
    portable manual hydraulic tools, 89–90
hydraulic valves, 85–86
manual effort tools, 62, 339–340
    cutting tools, 62
    disassembly tools, 65
    pulling tools, 63–65
    spreading tools, 62–63
pneumatic tools, 72–73, 345–347
    chisels, 74–75
    cutting tools, 76
    impact wrenches, 75–76
    tool systems, 73–74
ropes and related equipment
    rope-related equipment, 70–71
    types of rope, 65–69
    slings, 338–339
        roundslings, 338
    web sling configurations, 338–339
    wire rope, 340–343
eye injuries from hazardous materials, 222–223
eye protection, 39
    and litter transport, 308

fall zones, need for helmets in, 39
farm equipment. *See also* agricultural-rural incidents
    extrication from, 9–10, 11
farm equipment mechanic, role of, in extrication technique, 10, 20, 160, 165
field speed, 95, 99
fire fighting, protective clothing for, 37, 40, 41
fire-resistant fluids, 350
fires in silos, 201–203
fixed-line flyaway, 316, 323
fixed pulley, 60
flashlights, 42
flat-bladed pry bar, 62
flat chisel, 75
flighting, 120, 129, 151
flood, 24
flotation suit, 38
fluid-powered cylinders, 85
footwear, 40
four-wheel drive tractors, 99–102
fractures
    extremity, 287–291
    rib, 263
    skull, 281–282
    spinal, 283–287
friction, 46, 50–51
front-end loader, 95, 115–118
fulcrum, 48
fumigants, 215, 228–230

galvanized steel wire, 342

gas detector, 186
gear, 41–45
    turnout, 37
gloves, 40–41
goggles, 39
golden hour, 242, 246, 264, 272
Gore-Tex, 40
grab hooks, 72
grain and silage storage facility rescues
    hazards in confined spaces, 180
        atmospheric hazards, 180–187
    preincident planning for, 178–179
    special considerations, 178
grain tank, 129
grain tank augers, 128–129
    extrication technique for, 129–130
grain trailers, and use of air bags, 84
gramoxone, 231
gravity, law of, 50
grease gun injuries, 217
grief
    as crisis reaction, 329
    stress in coping with, 335
ground vehicle transportation, 317–318
    in transporting contaminated patients, 240

halocarbon fumigants, 229
hand tools, 339
hand winch. *See* come-along
hands
    decision to secure, in litter transport, 308
    hands-on stable, 286, 289
    protection of rescuer's, 40–41
harnesses, 70
hauling system, 303, 313–314
hazardous materials
    anhydrous ammonia
        management of exposure, 222–223
        mechanisms of injury, 221
        personal safety, 222
        physical properties, 220
        storage requirements, 220–221
    common classes of, 218
    decontamination, 236–238
    definition of, 215, 217
    hydraulic fluids, 231–232
        mechanisms of injury, 233–234
        personal safety, 234
    identification of, 217–220
    injuries associated with exposure to, 217, 271
    management of exposure, 239
        contamination control during transport, 240–241
        managing ill or injured patients, 239–240
        personal safety, 239
    pesticides, 224
        exposure to, 224–225
        major incidents, 227

personal safety, 225–226
    toxicity of, 224, 225
    protection from, 234–236
HBV exposure, 33–35
head injuries
  concussions, 280
  contusions, 280
  increased intracranial pressure
    assessment of, 278–280
    mechanism of injury, 278
    treatment of, 280
  intracranial hemorrhage, 280
  scalp lacerations, 280–281
  skull fractures, 281–282
header
  collapse of, 134–136
  definition of, 120, 134
headlamp, 42
healthcare workers, universal precautions for, 33–35
heart disease, chronic, 265
heat exhaustion, 258
helicopter transport, 304
  in air medical evacuation, 23, 318, 320
  landing zones for, 320–321
  nighttime landings for, 322
  packaging considerations for, 323–324
  personal safety, 23, 322–323
  type of litter in, 45
  wind direction, approach, and departure paths for, 321
helmets, 38–39
  in litter transport, 308
hematoma, 282
hemorrhage, intracranial, 280
high altitude cerebral edema (HACE), 278
high-angle/confined space, 38
high-angle work, 39
high-pressure air bags. *See* air bags
high-pressure injection injury, 296–297
high-speed circular cut-off saw, 76
high-test chain, 344
HIV exposure, 33–35
hook bill, 62
hooks, 72
  protection, maintenance, and storage of, 345
horizontal grain crusts, 192
horses, 208–210
"hot" aircraft, 316, 322
hydration, as physical threat to rescuer, 32–33
hydraulic cylinders, 85
hydraulic fluid, 86–87, 217
  mechanisms of injury, 233–234, 296–297
  personal safety, 234
  selecting appropriate, 87
  synthetic, 350
  toxic exposure to, 231–234
  types of, 349–352
hydraulic hoses and couplings, 87–88

hydraulic jacks
  in lifting front-end loaders, 118
  with self-contained pump, 88–89
hydraulic power, 59, 85
hydraulic system, failure of, and front-end loader incidents, 116
hydraulic tools
  operating, 88–90
  protection, maintenance, and storage of, 351–352
hydraulic valves, 85–86
hydrogen sulfide, 184
hyperventilation, 189
hypothermia, 33, 258
hypovolemic shock, 273, 274, 297
  treating, 275–276
hypoxia, effects of, 180

immediately dangerous to life and health (IDLH)
  atmospheric hazards as, 180
  definition of, 176, 179
immediate stress reaction, 327, 334
impaled objects, 296
implement input shaft, 139, 149
incident action plan, 21
incident commander
  definition of, 13, 16, 22
  leadership skills of, 26–27
  role of, 17, 20, 24–25
incident command post, 22
Incident Command System (ICS)
  and air medical evacuation, 23
  and change in nature of incidents, 27
  communication in, 20, 25–26
  definition of, 13, 19
  in disasters, 24
  equipment failure in, 27
  in extended incidents, 23–24
  functions in, 13–14, 19–20
  leadership in, 26–27
  logistic support in, 26
  multi-jurisdictional/multi-agency management in, 20
  mutual aid in, 19–20
  obstacles to overall coordination and leadership, 24–27
  personality conflicts in, 27
  span of control in, 27
  specialists untrained in rescue in, 20, 23
  and specific problem situations, 28–29
  terminology in, 21–22
incisions, 293
inclined plane, 46, 49
incomplete cord injury, 285–286
indirect injury, 292
inertia, 46, 50
infection control
  in burn patient, 297
  universal precautions for, 33–35
information flow in incident command system, 26

inhalation exposure to pesticides, 225
intermediate shaft on PTO, 139, 141–142
internal injury, 265
intracranial hemorrhage, 280
intracranial pressure, increased, 278–280
irrigation, for eye injury, 222–223
irrigation systems. *See* center pivot irrigation systems
ischemic tissue, 288
IV use/maintenance in litter transport, 309
IV volume replacement, in burns, 300–301

joule (J), 46, 48
jump kit, 316, 318, 319–320
jurisdictional, 22

kernmantle, 59, 66
Kinman rescue tool, 86

lacerations, 293
    scalp, 280–281
LAST, 242, 244
law enforcement personnel, at rescue scene, 9
leadership, in incident command system, 26–27
legal determination of death, 333
lever, 47, 48–49
levering injury, 264
lifting capacity of high-pressure air bags, 80
lifting force, 59, 77
lighting, 42
liquid manure storage, 203–204
litter team, 309–310
litter transport
    in air rescue, 45
    belaying litter in, 310
    in confined spaces, 311
    environmental protection for, 42–43, 307–308
    hauling systems in, 313–314
    lowering systems in, 311–313
    packaging for, 304–306
litters, 42–45
    semirigid, 45
    Stokes, 42–45
    types of, 304
living will, 333
load sling, 310
locking carabiners, 70–71
lockout, 176, 179
logistical support in incident command system, 26
lower explosive limit (LEL), 176, 184–185
lower extremity injuries, packaging patient for, 306–307
lowering, 303, 311
lowering systems, 311–313
low-pressure air bags. *See* air bags
lumbar spine injuries, 285–286

machine
    definition of, 47, 48
    inclined plane as, 49
    lever as, 48–49
Maillard reaction, 177, 201
manifold block, 86
manual effort tools, 339–340
manure decomposition, 181, 184
manure spreaders, 173–174
manure storage, liquid, 203–204
master links, 64, 72
Material Safety Data Sheet for hydraulic fluid, 87
mechanical advantage (MA), 60
    in classifying hauling systems, 314
    definition of, 47, 48
medical care, 244
    communications in, 248–249
        radio, 249
        written, 249
    deceased persons, 249–250
    extended transport, 245–247
    information gathering, 247
    personal safety, 247–248
medical facilities, problem of uneven distribution of patients to, 24
medical team, cooperation between rescue team and, 244
methane, 183–184
methyl bromide, 228, 229
minimum ultimate load, for chain, 344
mixing wagons, 170–171
    extrication technique for, 171–172
molasses tanks, 182
moment of force (torque), 47, 53–55
momentum, 47, 50
motion, laws of, 50
movable pulley, 60
multiple-tool operations, 86
multiple trauma, 261, 266
musculoskeletal injuries, 287
    extremity fractures, 287
        assessment of, 288–289
        treatment of, 289–291
mutual aid, 318
    agreements for, 16
    in agricultural-rural rescue, 19–20
    definition of, 13

National Association of Chain Manufacturers (NACM), 72, 344
Neill-Robertson litter, 45
nitric acid, 183
nitric oxide, 183
nitrogen dioxide, 183, 198
nitrogen tetroxide, 183
Nomex material, 235–236
nutrition, as physical threat to rescuer, 33

Occupational Safety and Health Administration (OSHA) standards,
    for rollover protective structure (ROPS), 98
omnivorous animals, 206, 211
operational period, 22
organochlorines, 230–231
organophosphates, 227–228
outer layer, 30, 35
overturns
    of combines, 123
        extrication technique for, 124–126
    rear, of tractors, 104–105
        extrication technique for, 106–114

packaging
    for air medical transport, 323–324
    considerations in, 304
    for litter evacuation, 304–306
        additional packaging, 307
        airway management, 307
        IV maintenance, 309
        IV use in rural areas, 309
        other types of litters, 307
        spinal, pelvic, or lower extremity injuries, 306–307
pain masking, 266
panel cutter chisel, 75
paraquat, 231
patient, communication with, in crisis intervention, 330–331
patient assessment
    in auger incidents, 154
    in burns, 297–300
    in combine incidents, 125–127, 128, 130, 132, 133
    in confined space incidents, 193–196, 199–200
    in dislocations, 292
    in head injuries, 278–280
    in mixing wagon incidents, 171–172
    in musculoskeletal injuries, 288–289
    in PTO entanglement, 145–146
    in shock, 274–275
    in spinal injuries, 284–286
    in tractor incidents, 109–114
    in wounds, 294–296
Patient Assessment System (PAS), 252, 253–254
    assessment, 259
    history, 259
    plan, 259
    primary survey, 255–256
    scene survey in, 254
    secondary survey, 256
    vital signs, 256–258
patient control, 301
patient removal. *See* extrication
pelvic injuries, packaging patient for, 306–307
penetrating trauma, 263–264
perfusion, 261, 273, 275
personal flotation devices (PFDs) in water rescues, 115
personality conflicts, in incident command systems, 27
personal safety, in agricultural-rural incidents, 10

personnel pool, 22
pesticides
    exposure to, 217, 224–225
    major incidents, 227
    personal safety, 225–226
    signs and symptoms of poisoning, 227–232
    toxicity of, 224, 225
petroleum oils, 349
phosphine fumigants, 228–229
physical threats
    atmosphere as, 32
    dehydration as, 32
    exercise as, 33
    nutrition as, 33
    temperature as, 32
pigs, 211–212
pit zips, 35
placards, 218
plane, inclined, 49
planning meeting, 22
plate hook, 72
pneumatic antishock garment (PASG), 42, 232, 246, 276, 294
pneumatic chisels, 74–75
pneumatic cutting tools, 76
pneumatic impact wrenches, 75–76
pneumatic tools, 72–74, 345–346
    protection, maintenance, and storage of, 346–347
polytrauma, 261, 266
portable manual hydraulic tools, 89–90
Porta-power spreader, 89
potato diggers, 173
    entanglement in, 175, 269
    extrication from, 173
power, 47, 48
power take-off (PTO), 140–143
    common injuries involving, 146, 268
    definition of, 139, 140
    disassembling, 149
    disentangling extremities or body from, 149–150
    entanglement, 143–144
        extrication technique for, 144–146
            minor, 146–148
            severe, 148–149
preincident plan, 239
    air medical evacuation in, 23
    for confined space rescue, 178–179
    information included in, 11, 15–17
    and jurisdictional disputes, 16
    for silo rescues, 198–199
    step-up plan in, 16
pressure relief valve for air bag, 81
primary driveline on PTO, 139, 143
primary survey, 252, 255–256
proof load for wire rope, 340
proof test
    for chains, 343–344
    for wire rope, 340
propane gas, 221

protective clothing, 35
  for agricultural-rural rescues, 10
  for cold weather, 35–36, 37
  decontamination of contaminated, 237–238
  EPA classifications of, 235
  footwear, 40
  hand protection, 40–41
  headgear, 38–39
  minimum clothing requirements, 36–37
  protection for dust and contaminants, 39
  skin protection, 41
  types of, 35–36
  in universal precautions, 33
pry bar, 339
  flat-bladed, 62
psychogenic shock, 277
psychological hazards, 188–189
  combating, 189
PTO. See power take-off
pulleys, 48–49, 60
  definition of, 47, 48
  fixed, 60
  movable, 60
pulling tools, 63–65
pulse, 257
puncture wounds, 293
purchase point, 59, 62–63
pyrolysis, 201

quadriplegia, 283, 285
quick-release retainer on pneumatic chisel, pull back to release, 74

rabies in cattle, 210–211
radio communications, 25–26, 249
ram cylinders, 85
rappel rack, 313
rated load, for wire rope, 340
rear overturns of tractor, 104–105
  extrication technique for, 106–14
    accessing patient, 109–111
    lifting tractor, 111–114
    securing scene, 106–109
  into water, 115
reciprocating hacksaw, 76
reflectorized tarp, 308
regulators, use of, for extrication, 73–74
remorse, as crisis reaction, 329
rescue operations. See also agricultural-rural rescues
  communications in, 248–249
  and deceased persons, 249–250
  and extended transport, 245–247
  information gathering for, 247
  and medical care, 244–245
  and personal safety, 247–248
rescue rope, 65–68
  characteristics of, 66
  safety inspection of, 67
rescue team
  cooperation between medical team and, 244
  makeup of, 9
  personal safety of, 10
rescue tools inventory, 92–93
rescuers
  deceased, 28
  exercise for, 33
  exposure to blood-borne pathogens, 33–35, 39, 40
  gear for, 41–45
  hydration of, 32–33
  injured, 28
  injury to patient caused by, 28
  nutrition for, 33
  overwhelmed, 28–29
  physical threats to, 32–33
  protective clothing for, 35–41
  safety of, 189
    in confined spaces, 179, 186–187
    ensuring, 247–248
    with hazardous materials, 225–226, 231, 234–236, 239
resource tracking system, 18–19
resources, 22
respiration, 257
respiratory arrest, 272–273
respiratory burn, 297
resuscitation, 272–273
  and universal precautions, 35
rib fractures, 263
RICE, 283
rigging, basic, 60–62
rigor mortis, 327, 333
rodenticides, 215, 231–232
rollover protective structure (ROPS), 95, 98
  and overturn fatalities, 105, 123
  straightening or cutting deformed cab, 111
rope handler, 303, 311
rope pads, 68
rope-related equipment, 70–71
ropes. See also rescue rope; utility rope; wire rope
  safe working capacities for, 67
  types of, 65–69
rotational injury, 264
Rule of Nines, 261, 298, 299

safety backup, 188
  in confined space rescue, 179
safety factor
  for rescue rope, 66
  for wire rope, 340
safety line handlers, 188
safety zone
  definition of, 6, 8
  escorting bystanders from, 8–9
    in baler incidents, 160, 163
    in combine incidents, 124, 128, 129, 131, 133

    in confined space incidents, 193, 199
    in ensilage cutter incidents, 168
    in mixing wagon incidents, 171
    in open auger entanglements, 158
    in portable auger entanglements, 153
    in PTO entanglements, 144–145
    in tractor incidents, 106
  establishing, 8
    in baler incidents, 160, 163
    in combine incidents, 124, 128, 129, 131, 133
    in confined space incidents, 193, 199
    in ensilage cutter incidents, 168
    in mixing wagon incidents, 171
    in open auger entanglements, 158
    in portable auger entanglements, 153
    in PTO entanglements, 144
    in tractor incidents, 106
scalp lacerations, 280–281
screw thread, 49
seat belts, cutting, 62
secondary driveline, 139, 143
secondary survey, 252, 256
self-contained breathing apparatus (SCBA)
  anxiety in wearing, 188–189
  in combating atmospheric hazards, 186–187
  in combating silo fires, 202
  in confined space rescue, 179
  and hazardous materials, 219, 222
  for high-pressure air bags, 78
  for pesticide exposure, 225–226, 230
  for pneumatic tool systems, 73
  for silo incidents, 198
self-contained underwater breathing apparatus (SCUBA) tanks, 73
  for high-pressure air bags, 78
semirigid litters, 44, 45
shackles, 72
sheet metal chisel, 75
shielding, 215, 234
shock
  anaphylactic, 274
  assessment of, 274–275
  cardiogenic, 274
    treating, 276
  definition of, 261, 273
  emotional, 328–329
  general treatment in, 275–277
  hypovolemic, 274, 297
    treating, 275–276
  mechanisms of injury, 273–274
  psychogenic, 277
  spinal, 283
  vascular, 274
    treating, 277
shock load, 59, 65
  for chains, 71
  for wire rope, 340
side rollovers, of tractors, 104–105
silo gas, 177, 183, 198, 248

silos, 196–199
  extrication technique for, 199–201
  fires in, 201–203
  hauling systems in rescues, 314
single-acting cylinders, 85
single basket hitch, 61
single choker hitch, 61
single rod cylinders, 85
situational crisis, 327, 328
skin protection, 41
skull fractures, 281–282
slings, 61–62
  definition of, 59, 61
  protection, maintenance, and storage of, 339
  roundslings, 338
  web sling configurations, 338–339
slip/sling hooks, 72
smoke ejector, 184
snapping rolls, 130–131
  definition of, 120, 130
  extrication technique for, 131–132
snap-ring tool, 149
SOAP format, 242, 249, 250
socks, 40
sodium bicarbonate, 236
sodium carbonate, 236
solids, elasticity of, 56–57
sorting hook, 72
span of control
  definition of, 13, 15
  loss of, at incident command system, 27
specialists untrained in agricultural-rural rescue, 20, 23
spinal fractures, 283
  assessment of, 284–286
  common mechanisms of injury, 283–284
  lifting, extricating, and moving patients with, 286–287
  treatment of, 286
spinal injuries, packaging patient for, 306–307
spinal shock, 283
spine board, 43–44
spleen, ruptured, 263
splinting, general principles of, 290–291
splint stable, 286, 290
spreading tools, 62–63
squeezing in animal incidents, 206, 208
stability, 51–52
  triangle of, 52–55
  and use of high-pressure air bags, 80
  and use of low-pressure air bags, 84
staging area, 22
stainless steel wire, 342
standard eye and eye sling, 339
status conditions, 19
  assigned, 19
  available, 19
  out-of-service, 19
step-up plan
  definition of, 13, 16

in preincident plan, 16
Stokes litter, 42–45
straw walkers, 133
    definition of, 120, 132
    extrication technique for, 133
stress, 333–334
    critical incident stress debriefing (CISD) for, 336–337
    definition of, 47, 57
    delayed reactions, 334
    effects of excessive, 334–335
    immediate reactions, 334
    recognizing excessive, 335–336
    traumatic, 336
strike team, 22
strike zone, 59, 80–81
strokes, 278
strychnine poisoning, 231–232
suffocation as danger in flowing grain entrapment, 190
sugar beet harvester, 173
    entanglement in, 175, 269
sunburn, 41
swivel connectors, 72
synthetic hydraulic fluids, 350

tandem disc, 165–166
T-card locator file, 18–19
technical specialist, 22
telescoping cylinders, 85
temperature as physical threat to rescuer, 32
tetanus, 208
thermal layer, 30, 35
thoracic spine injuries, 285
threaded quarter turn retainer on pneumatic chisel, 74
tissue necrosis, 288
torque, 139, 143
toxic gases, 221
    danger of, in liquid manure storage, 204
    in silos, 198
toxicity, of pesticides, 215, 224, 225
traction in position (TIP), 286, 289, 292
tractor
    articulated, 94, 99
    collisions with other vehicles, 115
    common injuries involving, 114, 267
    four-wheel drive, 99–102
    front-end loaders, 115–118
    gaining access to, 109–111
    history of design, 96–97
    lifting, 112–114
    rear overturns, 104–105
        extrication technique for, 106–114
        into water, 115
    rollover protective structure (ROPS), 98
    securing, 107–109
    side rollovers, 104–105
    stability of, 102
        ballast, 104
        center of gravity, 103
        drawbar pull, 104
        turning engine off, 106–107
tractor output shaft, 139, 142–143
transfer valve, 86
transport/binder chain, 344
transport layer, 30, 35
transport of patient, 244–245
transport. *See also* packaging
    extended, 245–247
    of patient with spinal injury, 286–287
transportation
    air medical evacuation, 23, 316, 318, 320
        landing zones, 320–321
        nighttime landings, 322
        packaging considerations, 323–324
        personal safety, 322–323
        wind direction, approach, and departure paths, 321
    ground-vehicle, 240, 317–318
traps, animal, 212–213
trauma, 261, 262
traumatic injuries, 262
triangle of stability (TOS), 52–55
trisodium phosphate, 236
tub grinders, 172–173
    fall into, 175, 269
turnout gear, 31, 37
twisted eye sling, 339

ultimate load for wire rope, 340
Union of International Alpine Associations (UIAA), 39
universal gravitation, 47, 50
universal joint, 139, 141
universal precautions, 31, 33–35
urination, as indicator of hydration, 33
utility rope, 69

vascular shock, 274
    treating, 277
vehicle lifting, mechanics of, 56
vehicle stabilization, mechanics of, 52–56
ventilation in combating atmospheric hazards, 184–185
venturi effect, 177, 184, 185
vital signs, 256–258

water
    in hydration, 32
    rear overturns into, 115
water glycol, 350
water-oil emulsions, 350
waterproof protection, 36
webbing, 70
webbing cutters, 62
windrow, 139, 160
wire beehive retainer, 74

wire rope, 68–69
    protection, maintenance, and storage of, 342–343
    selecting, 340
        rope lay in, 341
        rope strand in, 340–341
        wire core in, 342
        wire grade in, 341
        wire type in, 342
wire rope come-along, 64–65
wood cribbing
    as base for high-pressure air bags, 80
    with wire rope come-along, 64

work, 47, 48
working load limit for chains, 343
working pressure, 88
wounds, 293
    types of, 293–294
woven wire litter, 42
wrenches, pneumatic impact, 75–76
wristlet method, 187, 188
written communications, 249

zinc phosphate, 231